Prevention: What Works with Children and Adolescents?

'Alan Carr and his colleagues have been both thorough and systematic in their approach to the literature on prevention. Clinicians might well find it a useful resource for particular disorders or problems.'

Professor Sir Michael Rutter, Institute of Psychiatry, London

'This book reviews existing evidence on prevention in an up-to-date, thorough and methodical way. The summaries are concise and stimulating.'

Ian Wilkinson, Consultant Clinical Psychologist

'This is a much needed and excellently written book.'

Professor Martin Herbert

Prevention: What Works for Children and Adolescents? deals with the prevention of psychological problems which are of central concern to those who fund and develop health, social and educational services for children, adolescents and their families. Problems addressed in this book include developmental delay in low birth weight infants and socially disadvantaged children; adjustment problems in children with sensory and motor disabilities and autism; challenging behaviour in children with intellectual disabilities; physical and sexual abuse; bullying; adjustment problems in children with asthma and diabetes; teenage smoking; alcohol use and drug abuse; teenage pregnancy, STDs and HIV infection; post-traumatic adjustment problems; adolescent suicide. Conclusions drawn in this book are based on the results of over 200 rigorously conducted studies containing more than 70,000 children.

Alan Carr is Director of the Doctoral Programme in Clinical Psychology at University College Dublin. His other publications include *The Handbook of Child and Adolescent Clinical Psychology: A Contextual Approach* (1999), *What Works with Children and Adolescents?: A Critical Review of Psychological Interventions with Children, Adolescents and their Families* (2000) and *Abnormal Psychology* (2001).

Prevention: What Works with Children and Adolescents?

A Critical Review of Psychological Prevention Programmes for Children, Adolescents and their Families

Edited by Alan Carr

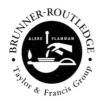

First published 2002 by Brunner-Routledge
27 Church Road, Hove, East Sussex BN3 2FA

Simultaneously published in the USA and Canada
by Taylor and Francis Inc
29 West 35th Street, New York, NY 10001

Brunner-Routledge is an imprint of the Taylor & Francis Group

© 2002 Selection and editorial matter, Alan Carr. Individual chapters,
the contributors

Typeset in Times by RefineCatch Limited, Bungay, Suffolk
Printed and bound in Great Britain by
Biddles Ltd, Guildford and King's Lynn
Cover design by Lou Page

British Library Cataloguing in Publication Data
A catalogue record for this book is available from the British Library

ISBN 1–58391–276–2 (hbk)

Contents

Contributors

Aoife Brinkley, MSc, D Psych Sc, Midland Health Board, Republic of Ireland

Alan Carr, MA, PhD, University College Dublin, Republic of Ireland

Barry J. Coughlan, PhD, D Psych Sc, Mid-Western Health Board, Republic of Ireland

Ruth Catherine Cullen, MSc, D Psych Sc, South Eastern Health Board, Republic of Ireland

Mairead Doyle, BSc, D Psych Sc, Midland Health Board, Republic of Ireland

Yvonne M. Duane, Dip Psych, D Psych Sc, North Eastern Health Board, Republic of Ireland

Siofradh Enright, M Psych Sc, D Psych Sc, Midland Health Board, Republic of Ireland

Aine Fahey, BA, D Psych Sc, South Eastern Health Board, Republic of Ireland

Eimear Farrell, MSc, D Psych Sc, North Western Health Board, Republic of Ireland

Linda M. Finnegan, MA, D Psych Sc, South Eastern Health Board, Republic of Ireland

Deirdre Hickey, MA, D Psych Sc, South Eastern Health Board, Republic of Ireland

Bronagh Kennedy, MEd, D Psych Sc, North Western Health Board, Republic of Ireland

Gregor Lange, MSc, D Psych Sc, North Eastern Health Board, Republic of Ireland

Orna P. McCarthy, MA, D Psych Sc, South Eastern Health Board, Republic of Ireland

Attracta A. McGlinchey, PhD, D Psych Sc, Southern Health Board, Republic of Ireland

Nodlaig Moore, MSc, D Psych Sc, Midwestern Health Board, Republic of Ireland

Beth O'Riordan, MA, D Psych Sc, Midland Health Board, Republic of Ireland

Anna-Marie O'Sullivan, MA, D Psych Sc, North Eastern Health Board, Republic of Ireland

Brian Waldron, MSc, D Psych Sc, North Western Health Board, Republic of Ireland

Foreword

In these times of increasing insistence, much overdue, on empirically supported psychological treatments, there is a welcome burgeoning of publications of the "What works?" variety. Alan Carr's earlier edited volume in this
tradition provided one of the seminal contributions. However, there is an
equally important, perhaps even more significant question, to answer. What
works in the area of preventive work? Here there is a much more sparse
literature to consult, a fact that makes the present volume – with its review of
empirically rigorous prevention programmes in15 problem areas – a ground-
breaking addition to the clinician's knowledge base. A bonus in the book
is the detailed explanation of the methodology for selecting and evaluating
the prevention investigations (involving 70,000 participants) culled from 23
years of publications in English language journals. Eighteen experts have
co-written with Alan Carr the 17 chapters dealing with a variety of
heterogeneous problems ranging from low birth weight, cognitive delays,
adjustment difficulties in children with autism, cerebral palsy and sensory
disabilities, to drug abuse, suicide, bronchial asthma, and teenage pregnancy.
In other words, it is comprehensive; and in addition, lucidly written. To sum
up, this is an invaluable reference and study text, a 'must' for the clinician's
bookshelf.

Martin Herbert
Emeritus Professor, Exeter University

Preface

'Life . . . there is queer small utility in it. You cannot eat it or drink it and it does not keep the rain out. Many a man has spent a hundred years trying to get the dimensions of it and when he understands it at last and entertains the certain pattern of it in his head, he takes to his bed and dies. It is a queer contraption and a certain death-trap. Life.' said Martin Finnucane.

'There are five rules of wisdom' said the Sergeant.
'1. Always ask any questions that are to be asked and never answer any.
2. Turn everything you hear to your own advantage.
3. Always carry a bicycle repair outfit.
4. Take left turns as much as possible.
5. Never apply your front brake first.
If you follow these rules you will save your soul and you will never get a fall on a slippery road.'

(Flann O'Brien (1967) *The Third Policeman*. London: Flamingo. pp. 46–47 and 62–63.)

In this era of increased demands for evidenced-based-practice and the use of empirically supported psychological interventions there has been a clear need for a concise, empirically based statement of the types of psychological prevention programmes that may be effective in preventing common psychological problems in childhood and adolescence. Our aim in writing this text has been to meet this need. In certain respects we were faced with Martin Finnucane's dilemma and went looking for a set of guidelines like the Sergeant's five rules of wisdom in Flann O'Brien's celebrated tale of *The Third Policeman*.

Empirical evidence from rigorously conducted research trials in each of fifteen problem areas is reviewed by a team of nineteen psychologists in this volume. This evidence was culled from thorough literature searches for psychological prevention programme evaluation studies that had been published in English language journals in the period from 1977 to 2000. From this enormous body of literature, only those studies which met stringent methodological criteria were selected for inclusion in the database for this book. In all, over 200 well-conducted studies were identified and these contained over 70,000 participants. Thus, the conclusions reached in this volume are based on a solid bedrock of rigorous empirical evidence.

Prevention: What Works with Children and Adolescents? complements our previous text – *What Works with Children and Adolescents?* (Carr, 2000, published by Routledge) – insofar as it provides a review of the evidence on prevention programmes while our last volume focused on treatment programmes. In selecting chapter topics, we focused on problems which are of particular concern to health care professionals and educationalists. We have omitted chapters on some important topics, such as the prevention of serious antisocial behaviour in adolescence, because to some degree, this literature has already been addressed in the chapter on behavioural parent training for oppositional defiant disorder in our previous book on evidence-based practice *What Works with Children and Adolescents?*. We have also included in the current volume chapters on topics, such as autism, that could arguably have been better placed in our previous text. However, studies of programmes which aim to prevent adjustment difficulties in youngsters with autism are included in this volume because such programmes are probably better conceptualized as prevention programmes than treatment programmes.

We are grateful to the many people who have helped develop the ideas presented in this book. A particular debt of gratitude is due to Professor Ciarán Benson, Professor Patricia Noonan Walsh, Dr Muireann McNulty, Dr Barbara Dooley, Dr Teresa Burke, Dr Gary O'Reilly and Muriel Keegan, MA, who have been very supportive during our efforts to write this text. The research on which this book is based has been supported, in part, by funds from the Midland Health Board, the North Eastern Health Board, the North Western Health Board, the South Eastern Health Board, and the Midwestern Health Board in the Republic of Ireland.

AC
October 2001

1   Introduction

Alan Carr

Between 10% and 20% of youngsters suffer from psychological problems serious enough to warrant psychological treatment (Carr, 1999). There is now an impressive body of research which shows that psychological interventions for many of these problems are highly effective (Carr, 2000). However, for all who work in child and adolescent health, education, and social services a central concern is how these psychological problems might be prevented in the first place. Our book aims to answer this question. Our answer is based on a thorough, critical review of rigorously conducted prevention programme evaluation research.

Selection of areas for review

In structuring the review process, we decided to focus on groups of children who, because of biological or psychosocial adversity, are vulnerable to developing adjustment problems which entail particularly negative outcomes. For example, children with diabetes, because of biological adversity, are vulnerable to a range of serious medical complications if they do not strictly adhere to their illness management regime. Socially disadvantaged youngsters, because of environmental adversity, are vulnerable to cognitive and language developmental delays and school-based attainment difficulties. We also decided to focus on problems which may affect all youngsters and which can lead to particularly negative outcomes, for example sexual risk-taking which can lead to teenage pregnancy and infection with sexually transmitted diseases including HIV. Our selection of areas for review was limited by the availability of methodologically robust prevention programme evaluation studies. Finally, for the most part, we excluded populations and problems considered in our recent critical review of the child and adolescent psychological treatment outcome literature: *What Works with Children and Adolescents?* (Carr, 2000). So, for example, because behavioural parent training for youngsters with oppositional defiant disorder was covered in *What Works with Children and Adolescents?*, the same literature is not reviewed here in a chapter on the prevention of conduct disorder. Using these inclusion and exclusion criteria the following problem areas were selected and a chapter is devoted to each in this volume:

- developmental delay in low birth weight infants
- cognitive delays in environmentally disadvantaged children
- adjustment problems in children with cerebral palsy
- adjustment problems in children with sensory disabilities
- adjustment problems in children with autism
- challenging behaviour in children with intellectual disabilities
- physical abuse
- sexual abuse
- bullying
- adjustment problems in children with asthma
- adjustment problems in children with diabetes
- teenage smoking, alcohol use and drug abuse
- teenage pregnancy, sexually transmitted diseases and HIV infection
- post-traumatic adjustment problems in children and adolescents
- suicide in adolescence

While the empirical literature on the effectiveness of intervention programmes for some of these problems has been reviewed previously, all of these areas have never been considered in a single volume in a uniform way (Ammerman & Hersen, 1997; Guralnick & Bennet, 1987; Guralnick, 1997; Di Clemente et al., 1996). In this sense the present volume is unique.

Overall review strategy

For each of the 15 problem areas listed in the previous section, the following review strategy was used for the period 1977–2000. First, a PsychLit search of English language journals and book chapters was conducted using the core problem term and variations of it combined with terms such as *prevention*, *intervention*, *evaluation* and related phrases to identify potential programme evaluation studies. Second, a PsychLit search was conducted using the core problem term combined with the term *review*, to identify review papers. Third, the bibliographies of review papers, treatment outcome studies and relevant journals were manually searched. Fourth, in certain instances investigators were contacted directly to solicit copies of recent articles, although only in exceptional circumstances where very few high quality published studies were available were unpublished studies included in reviews. Fifth, with a couple of exceptions mentioned below, studies were selected for inclusion if they met the following stringent methodological criteria: a randomized or matched comparative group outcome design was used; cases were diagnostically homogeneous; at least five cases were included in each group; reliable and valid pre- and post-programme measures were used. Sixth, if these stringent methodological criteria yielded a particularly small pool of studies, the criteria were relaxed and less methodologically robust studies were included for review. These procedures ensured that for each problem area, a pool of the most methodologically robust available studies containing at least 50 treated cases was reviewed. Seventh, for each group of studies wherever possible at least four types of tables were drawn up to summarize key features. These tables covered (1) general characteristics; (2) methodological features; (3) effect sizes and outcome rates; and (4) key findings. The structure of these tables and definitions of the terms included in them are given below. Eighth, narrative accounts were written summarizing the main trends in each of the tables, with one section giving an overview of the characteristics of the studies; a further section commenting on their methodological features; and the third section summarizing the substantive findings. Ninth, in constructing tables and writing sections on substantive findings, studies were grouped by problem subtype (e.g. deaf children, blind children, deaf-blind children) and type of intervention programme (e.g. psychoeducation only; psychoeducation and communication skills training only; psychoeducation, communication and behavioural skills training). In outlining substantive findings reference was made to the results of each study or group of studies on a range of relevant outcome measures which varied from study to study. For example, in studies of low birth weight children, cognitive functioning was one of the widely used outcome measures whereas for adolescent sexual risk-taking frequency of condom use was one of the outcome measures commonly reported. Tenth, a summary of the main conclusions and the confidence with which these were drawn was outlined before highlighting the implications for future policy, practice and research. Finally, for each problem area resources for assessment, intervention, and informing clients about the area or problem were listed.

There were a number of exceptions to this overall strategy. All of the empirical studies of the impact of psychological interventions to prevent challenging behaviour in children with intellectual disabilities which were identified were experimental single case designs. Rather than omit this important area, we selected and reviewed a representative group of these experimental single case design studies. In most of the studies of bullying prevention programmes there were no control groups and conclusions about programme effectiveness were based on time-lagged contrasts between age-equivalent groups, i.e. data from Time 1 were used as a baseline against which data from Time 2, and in some instances Time 3, could be compared. In the area of sensory disabilities a number of studies lacked control groups and statistical procedures were used to control for maturational processes. We therefore included these types of studies in our review.

To orient readers at the outset of each chapter definitions of core problems addressed within the chapter are given along with epidemiological information, a summary of the main aetiological theories and the principal conclusions of previous reviews. In instances where the programme evaluation literature was very large, and where previous reviews clearly indicated that certain types of intervention programmes were particularly effective, while others were clearly ineffective, we confined our review to studies of intervention programmes that previous reviewers identified as being particularly effective. For example, within the substance use prevention literature we confined our review to resistance skills training, life skills training and multisystemic, multimodal programmes, since there is some consensus within the literature that these can be effective. However, we did not review the voluminous literature on psychoeducational and affectively oriented programmes, which have been shown repeatedly to be ineffective. In instances where very large numbers of methodologically robust studies of effective programmes were identified, we confined our review to a representative group of 10–20 studies.

Strategy for tabulating general characteristics of studies

To provide an overview of the general characteristics of studies reviewed, a table containing the following headings was constructed for problems addressed in each chapter.

- *Authors*.
- *Year*: The year of publication is given under this heading.
- *N per group*: The number of cases in each group is given under this heading.
- *Age*: The mean age and age range of participants are given under this heading.
- *Gender*: The number of males and females is given under this heading.
- *Family characteristics*: Descriptions of the structure, socioeconomic status (SES) and ethnicity are given under this heading.
- *Programme setting*: Distinctions are made between hospital inpatient settings, community outpatient and day programme settings, preschools, primary schools and secondary school.
- *Programme duration*: The average number of sessions or hours of intervention and the time period over which this occurred are given under this heading, e.g. 20 hourly sessions over 1 year.

Where all studies shared a particular characteristic or where information on a particular characteristic was unavailable for most studies, then a column for categorizing that characteristic was eliminated from the table so as to simplify the overall presentation of information. Additional column headings were added if all studies in a particular group provided important information on that variable.

Strategy for tabulating methodological features

Different strategies were used for tabulating methodological features for comparative group outcome designs and single case designs, so each will be addressed in separate sections below.

Methodological features of comparative group outcome studies

To provide an overview of the methodological features of comparative group outcome studies, a table containing categories listed below was constructed in each chapter and the presence or absence of each methodological feature for each study was noted. These categories collectively constitute a checklist for assessing methodological robustness. The checklist represents a synthesis of other similar checklists (Carr, 2000). In interpreting tables based on this checklist, attention was paid to both profiles and total scores. Examination of each study's profile on this checklist threw light on its methodological strengths and weaknesses. Greater confidence was placed in the results of studies that obtained higher total scores. What follows are definitions of items in the checklist.

- *Control group*. A control group was used.
- *Random assignment*. Cases were randomly assigned to treatment and control groups.
- *Diagnostic homogeneity*. All cases in treatment and control groups had the same diagnosis or problem profile.
- *Demographic similarity*. Cases in treatment and control groups did not differ significantly in terms of the children's age or gender.
- *Pre-treatment assessment*. Cases were assessed before the intervention programme.
- *Post-treatment assessment*. Cases were assessed after the intervention programme.
- *Follow-up assessment*. Cases were assessed at some specified period after the treatment group had completed the prevention programme.
- *Children's self-report*. Children's self-report instruments were used to assess children's adjustment before and after intervention.
- *Parents' ratings*. Instruments that yielded parents' ratings of children's adjustment were used to assess children's pre- and post-intervention status.
- *Teachers' ratings*. Teachers' ratings of children's adjustment were used to assess children's pre- and post-intervention status.
- *Therapist or trainer ratings*. Instruments that yielded therapists' or trainers' ratings of children's adjustment were used to assess children's pre- and post-intervention status. Trainers were staff who implemented programmes.
- *Researcher ratings*. Instruments that yielded researchers' ratings of

children's adjustment were used to assess children's pre-treatment and post-treatment status.

- *Standardized psychometric tests.* Standardized psychometric tests to measure cognitive or language functioning were used. This item was only included in those chapters where it was appropriate to do so.
- *Deterioration assessed.* Deterioration following intervention was evaluated in those cases where it occurred.
- *Drop-out assessed.* The number of drop-outs from the intervention and control groups was reported.
- *Clinical significance of change assessed.* Cases were classified as clinically improved following treatment using cut-off scores on standardized instruments or Reliable Change Indices (Jacobson et al., 1984; Hageman & Arrindell, 1993) and the frequency of improved cases in intervention and control groups was compared using appropriate non-parametric statistics.
- *Experienced trainers used for all treatments.* Experienced trainers with formal training or qualifications delivered the intervention programme.
- *Programmes were equally valued.* Where two intervention programmes were compared, skilled trainers committed to their model of intervention delivered both programmes.
- *Programmes were manualized.* Intervention was guided by a manual that was either flexibly or rigidly adhered to by trainers.
- *Supervision was provided.* All trainers participating in the study received ongoing supervision to ensure that a high quality of intervention was offered to clients.
- *Programme integrity checked.* The integrity of each programme was checked by, for example, observing or recording a selection of sessions and using a checklist to assess the degree to which trainers' behaviour conformed to the guidelines laid down in the programme implementation manual.
- *Data on concurrent treatment given.* Information was given on whether or not children or other family members were receiving concurrent psychological or pharmacological treatment for the core problem or related difficulties.
- *Data on subsequent treatment given.* Information was given on whether or not children or other family members engaged in further treatment following the intervention assessed in the study.

Methodological features of experimental single case designs

To provide an overview of the methodological features of studies in which experimental single case designs were used, a table containing categories listed below was constructed for the chapter on prevention programmes for challenging behaviour and the presence or absence of each methodological feature for each study was noted. This table is based on a synthesis of guidelines from other sources (Kazdin, 1982; O'Neill et al., 1997; Iwata, 1994a,b). Examination of each study's profile on this checklist threw light on its methodological strengths and weaknesses. Greater confidence was placed in the results of studies that obtained higher total scores. What follows are definitions of items in the checklist.

- *Operational definitions of target behaviour.* A detailed description of the target behaviour or dependent variable was given.
- *Operational procedural descriptions.* A detailed description of the treatment procedures or independent variable was given.
- *Structured behavioural interview.* A formal structured behavioural assessment interview was conducted to identify target behaviours and both proximal and distal antecedents and consequences.
- *Motivation assessment scale.* This scale for assessing the likelihood of a particular behaviour occurring in different situations was used. In all sixteen questions about situations involving social attention, presentation of tangible objects, sensory feedback and demands are contained in the instrument and responses are rated on seven-point Likert scales (Durand & Crimmins, 1992).
- *Analogue functional analysis.* This type of assessment was used in which behaviour reactions in experimentally controlled conditions were tested including: demand, social attention, play and tangibles to find out what types of situations tend to maintain the problem behaviour (Iwata, 1994a,b).
- *ABC analysis.* Antecedents, target behaviours and consequences were assessed.
- *Scatterplot observational assessment.* A scatterplot of target behaviours and contingencies was used for assessment.
- *Pre-experimental informal observation or interview.* These informal procedures were used.
- *Experienced observers or trainers used.* Observers who rated dependent or independent variables and staff who implemented the programme were trained.
- *Inter-observer reliability for assessment > 80%.* For the independent and dependent variables, there was agreement for 80% or more of ratings made by two independent observers.
- *Implementation reliability checks.* The degree to which staff implementing the programme did so according to the programme guidelines was formally checked.
- *Generalization probe.* The degree to which gains made in the programme implementation setting generalized to other settings was formally checked.
- *Follow-up.* Long-term follow-up data were reported.
- *Supplementary objective.* Additional positive behaviour changes (other than changes in the target behaviour) were reported.

Strategy for tabulating quantitative results

In tabulating effect sizes and outcome rates, a framework was drawn up which takes account of a number of important distinctions that have been established in the literature on early intervention and prevention programme evaluation. Distinctions were made between improvements shown immediately following intervention and improvement shown at various follow-up time points. For each of the fifteen problem areas addressed in the chapters in the body of this book, the range of domains on which effect sizes were calculated was decided on the basis of the measures most commonly reported in programme evaluation studies. Provision was made for reporting both effect sizes and percentages of cases showing clinically significant improvement, deterioration and drop-out or attrition. Finally, provision was made for identifying whether the source of outcome data was a child, parent, teacher, trainer/therapist, or researcher.

This overall strategy was used in tabulating quantitative results from comparative group outcome studies. It was also used in those infrequent instances where results from single group outcome studies involving predictive designs were used. However, for single case designs only effectiveness ratings were tabulated. Methods for calculating effect sizes from group studies and effectiveness ratings from single case designs are considered below.

Calculating effect sizes for comparative group outcome studies

For readers unfamiliar with the statistical concept of effect size, a graphic explanation is given in Figure 1.1. Where possible, effect sizes were calculated for outcome measures using the methods set out in Table 1.1 (Shadish, 1993). These were interpreted using Figure 1.2.

Where studies contained a single intervention group and a single control group, effect sizes were based on a comparison of the two groups. Where studies contained more than two intervention groups and a control group, effect sizes were calculated for comparisons of one or more active treatment groups with the control group. Where other comparisons were made, these are clearly specified in the table of quantitative results.

Where studies contained many outcome measures or dependent variables in a single domain, in most instances effect sizes were calculated on all variables within a domain and averaged.

Calculating effect sizes in single group studies with predictive designs

In a number of longitudinal studies of children with developmental disabilities where control groups were not employed, effect sizes were based on hypothetical post-intervention scores predicted by children's pre-intervention scores on standardized developmental ability tests. For example, Sheehan

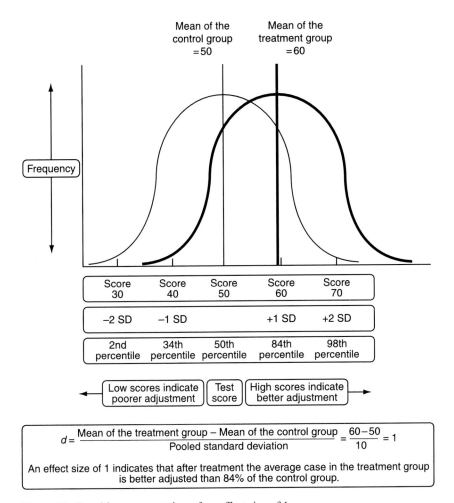

Figure 1.1 Graphic representation of an effect size of 1.

(1979) proposes that the impact of treatment may be evaluated by calculating predicated post-intervention developmental age scores using the formula in Table 1.2 and comparing these to actual developmental age scores using the effect size equation in Table 1.2. Effect sizes are calculated by subtracting actual and predicted post-intervention means and dividing by the standard deviation of the predicted post-intervention scores. Where interventions are effective the actual developmental age mean score is greater than the mean predicted developmental age score and the effect size is large. This procedure was used in studies of children with sensory impairments described in Chapter 5.

Table 1.1 Calculation of effect sizes

Conditions where suitable	Formula	Definition of terms
1 Means and standard deviations are given	$d = \dfrac{M1 - M2}{SD}$	SD = Standard deviation of the control group or the pooled standard deviation Pooled $SD = \dfrac{\sqrt{(n1 - 1)SD1^2 + (n2 - 1)SD2^2}}{(n1 + n2 - 2)}$ M1 = Mean of the treatment group M2 = Mean of the control group n1 = no. of cases in treatment group n2 = no. of cases in control group SD1 = Standard deviation of treatment group SD2 = Standard deviation of control group If only SE is given, $SD = SE \times \sqrt{N} - 1$
2 Frequency of improved cases in treatment and control groups is given	$d = [\ln (AD/CB)]\sqrt{3}/\pi$	$\sqrt{3}/\pi = 0.55$ ln = natural log A = no. of improved treated cases B = no. of unimproved treated cases C = no. of improved untreated cases D = no. of unimproved untreated cases
3 t-test result on raw post-treatment scores is given	$d = t \sqrt{1/n1 + 1/n2}$	t = t value from t-test on raw post-treatment scores n1 = no. of cases in treatment group n2 = no. of cases in control group
4 For 2-group studies ANOVA F statistic on raw post-treatment scores is given	$d = \sqrt{F(1/n1 + 1/n2)}$	F = F value from t-test on raw post-treatment scores n1 = no. of cases in treatment group n2 = no. of cases in control group

5	For studies with more than 2 groups ANOVA F statistic on raw post-treatment scores is given along with means	$d = \dfrac{M1 - M2}{\sqrt{[\Sigma\, ni(Mi - GM)^2/(k-1)]}\, F}$	M1 = Mean of the treatment group M2 = Mean of the control group ni = no. of cases in group i Mi = mean of group i GM = grand mean k = number of groups F = F statistic
6	ANCOVA F statistic on adjusted post-treatment scores is given	$d = \sqrt{F(1/n1 + 1/n2)\,(1 - rxx)}$	F = F value from t-test on raw post-treatment scores n1 = no. of cases in treatment group n2 = no. of cases in control group rxx = test–retest correlation of covariate if reported. If not reported assume it is 0.5
7	Probability level ($p < 0.05$ or $p < 0.01$), n1 and n2 only are given	$d = t\ (\text{estimated})\sqrt{1/n1 + 1/n2}$	t (estimated) = is taken from a table of t values for 2-tailed tests for the reported p value and df value. df = (n1 + n2) − 2 n1 = no. of cases in treatment group n2 = no. of cases in control group
8	Results are described as non-significant and no data are given	$d = 0$	Assume $d = 0$ if results are reported to be non-significant and no other data are available

Source: Adapted from Shadish (1993).

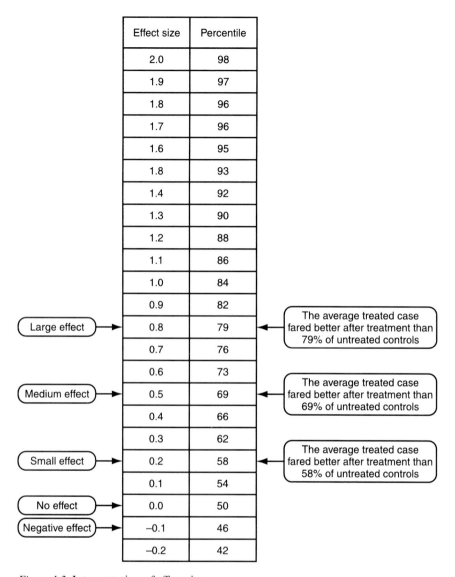

Effect size	Percentile
2.0	98
1.9	97
1.8	96
1.7	96
1.6	95
1.8	93
1.4	92
1.3	90
1.2	88
1.1	86
1.0	84
0.9	82
0.8	79
0.7	76
0.6	73
0.5	69
0.4	66
0.3	62
0.2	58
0.1	54
0.0	50
−0.1	46
−0.2	42

Large effect → 0.8 ← The average treated case fared better after treatment than 79% of untreated controls

Medium effect → 0.5 ← The average treated case fared better after treatment than 69% of untreated controls

Small effect → 0.2 ← The average treated case fared better after treatment than 58% of untreated controls

No effect → 0.0

Negative effect → −0.1

Figure 1.2 Interpretation of effect sizes.

Calculating effectiveness ratings in single case designs

In order to quantitatively compare and synthesize the results of studies in which quantitative single case designs were used, treatment effectiveness ratings may be calculated using data from baseline and intervention phases of case studies. In Chapter 7 on challenging behaviour these procedures were

Table 1.2 Calculation of effect sizes in single group predictive designs

	Conditions where suitable	Formula	Definition of terms
1	In single group outcome studies, PPIDA scores can be calculated from raw data using this formula	PPIDA = (Time 1 DA/ Time 1 CA) × Time 2 CA	PPIDA = the predicted post-intervention developmental age score Time 1 DA = developmental age score on a test before the intervention Time 1CA = chronological age before the intervention Time 2 CA = chronological age after the intervention
2	In single group outcome studies effect sizes can be calculated if the mean and standard deviations of treatment groups actual and predicted post-intervention developmental age scores are given	$d = \dfrac{AM - PM}{PSD}$	AM = actual mean post-intervention developmental age score PM = predicted mean post-intervention developmental age score PSD = standard deviation of predicted post-intervention developmental age scores

used, since available data in this come from experimental single case design studies. Three types of effectiveness ratings are now widely used:

- percentage non-overlapping data
- the percentage zero data
- mean percentage reduction in challenging behaviour

Percentage non-overlapping data (PND)

PND is calculated by counting the number of data points in the treatment phase that exceed the value of the data point in the baseline condition with the highest value. This procedure yields the number of non-overlapping data points. This is expressed as a percentage by using the first equation in Table 1.3. With ABAB designs, a PND is calculated for each pair of baseline and treatment phases and the final PND is the obtained by averaging all of these PND values. If a baseline phase contains one or more zero data points, then a PND of zero would occur, even if all remaining treatment phase data points are below non-zero baseline data points. To deal with the problem of such spurious effectiveness ratings, all baseline zero data points are excluded from calculations of PND. In order to counterbalance for the effect of this

Table 1.3 Calculation of effectiveness ratings in experimental single case designs

Formula	Definition of terms
PND = (ND/TD) × 100	PND = percentage non-overlapping data ND = number of non-overlapping data points (number of data points in the treatment phase that exceed the value of the data point in the baseline condition with the highest value) TD = total number of data points in treatment phase
PZD = (ZD/TD) × 100	PZD = percentage zero data ZD = number of zero data points in the treatment phase TD = total number of data points in treatment phase
MPR = ((BLM – TPM)/ BLM) × 100	MPR = mean percentage reduction in challenging behaviour BLM = baseline mean based on all baseline data points TPM = treatment phase mean based on the last 5 data points of the treatment phase

Sources: PND is adapted from Scruggs et al. (1987). PZD is adapted from Scotti et al. (1991). MPR is adapted from Hagopian et al. (1998).

operation, one data point must be withdrawn from the treatment phase for each zero data point excluded from the baseline phase before calculating PND. In such instances when applying the first formula in Table 1.3, ND is the number of non-overlapping data points after zero data points have been excluded from the baseline phase and an equivalent number of data points have been excluded from the treatment phase, and TD is the total number of data points in the treatment phase minus the number of data points excluded from the treatment phase to counterbalance for excluding zero data points from the baseline phase. This method has been described by Scruggs et al. (1987) and used by Didden et al. (1997) in a major meta-analysis of treatment methods for challenging behaviour. PND is a measure of treatment effectiveness based on the assumption that if performance during an intervention phase does not overlap with performance during the baseline phase then the effects in the predicted direction can usually be regarded as reliable. In addition, the replication of non-overlapping distributions during different treatment phases strengthens the reliability of the treatment effect (Scruggs et al., 1987). Didden et al. (1997) interpreted different PND results using the following criteria:

- highly effective treatment: PND >90%
- fairly effective treatment: PND between 70% and 90%
- questionable treatment: PND between 50% and 70%
- unreliable treatment: PND <50%

The percentage zero data (PZD)

PZD is calculated by counting the number of zero data points in the treatment phase and expressing this as a percentage using the second formula in Table 1.3. With ABAB designs, a PZD is calculated for each treatment phase and the final PZD is then obtained by averaging all of these PZD values. PZD is a measure of treatment effectiveness developed by Scotti et al. (1991) which is based on the assumption that the goal of interventions is to reduce target challenging behaviours to zero levels. PZD is a very stringent index of treatment effectiveness and so should be interpreted using more lenient criteria than those appropriate for PND. The following criteria may be used:

- highly effective treatment : PZD >75%
- fairly effective treatment: PZD between 50% and 75%
- questionable treatment: PZD between 25% and 50%
- unreliable treatment: PZD <25%

The mean percentage reduction in challenging behaviour (MPR)

MPR is calculated by averaging, the values of the data points in the initial baseline phase to get the baseline mean (BLM), averaging the values of the last five data points from each treatment phase to get the treatment phase mean (TPM), and then expressing the mean reduction in challenging behaviour from baseline to treatment using the third formula in Table 1.3. Hagopian et al. (1998), who have used MPR as an effectiveness rating in a quantitative review of functional communication training, advise that interventions which show an MPR of 90% or more may be considered to be highly effective.

Strategy for tabulating key findings

For each study in which a group design was used, statistically and clinically significant differences between treatment and control or comparison groups after treatment and at follow-up were tabulated as bullet points. In addition, the performance of the treated group or groups with respect to control or comparison groups was given in shorthand, using mathematical symbols. For example, $1 > 2 = 3$, means that following treatment group 1, overall, fared better than groups 2 and 3 whose levels of improvement were similar. For single case designs, simple statements about treatment effects were tabulated as bullet points.

Reader's guide

Each chapter in this volume closes with a statement of the implications of the results of the studies reviewed within it for policy, clinical practice and further research. From a service development perspective, our intention has been to provide an empirical basis from which well-founded arguments may be made about the development of prevention services for children and adolescents. While reference is made to the main components of effective prevention programmes, the level of detail concerning prevention procedures is insufficient for professionals to use this text as an intervention manual. However, references to programme manuals are given at the end of each chapter, where appropriate.

From a research perspective, the level of detail given throughout the text, particularly in the sections on substantive findings, is sufficient to provide the basis for designing new methodologically robust studies. In pitching the overall level of detail given about studies reviewed within each chapter, we have intentionally opted to give more, rather than less detail, so that this text may be used as a source book for researchers seeking information on the nitty-gritty of designing and conducting studies on the effectiveness of prevention programmes for problems of childhood and adolescence. The text is replete with references to specific intervention programmes, specific assessment instruments, specific approaches to data analysis and detailed consideration of important methodological issues. Hopefully advanced postgraduate students and researchers will find this level of detail helpful and will find it useful to study particular sets of substantive findings in depth.

On the other hand, professionals, clinicians, and those involved in service development or funding, may find it more useful to read the opening and closing sections of each chapter in detail, and skim through the intervening sections on substantive findings. Most readers will find the final chapter of interest, since it offers a summary of the central findings of the entire project.

Further reading

Ammerman, R. T. & Hersen, M. (1997). *Handbook of Prevention and Treatment with Children and Adolescents*. New York: Wiley.

Di Clemente, R., Hansen, W. & Ponton, L. (1996). *Handbook of Adolescent Health Risk Behaviour*. New York: Plenum.

Guralnick, M. (1997). *The Effectiveness of Early Intervention*. Baltimore: Brookes.

Guralnick, M. & Bennet, F. (1987). *The Effectiveness of Early Intervention for at Risk and Handicapped Children*. New York: Academic Press.

2 Prevention of developmental delay in low birth weight infants

Anna-Marie O'Sullivan and Alan Carr

Low birth weight is a problem that places infants at risk for developmental delay. Infants are classified as low birth weight (LBW) if they are less than 2,500 grams (about five and a half pounds) at birth. If at birth they weigh less than 1,500 grams (about three and a half pounds), they are classified as very low birth weight (VLBW) (Stevens-Simon & Orleans, 1999). The psychological development of low birth weight infants frequently lags behind that of infants whose body weight falls within normal limits. Low birth weight is a biological vulnerability which is commonly associated with other psychosocial risk factors, such as poverty, and collectively these factors place infants at risk for developmental delay. A number of early intervention programmes for low birth weight infants have been developed, the aim of which is to prevent developmental delays. The effectiveness of many of these remains untested. The aim of this chapter is to review methodologically robust research studies on the effectiveness of early intervention programmes for low birth weight infants, draw reliable conclusions about the effectiveness of these, and outline the implications of these conclusions for policy and practice.

Epidemiology

About 7% of all newborns in industrialized countries have low birth weights and 1% of children at birth meet the criterion for very low birth weight (Blair & Ramey, 1997). Low birth weight infants are twice as likely to die within the first 28 days of life as infants of normal weight (Institute of Medicine, 1985). Results of a meta-analysis of longitudinal studies showed that the mean IQ of low birth weight infants was half a standard deviation (or 8 IQ points) below the norm (Aylward et al., 1989). About 10% of low birth weight children and more than 20% of very low birth weight children develop a major handicapping condition such as moderate or severe intellectual disability, cerebral palsy, blindness and deafness. Findings from the control group of the Infant Health and Development Study indicate that by three years of age, low birth weight children are 2.7 times more likely to develop mild intellectual disability and 1.8 times more likely to develop significant behaviour problems

(Infant Health and Development Program, 1990). At primary and second-ary school low birth weight children have significant problems with academic attainment.

Aetiology

Poverty is the single overarching social risk factor associated with low birth weight (Blair & Ramey, 1997). Other risk factors for low birth weight, entailed by poverty, include mother's membership of a low SES group, membership of a disadvantaged ethnic minority group, limited access to health care, and poor health behaviour. Mothers with poor health behaviour during pregnancy have inadequate diets, smoke, drink alcohol and may use other non-prescription drugs.

Preterm birth is the major medical risk factor for low birth weight (Institute of Medicine, 1985). Preterm birth refers to gestational age, and is applied to pregnancies of less than 37 weeks. Infants at gestational ages less than 34 weeks commonly have very low birth weights. Some of these infants have medical complications such as respiratory distress syndrome, bronchopulmonary dysplasia, and intraventricular haemorrhage, all of which can lead to adverse outcomes.

While there has been little change in the rate of preterm births over the past 20 years, there has been considerable increase in the survival rate of preterm infants (McCarton et al., 1995). This increased rate of survival has been due to the development of effective prenatal and neonatal intensive care techniques.

Being a twin is also a biological risk factor for low birth weight.

Intervention

Low birth weight and very low birth weight infants require intensive medical care, including being placed under a radiant heater, monitoring of respiration and heart rate, and in those instances where they are unable to feed from the nipple, feeding through nasogastric tubes with special formula or breast milk supplemented with human milk fortifier (Bernbaum & Batshaw, 1997).

Three broad types of early intervention programmes have been developed for low birth weight infants: programmes which focus exclusively on the needs and requirements of infants for an optimal level of stimulation; programmes which aim to help socially disadvantaged parents understand and meet the needs of their biologically vulnerable children; and multisystemic programmes which aim to focus on the child's needs for stimulation, the parents' needs for training and support and the dyad's needs for developing a secure attachment (Bennett, 1987; Guralnick, 1997; McCarton et al., 1995). The main elements of these three types of programmes are summarized in Table 2.1.

Table 2.1 Components of early intervention programmes for low birth weight infants

Child-focused programmes	**Postnatal stimulation**	<ul><li>Introduce diurnal rhythms and avoid overstimulation during periods where rest or sleep</li><li>Facilitate reciprocal tactile, kinaesthetic, auditory and visual stimulation during periods of alertness</li><li>For tactile stimulation engage infant in handling, stroking, massaging, flexing, positioning, and non-nutritive sucking</li><li>For kinaesthetic and vestibular stimulation place child on waterbed continually and during simulation episodes engage child in rocking in the arms</li><li>For auditory stimulation talk or sing to the infant and provide tap recordings of mother's heartbeat, mother's voice and music</li><li>For visual stimulation interact with the child in moderately lit room and introduce mobiles with brightly coloured objects into environment</li><li>Terminate all stimulation that leads to avoidance or distress due to overstimulation</li></ul>
	Special early education	<ul><li>Provide preschool children with enriched preschool environment</li><li>Use low infant:carer ratio.</li><li>Match curriculum to child's developmental stage</li><li>Involve parents in home activities based on school curriculum</li></ul>
Parent-focused programmes	**Parent training**	<ul><li>Educate parents about physical and psychological development of LBW children</li><li>Train parents to understand child's signals</li><li>Train parents to become attuned to child's communications about needs for feeding, toileting, comfort, sensory stimulation, communication and routine</li><li>Train parents to meet children's needs promptly and appropriately</li></ul>

Table 2.1 continued

Parent support groups	• Arrange for groups of parents of low birth weight infants to meet to discuss parenting and self-management issues • Provide parent education in a group setting • Train parents in systematic problem-solving skills for resolving personal and parenting problems • Provide life skills training to help parents manage family socio-economic difficulties • Provide stress management training to help parents deal with parental negative mood states
Parent–child focused programmes **Conjoint parent–child sessions**	• Conduct coaching in conjoint mother–infant sessions • Coach mothers and infants in optimal patterns of interaction for secure attachment • Use instruction, shaping and social reinforcement during coaching to promote new interaction patterns
Individual child- and parent-focused interventions	• Child-focused postnatal stimulation and special early education • Parent training and parent support groups

Programmes which focus exclusively on meeting the child's needs for an optimal level of stimulation are based on the premise that the premature low birth weight child in a neonatal intensive care unit requires compensation for lost intrauterine experiences and correction for sensory deprivation or over-stimulation while isolated in a neonatal intensive care unit. Programmes which focus exclusively on the mother are based on the premise that low birth weight infants place considerable demands upon parents, particularly socially disadvantaged parents, and so the needs of the infant may best be met by providing mothers with parent education and support. Programmes that focus on both mothers and infants combine the rationales of programmes exclusively for infants and mothers and augment these with the premise that secure mother–infant attachment is essential for optimal infant development. For this reason many programmes that focus on mothers and infants include conjoint training sessions for mothers and infants in optimal mother–infant interaction patterns in addition to parent education and child stimulation interventions.

Previous reviews

Previous reviews of early intervention studies for low birth weight infants have reached a number of important conclusions (Bennett, 1987; Blair & Ramey, 1997; Stevens-Simon & Orleans, 1999; McCarton et al., 1995). First, early intervention programmes can have a significant and positive effect on the development of low birth weight infants. Second, effective programmes have been delivered in a number of locations including maternity hospitals, on a home visiting basis, and in special paediatric treatment centres Third, effective programmes may be classified by their focus of intervention into three groups: those that focus exclusively on the infant and involve sensory stimulation; those that focus on the parents and involve parent training; and multisystemic programmes which focus on both the infant and the parents. Fourth, there has been considerable vari-ability in the intervention procedures used in each of the three types of programmes. Fifth, there has been considerable variability in the intensity and duration with which programmes have been offered. Some hospital-based programmes last no more than a few hours while other multisys-temic programmes involve both hospital-based and home-visiting-based intervention spanning a number of years. Sixth, there is some evidence to show that multisystemic programmes of longer duration and greater inten-sity may be the most effective. Seventh, effective programmes lead to increased IQ and fewer behavioural difficulties in low birth weight children along with improvements in parents' child development knowledge, atti-tudes and skills. Eighth, the mechanisms underpinning effective early intervention programmes are not fully understood, but programme effective-ness may be moderated by certain features of the child, family and wider social context within which the intervention programme is offered. All reviewers expressed concerns about methodological features of some studies reviewed.

Method

The aim of the present review was to identify effective early intervention programmes for low birth weight infants. PsychLit and Medline database searches of English language journals for the years 1967 to 2000 were conducted to identify studies in which early intervention programmes for low birth weight infants were evaluated. The terms *low birth weight* and *preterm* were combined with terms such as *early intervention, prevention programme, study, evaluation* and *effect*. A manual search through the bibliographies of all recent reviews, and relevant psychological and paediatric journals, was also conducted. Studies were selected for review if they had a group design, which included treatment and control or comparison group; if at least ten cases were included in each group; and if reliable post-intervention measures were included. A large number of studies which evaluated brief exclusively child-focused or exclusively parent-focused interventions were identified. Three examples of studies of effective brief early intervention programmes in each of these domains were selected for review. We also selected for review all studies of more intensive and comprehensive multisystemic prevention programmes which included medium- or long-term interventions targeting infants and mothers.

Characteristics of the studies

The main characteristics of the twelve studies are presented in Table 2.2. In three studies child stimulation programmes were evaluated; in a further three, behavioural parent training programmes were evaluated; and in six, complex multisystemic programmes were evaluated. The three child stimulation studies were exclusively hospital based. In the three behavioural parent training studies, programmes were offered in whole or in part within maternity hospitals and in one study home visiting was also included. In the six multisystemic studies, programmes were offered in whole or in part on a home visiting basis. In three of these, the programme was initiated in a hospital setting and in one study the programme involved attendance at a day programme in a child development centre. All of the studies were conducted in North America between 1971 and 1998. In all 1,600 families were involved in these twelve studies; 782 cases participated in prevention programmes and 818 cases were in routine-medical-management control groups. Data on gender were available for eight of the twelve studies and averaging across these, 55% of infants were male and 45% were female. In ten studies gestational age data were available and in these gestational ages ranged from 29 to 36 weeks with a mean of 32 weeks. Mean birth weights or ranges were given in all studies and across all studies the average birth weight was 1,452 g. The socioeconomic

Table 2.2 Summary of key findings of early intervention programmes for low birth weight children

No	LOC	Focus	Authors	Year	N per group	Gender	Age	Birth weight	Mother's age	SES and ethnicity	Duration and setting
1	H	C	Field et al.	1986	1. CS-H = 20 2. C = 20	—	31 wGA	1,280 g	—	—	75 mpd for 10 d in H
2	H	C	Powell	1974	1. CS-H = 13 2. CS-H-P = 11 3. C = 12*	—	—	1,000–2,000 g	—	Low SES Black	2 × 20 mpd for 1m in H
3	H	C	Leib et al.	1980	1. CS-Hp = 14 2. C = 14	1. M 50% F 50% 2. M 57% F 43%	36 wGA	1,200–1,800 g	—	White Mid SES	5 hpd for 2 w in H
4	H	P	Parker et al. Zahr et al.	1992 1992	1. BPT-H = 30 2. C = 30	—	32 wGA	1,527 g	21 y	Low SES Black and Hispanic	4 × 90 min H
5	H	P	Meyer et al.	1994	1. BPT-H = 18 2. C = 16	1. M 56% F 64% 2. M 69% F 31%	29 wGA	1,191 g	28 y	Mid SES White Married 76%	17 × 90 min in H
6	H HV	P	Rauh et al. Achenbach et al. Achenbach et al.	1988 1990 1993	1. BPT-H + HV = 38 2. C = 40	1. M 44% F 56% 2. M 36% F 64%	32 wGA	1,599 g	27 y	Mid-Low SES	7 × 1 h in H 4 × 1 h in HV over 3 m
7	H HV	P + C	Scarr-Salapatek & Williams	1973	1. CS-H + BPT-HV = 15 2. C = 15	1. M 47% F 53% 2. M 27% F 73%	33 wGA	1,572 g	21 y	Low SES Black Unmarried	8 × 30 min pd for 6 w in H 52 × 1 h in HV over 1 y
8	H HV	P + C	Resnick et al.	1988	1. CS-H + BPT-HV + EM = 21 2. C = 20	1. M 52% F 48% 2. M 40% F 60%	31w GA	1,374 g	24 y	Low SES Rural North Florida	2 hpd for 6 w in H 48 × 1 h in H over 1 y
9	H HV	P + C	Resnick et al.	1987	1. CS-H + BPT-HV + EM = 107 2. C = 114	1. M 49% F 51% 2. M 39% F 61%	32 wGA	1,414 g	—	Low SES Black 59%	2 × 20 min pd for 4 w in H 48 × 1 h in HV over 2 y
10	HV	P + C	Williams & Scarr	1971	1. CS-HV + BPT-HV + EM = 40 2. EM = 40 3. C = 40	—	0–1 y = 30 1–2 y = 30 2–3 y = 30 3–4 y = 30	1,380 g	—	Low SES Unmarried 45%	0–1y = 32 sess over 4 m 1–3y = 16 sess over 4 m 3–4y = 48 sess over 4 m
11	HV	P + C	Barrera et al.	1986	1. BPT-HV = 22 2. CS-HV = 16 3. C = 21	1. M 55% F 45% 2. M 53% F 47% 3. M 57% F 43%	33 wGA	1,677 g	27 y	Mixed SES	HV 30 sess over 1 y
12	HV DP	P + C	IHDP Brooks-Gunn et al. McCarton et al. Ramey et al. Casey et al. Berlin et al. McCormick	1990 1994 1997 1992 1994 1998 1993	1. CS-DP-HV + BPT-HV-G-EM = 377 2. C = 608	M 50% F 50%	33 wGA	1,819 g	24 y	Mixed SES Black and Hispanic 63%	HV104 sess over 3 y DP over 2 y

Notes

H = Hospital-based programme. HV = home-visiting-based programme. DP = day programme. P = parent. C = child. ST = short term, less than 6 weeks. MT = medium term, between 6 weeks and a year. LT = long term, more than a year. CS = child stimulation programme. BPT = behavioural parent training. EM = provision of educational materials. sess = session. min = minute. h = hour. d = day. w = week. m = month. y = year. hpw = hours per week. hpd = hours per day. hpm = hours per month. wGA = weeks gestational age. SES = socioeconomic status. g = gram.

status of participants ranged across the entire social spectrum. However, in six studies participants were from predominantly low socioeconomic groups. In five studies the majority of participants were from ethnic minority groups (black or Hispanic). Mean ages of mothers in these programmes ranged from 21 to 28 years. Programme duration ranged from four 90-minute sessions over a couple of weeks to 104 home visits over three years combined with regular attendance at a day programme over two years.

Methodological features

Methodological features of the studies are outlined in Table 2.3. In all studies cases were randomly assigned to intervention groups and control groups to whom routine medical services were offered. All studies included low birth weight as a primary diagnostic criterion for selection and so all studies included diagnostically homogeneous groups. Randomization ensured a considerable degree of demographic similarity across all studies. In seven studies pre-programme assessments were conducted and in all studies assessments were conducted shortly after programme completion. In six studies follow-up data were collected when infants were at least a year old and in two of these studies data were collected right up to middle childhood when children were aged eight or nine years. Intelligence or cognitive functioning test data were collected in ten of the twelve studies. In seven studies parental self-report data were collected and in eleven studies researcher ratings of infants' or mothers' behaviour were taken. Deterioration was evaluated in all studies and drop-out rates were reported in six. Experienced trainers or therapists were involved in eleven studies. In the two studies where two different treatment programmes were compared, both programmes were apparently equally valued by the research team. There was some degree of manualization in six of the twelve studies. There was evidence that supervision was provided to those implementing the programmes in nine of the twelve studies. Reports of integrity checks for programme implementation were included in none of the studies. Data on concurrent or subsequent intervention were given in none of the studies.

Overall this group of studies were fairly methodologically robust.

Outcome measures

In these studies weight gain, general neonatal development, motor and mental development, psychosocial adjustment and maternal behaviour were among the more important outcome measures. The Brazelton (1973) Neonatal Behaviour Assessment Scale was widely used to evaluate neonatal development. For infants the Bayley (1969) Scales of Infant Development was used to evaluate mental and motor development and the Infant Behaviour Record which accompanies this scale was used to evaluate psychosocial adjustment. For older children, the Stanford Binet Intelligence Test

Table 2.3 Methodological features

	Study number											
	S1	S2	S3	S4	S5	S6	S7	S8	S9	S10	S11	S12
Control or comparison group	1	1	1	1	1	1	1	1	1	1	1	1
Random assignment	1	1	1	1	1	1	1	1	1	1	1	1
Diagnostic homogeneity	1	1	1	1	1	1	1	1	1	1	1	1
Demographic similarity	1	1	1	1	1	1	1	1	1	1	1	1
Pre-treatment assessment	0	0	1	0	1	1	1	1	0	1	0	1
Post-treatment assessment	1	1	1	1	1	1	1	1	1	1	1	1
1-year follow-up assessment	0	0	0	1	0	1	1	1	1	1	1	1
Intelligence or cognitive development test	0	1	1	1	1	1	1	1	1	1	1	1
Parent reports	0	1	0	1	0	1	0	0	1	0	1	1
Researcher ratings	1	1	1	1	1	1	1	1	0	0	1	1
Deterioration assessed	1	1	1	1	1	1	1	1	1	1	1	1
Drop-out assessed	1	1	0	1	1	1	1	1	1	1	1	1
Clinical significance of change assessed	1	0	1	1	1	1	1	1	1	0	1	1
Experienced therapists or trainers used	1	1	1	0	1	0	1	1	0	0	1	0
Programmes were equally valued	0	1	0	0	0	0	0	0	0	1	1	1
Programmes were manualized	0	0	0	0	1	0	0	1	1	1	1	1
Supervision was provided	0	1	1	0	1	1	0	1	1	0	1	1
Programme integrity checked	0	0	0	0	0	0	0	0	0	0	0	0
Data on concurrent treatment given	0	0	0	0	0	0	0	0	0	0	0	0
Data on subsequent treatment given	0	0	0	0	0	0	0	0	0	0	0	0
Total	10	13	12	12	14	14	13	15	13	12	16	16

Note
S = study. 1 = design feature was present. 0 = design feature was absent.

(Terman & Merrill, 1972; Thorndike et al., 1986) and the Wechsler Intelligence Scale for Children and its revised versions (Wechsler, 1989, 1991) were used to evaluate intelligence. A wide range of measures was used to evaluate parental well-being, knowledge, attitudes, behaviour and skills.

Substantive findings

Treatment effect sizes and outcome rates for the twelve studies are presented in Table 2.4. A narrative summary of key findings from each study is given in Table 2.5.

Child-focused interventions

Three studies evaluate child-focused programmes and in each of these the intervention programme involved sensory stimulation (Field et al., 1986; Powell, 1974; Leib et al., 1980). In a study of low birth weight, preterm neonates, Field et al. (1986) found that compared with controls who received routine treatment, a programme of tactile and kinaesthetic stimulation led to increased daily weight gain (25 g v 17 g), greater maturity on the habituation, orientation, motor behaviour, and range of state dimensions of the Brazelton (1973) Neonatal Behaviour Assessment Scale and a six-day reduction in the duration of hospitalization. Each infant in this child stimulation programme received 15 minutes of tactile stimulation at the beginning of three consecutive hours beginning after the morning feed for 10 days. In the first and third 5-minute period of each 15-minute episode, the nurse stroked and massaged the child through the isolette portholes. In the middle 5-minute period of each 15-minute episode, the infant received kinaesthetic stimulation in which the nurse flexed and extended each of the arms and legs in sequence a number of times.

In a study of low birth weight black infants Powell (1974) found that compared with infants who received routine treatment, those who received regular handling (stroking, holding and rocking) from either the mother or nurses for 20 minutes twice a day from three days of age until discharge showed more favourable development on the mental and motor dimensions or the Bayley (1969) Scales of Infant Development at four months, but not two or six months, and improvement of the Infant Behaviour Record at six months. Also handling did not accelerate weight gain and maternal handling did not lead to improvements in mother–infant interaction or parenting skill as rated by independent observers.

In a study of low birth weight, high-risk preterm infants, Leib et al. (1980) found that compared with controls who received routine treatment, infants who received a multimodal sensory enrichment programme showed significant improvement on the interactive processes dimension of the Brazelton (1973) Neonatal Behaviour Assessment Scale after intervention and had higher mental and motor developmental scores on the Bayley (1969) Scales

Table 2.4 Summary of results of treatment effects and outcome rates

| | Child focused | | | | Parent focused | | | Child + parent focused | | | | | | | |
| | Study 1 | Study 2 | | Study 3 | Study 4 | Study 5 | Study 6 | Study 7 | Study 8 | Study 9 | Study 10 | Study 11 | | Study 12 | |
Variable	CS-H v C	CS-H v C	CS-H-P v C	CS-H v C	BPT-H v C	BPT-H v C	BPT-HV + HV v C	CS-H + BPT-HV v C	CSH + BPT-HV + EM v C	CS-H + BPT-HV + EM v C	CS-HV + BPT-HV + EM v C	BPT-HV v C	CS-HV v C	LBW CS-DP-HV + BPT-HV-DP-EM v C	VLBW CS-DP-HV + BPT-HV-DP-EM v C
Weight after programme	1.2	0.0	0.0	0.0	0.3			0.7						0.0	0.0
Brazelton NBAS after programme	1.2			0.4				0.0							
Motor development															
After programme		0.3	0.3		0.6				0.0			0.0	0.0		
After 6 months		0.4	0.4	1.4	0.1				0.0	0.6		0.0	0.0		
IQ and mental development															
After programme (0–6 m)		0.6	0.6		0.6		−0.1		0.0		1.2*				
After 6 months		−0.5	−0.5	1.4	0.7		0.0		0.6						
After 1 year								0.6	0.6			0.6	0.6		
After 2 years							0.5			0.7					
After 3 years							0.6			0.6				0.8	0.4
After 4 years							0.8								
After 5 years														0.1	0.0
After 6 years															
After 7 years							0.9							0.1	0.0
After 8 years															
After 9 years							1.0								
Child's psychosocial development															
After programme (0–6 m)		0.1			0.3						2.6†				
After 6 months		1.4			0.3										
After 1 year												0.6	0.6		
After 3 years															
After 5 years															
After 8 years															
Mother's status after programme															
Well-being						1.0									
Parenting knowledge and attitudes					0.2	0.3	0.8					0.6	0.0		
Quality of mother-child interaction	0	0				1.1			0.8			0.7	0.7		
Parenting skills															
Drop-out	0%	0%	0%		0%	0%	6% v 27%			82% v 81%				7%	7%

Notes

H = hospital based programme. HV = Home visiting-based programme. DP = day programme. P = parent. C = child. ST = short term, less than 6 weeks. MT = medium term, between 6 weeks and a year. LT = long term, more than a year. CS = child stimulation programme. BPT = behavioural parent training. EM = provision of educational materials. NBAs = neonatal behavioural assessment scale. *Effect size calculated for neurologically impaired cases only. †Effect size calculated for non-neurologically impaired cases only.

Table 2.5 Summary of key findings of early intervention programmes for low birth weight children

No	LOC.	Focus	Authors	Year	N per group	Duration and setting	Group differences	Key findings
1	H	C	Field et al.	1986	1. CS-H = 20 2. C = 20	75 min pd for 10 d in H	1 > 2	• Compared with controls, infants who received tactile and kinaesthetic stimulation (stroking and limb movement) for 75 minutes per day over 10 days showed greater weight gain and maturity on the Brazelton Neonatal Behaviour Assessment scale and were discharged 6 days earlier
2	H	C	Powell	1974	1. CS-H = 13 2. CS-H-P = 11 3. C = 12	2 × 20 min pd for 1 m in H	1 > 2 > 3	• Low birth weight infants who were given extra stimulation through stroking, holding and rocking in the hospital during the first month of life had significantly higher Bayley Mental and Motor Scale scores at 4m, and higher Infant Behaviour Record scores at 6m of age than controls
3	H	C	Leib et al.	1980	1. CS-Hp = 14 2. C = 14	5 hpd for 2 w in H	1 > 2	• At 6 months, preterm infants who received intensive daily perceptual and tactile stimulation for 2 weeks following birth showed significantly higher developmental status than controls. • Treated infants scores on the Bayley Scales of Infant Development were 15–20 points higher
4	*H	P	Parker et al. Zahr et al.	1992 1992	1. BPT-H = 30 2. C = 30	4 × 90min H	1 > 2	• Compared with controls, infants of mothers who received 4, 90 minute parent training sessions while in hospital showed better cognitive development at 4 and 8 months and better motor development at 4 months • Mothers who participated in the programme showed better parenting care at 4 but not 8 months • VLBW infants derived more benefit from the programme than LBW infants and showed better mental and motor development at 4 and 8 months and their mothers showed better knowledge, attitudes and parenting skills at 4 months
5	H	P	Meyer et al.	1994	1. BPT-H = 18 2. C = 16	17 × 90m in H	1 > 2	• Compared with controls, mother-infant dyads who received up to 17 90 minute behavioural parent training sessions while in hospital showed better adjustment at discharge • Improvements in mother–infant interaction particularly during feed in occurred in the intervention group • Mothers who participated in behavioural parent training reported less parental stress and depression

No.	Type	Design	Author	Year	Groups	Intervention details	Comparison	Findings
6	*H HV	P	Rauh et al. Achenbach et al. Achenbach et al.	1988 1990 1992	1. BPT-H + HV = 38 2. C = 40	7 × 1 h in H 4 × 1 h in HV over 3 m	1 > 2	• Compared with controls, infants whose parents received an 11 session parent training programme (7 in hospital 3 in the home over 3 months) showed better cognitive development at 3 y; 4 y; 7 y and 9 y • Compared with controls, parents who received training showed improvements in parenting attitudes and skills
7	H HV	P + C	Scarr-Salapatek & Williams	1973	1. CS-H + BPT-HV + EM = 15 2. C = 15	8 × 30 min pd for 6 w in H 52 × 1 h in HV over 1 y	1 > 2	• Following 6 weeks of stimulation after birth in the nursery and weekly home visits for one year, infants participating in the programme displayed greater developmental progress and had IQs on the Cattell Infant Development scale which were 10 points higher than those in the control group
8	*H HV	P + C	Resnick et al.	1988	1. CS-H + BPT-HV + EM = 21 2. C = 20	2 hpd for 6 w in H 48 × 1 h in H over 1 y	1 > 2	• Following twice daily stimulation sessions after birth until discharge and fortnightly home visits for a year infants showed better cognitive development and parent–child interaction than controls who received routine care at 1 year
9	H HV	P + C	Resnick et al.	1987	1. CS-H + BPT-HV + EM = 107 2. C = 114	2 × 20 min pd for 4 w in H 48 × 1 h in HV over 2 y	1 > 2	• At 1 and 2 y, infants who received an intensive hospital and home-based programme focused on children and parents showed a lower incidence of developmental delay and obtained higher scores on the Bayley Scales of Infant Development than controls
10	HV	P + C	Williams & Scarr	1971	1. CS-HV + BPT-HV + EM = 40 2. EM = 40 3. C = 40	0–1 y = 32 sess over 4 m 1–3 y = 16 sess over 4 m 3–4 y = 48 sess over 4 m	1 > 2 > 3	• Following a home-based developmentally staged information and education programme LBW children with neurological impairment showed greater social maturity than matched no-treatment controls and controls who received educational materials only • Following a home-based developmentally staged information and education programme LBW children without neurological impairment returned higher IQ scores on the Peabody Picture Vocabulary Test than the matched no-treatment controls and controls who received educational materials only • Following a home-based developmentally staged information and education programme 3–4-year-old LBW children with and without neurological impairment showed better language development on the Illinois Test of Psycholinguistic Abilities than matched no-treatment controls and controls who received educational materials only
11	HV	P + C	Barrera et al.	1986	1. BPT-HV = 22 2. CS-HV = 16 3. C = 21	HV 30 sess over 1 y	1 = 2 > 3	• Compared with controls, infants and mothers in both intervention groups showed better adjustment after 1 year • Infants showed better verbal development and independent play • Mothers showed better responsiveness and parent–child interaction

Table 2.5 continued

No	LOC.	Focus	Authors	Year	N per group	Duration and setting	Group differences	Key findings
12	HV DP	P + C	IHDP Brooks-Gunn et al. McCarton et al. Ramey et al. Casey et al. Berlin et al.	1990 1994 1997 1992 1994 1998	1. CS-DP-HV + BPT-HV-DP-EM = 377 2. C = 608	HV104 sess over 3 y DP over 2 y	1 > 2	• The LBW and VLBW children from mixed SES families who participated in the child stimulation and parent training programme involving home visiting and attendance at a day programme over the child's first 3 years of life benefited from the programme but the benefits diminished over time • At 3 y, compared with controls, low birth weight children's mean IQ was 13 points higher and very low birth weight children's IQs were 7 points higher than controls' • At 5 and 8 y the low birth weight children's mean IQ was 4 points higher than controls' but the VLBW children's IQs did not differ from controls' • Compared with controls at 3 y, infants in the intervention group showed better psychosocial adjustment but no intergroup differences occurred in psychosocial adjustment at 5 y • Heavier infants (over 2,000 g) and children from poorer families made the greatest and longest lasting gains in IQ and psychosocial development • VLBW and low levels of programme participation were associated with poorest outcome • At 3 y, very low birth weight infants who participated in the programme had IQs that were 7 points higher than very low birth weight children from the control group • At 3 y, children with failure to thrive whose families were highly involved in the programme and showed good compliance had higher IQs than families of failure to thrive children who showed low compliance

Note:
H = hospital-based programme. HV = home-visiting-based programme. DP = day programme. P = parent. C = child. ST = short term, less than 6 weeks. MT = medium term, between 6 weeks and a year. LT = long term, more than a year. CS = child stimulation programme. BPT = behavioural parent training. EM = provision of educational materials. sess = session. min = minute. h = hour. d = day. w = week. m = month. y = year. hpw = hours per week. hpd = hours per day. hpm = hours per month.

of Infant Development at six months. The intervention did not lead to accelerated weight gain or growth. The sensory enrichment programme involved visual stimulation (bright coloured mobile), tactile stimulation (rubbing, stroking), kinaesthetic stimulation (being fed by a nurse in a rocking chair), and auditory stimulation (talking and singing during periods of interaction).

From the results of the three studies summarized above and in Tables 2.4 and 2.5, the following conclusions may be drawn. First, programmes for preventing developmental delay in low birth weight infants in which child stimulation is a central component have a positive effect, of moderate size, on infant development.

Second, child stimulation had a positive effect on infant growth in only one out of three studies. Averaging across the three studies, the effect size for weight gain was only 0.3, indicating that the average infant who participated in a child stimulation programme fared better afterwards than only 62% of controls.

Third, child stimulation had a positive effect on neonatal development as assessed by the Brazelton Neonatal Behaviour Assessment Scale. Averaging across the two studies where infants were assessed on this scale, the effect size was 0.8, indicating that the average infant who participated in a child stimulation programme fared better afterwards than 79% of controls.

Fourth, child stimulation had a positive effect on post-programme cognitive development as assessed by the Bayley Scale of Infant Development. In the single study where data were available, the effect size was 0.6, indicating that the average infant who participated in a child stimulation programme fared better afterwards than 73% of controls. At six months, however, an effect size of -0.5 was obtained in a study of disadvantaged families and an effect size of 1.4 was obtained in a study of middle-class families, suggesting that gains in cognitive development are maintained in families where infants are not exposed to social disadvantage.

Fifth, child stimulation had a positive effect on post-programme psychosocial development at six months. In the single study where data were available the effect size was 1.4, indicating that the average infant who participated in a child stimulation programme showed better psychosocial adjustment at six months than 92% of controls.

Sixth, programmes for preventing developmental delay in low birth weight infants in which child stimulation is a central component had no impact on mother–child interaction or parenting skills.

Seventh, all families completed these hospital-based child stimulation programmes without dropping out. Unfortunately long-term follow-up data were not reported in any of these studies so the durability of the positive effects remains a matter of conjecture and a potential focus for future research.

Parent-focused interventions

In three studies parent-focused interventions were evaluated (Parker et al., 1992; Meyer et al., 1994; Rauh et al., 1988). In a study of low birth weight premature infants, Parker et al. (1992) found that compared with controls, infants of mothers who received four 90-minute parent training sessions while in hospital showed better cognitive development at four and eight months and better motor development at four months on the Bayley Scales of Infant Development. Mothers who participated in the programme showed better parenting care on the HOME Scale at four but not eight months. Intervention and control groups did not differ in rates of weight gain or weight gain at discharge. Very low birth weight infants derived more benefit from the programme than low birth weight infants (Zahr et al., 1992). The very low birth weight children showed better mental and motor development at four and eight months and their mothers showed better knowledge, attitudes and parenting skills at four months. The parent training programme involved the mother having weekly sessions in hospital with an infant development specialist in which they observed and assessed the child using a version of the Brazelton Neonatal Behaviour Assessment Scale and the mother was taught how to interpret her infant's behaviour and appropriately modify her care-taking to meet her child's needs.

In a study of preterm low birth weight infants Meyer et al. (1994) found that compared with controls, mother–infant dyads who received up to seventeen 90-minute behavioural parent training sessions while in hospital showed better adjustment at discharge. Improvements in mother–infant interaction particularly during feedings occurred in the intervention group. Mothers who participated in behavioural parent training reported less parental stress and depression on the Beck Depression Inventory (Beck et al., 1961). The behavioural parent training programme was based on detailed assessment of the infant and the family and while each programme was tailored to the needs of each family, specific interventions fell into four main categories: parent education about infants' behaviour characteristics and special needs; parent training to identify and meet infant needs; parent and family counselling to facilitate coping with individual and marital stress associated with the demands of caring for a high-risk infant; and practical assistance with accessing community resources and services.

In a study of preterm low birth weight infants, Rauh and Achenbach (Rauh et al., 1988; Achenbach et al., 1990, 1993) found that compared with controls, infants whose parents received an eleven-session parent training programme (seven in hospital and four in the home over three months) showed better cognitive development at three, four, seven and nine years. Cognitive development was assessed with the Bayley (1969) Scales of Infant Development at six, twelve and twenty-four months, the McCarthy (1972) Scales of Children's Abilities at three and four years and the Kaufman Assessment Battery for Children at seven and nine years (Kaufman &

Kaufman, 1983). Compared with controls, parents who received training showed improvements in parenting attitudes and skills at six months. The mother–infant transaction programme was designed to help mothers appreciate their infants' unique behavioural characteristics; sensitized them to infants' cues, particularly those that signal distress, stimulus overload and readiness for interaction; and helped them to develop skills for responding to these cues so as to promote satisfying interactions.

From the results of the three studies summarized above and in Tables 2.4 and 2.5, the following conclusions may be drawn. First, programmes for preventing developmental delay in low birth weight infants in which behavioural parent training is a central component have a positive and sustained effect on infant development.

Second, parent training had a moderately positive effect on infant growth in the only study in which this was evaluated. The effect size for weight gain was only 0.3, indicating that the average infant whose mother participated in the parent training programme fared better afterwards than only 62% of controls.

Third, parent training had a positive effect on cognitive or mental development and in both studies where cognitive development was assessed at two or more time points, the effects of the programme intensified with the passage of time. For example, in the study by Rauh and Achenbach's team, the effect size at one year was 0, at two years was 0.5, at three years was 0.6, at four years was 0.8, at seven years was 0.9 and at nine years was 1.0 (Rauh et al., 1988; Achenbach et al., 1990, 1993). Thus, at nine years the average child whose mother participated in the parent training programme fared better than 84% of controls.

Fourth, parent training had a moderately positive effect on psychosocial adjustment in the only study in which this was evaluated. The effect size for psychosocial adjustment was only 0.3 after treatment and at six-month follow-up, indicating that the average infant whose mother participated in the parent training programme fared better afterwards than only 62% of controls.

Fifth, parent training programmes had a positive impact on maternal well-being, parenting knowledge and attitudes, and parenting skills. Effect sizes in these areas ranged from 0.2 to 1.1 with an average of 0.9, indicating that the average mother who participated in a parent training programme fared better than 82% of controls afterwards.

Sixth, all families completed these hospital-based behavioural parent training programmes without dropping out.

Multisystemic parent- and child-focused interventions

In six studies complex multisystemic intervention programmes which focused on parents and children were evaluated (Scarr-Salapatek & Williams, 1973; Resnick et al., 1987, 1988; Williams & Scarr, 1971; Barrera et al., 1986; Infant Health and Development Programme, 1990).

In a study of low SES, preterm low birth weight children Scarr-Salapatek & Williams (1973) found that following six weeks of stimulation after birth in the nursery and weekly home visits for one year, infants participating in the programme displayed greater developmental progress and had IQs on the Cattell Infant Development scale which were ten points higher than those in the control group. In hospital the infants received visual, tactile and kinaesthetic stimulation for eight 30-minute periods per day. After discharge, mothers were visited weekly for a year by a social worker who conducted behavioural parent training and encouraged mothers to follow the Gordon and Lally (1967) manual, which describes principles of child development and stimulation procedures that promote optimal cognitive and psychosocial development. The curriculum covers cognition, communication, motor development, socioemotional development, and self-help skills. Mothers were also provided with educational materials including mobiles, wall posters and appropriate toys.

In a study of low SES, preterm low birth weight children Resnick et al. (1988) found that at one year, following twice-daily stimulation sessions after birth until discharge and fortnightly home visits for a year, infants showed better cognitive development on the Bayley (1969) Scales of Infant Development and more positive parent–child interaction as evaluated by independent observers than did controls who received routine care.

In a subsequent study of low SES, preterm low birth weight children Resnick et al. (1987) found that at one and two years, infants who received an intensive hospital and home-based programme which focused on children and parents showed a lower incidence of developmental delay and obtained higher scores on the Bayley (1969) Scales of Infant Development than controls. Attrition was a major problem in this study. At one year 61% of cases in the intervention group were still in the programme, but at two years this had fallen to 18%. There was comparable drop-out from the control group.

In both of these studies Resnick used the following programme. While in the neonatal intensive care unit, infants were placed on water mattresses to receive continual vestibular stimulation. Their environment contained mobiles and coloured patterns for visual stimulation. During the hospital-based stimulation periods they were massaged, engaged in passive motion exercises and heard tape recordings of their mother's heartbeat, voice and music. They also received oral stimulation to prepare them for feeding. During the home visits, the nurse trained the mother to engage the child in a series of exercises to promote development in a number of domains including: physical development, visual development, auditory development, language, social development, memory and perceptual and motor skills. Specific sets of exercises were set for each of the developmental stages through which infants passed during the extended period of home visiting. In addition parents were trained to keep detailed records of infant development in a baby book provided by the home-visiting nurse.

In a study of low birth weight children aged 0–48 months, Williams &

Scarr (1971) found that following a home-based developmentally staged information and education programme, low birth weight children with neurological impairment showed greater social maturity than matched no-treatment controls and controls who received educational materials only. In the intervention group low birth weight children without neurological impairment returned higher IQ scores on the Peabody Picture Vocabulary Test than matched no-treatment controls and controls who received educational materials only. Low birth weight children with and without neurological impairment showed better language development on the Illinois Test of Psycholinguistic Abilities than matched no-treatment controls and controls who received educational materials only. Within the programme, children aged two, three and four years received direct stimulation and education from home-visiting tutors over a four-month period and mothers received both child development education and behavioural parent training. Where children were under a year old, only parent education and training were offered. For children aged three and four years tutors used the Bereiter–Engleman direct verbal training method (Berieter & Engleman, 1966).

In a study of low birth weight infants Barrera et al. (1986) found that compared with controls, infants and mothers who participated in a home-visiting programme involving coaching in parent–child interaction and those who participated in a home-visiting child stimulation programme showed better adjustment after one year. Infants showed better cognitive development on the Bayley (1969) Scales of Infant Development and more independent play as rated by observers. Mothers showed better parenting knowledge, attitudes and skills and better responsiveness. In the parenting skills training, mothers were trained to recognize and interpret their infant's cues and respond to their needs contingently. In the child stimulation programme mothers implemented a curriculum of exercises with their infants that covered cognition, communication, motor development, socioemotional development, and self-help skills.

In the Infant Health and Development Program a complex multisystemic intervention for premature low birth weight infants and their mothers was evaluated (Berlin et al., 1998; Brooks-Gunn et al., 1994; Casey et al., 1994; Infant Health and Development Program, 1990; McCormick et al., 1993; McCarton et al., 1997; Ramey et al., 1992). The intervention included a child stimulation programme and a parent training programme offered both within a home-visiting context and within a child development centre. The child stimulation programme included a series of developmentally staged exercises and activities to promote physical, cognitive, linguistic and social development (Sparling & Lewis 1984a; Sparling et al., 1988, 1991). Mothers were helped to implement the programme at home by home visitors and the programme was followed and extended in visits to a day programme run at child development centres. Home visiting began following discharge from neonatal intensive care units and attendance at child development centres began when infants reached their first birthday. The parent training programme involved training mothers in systematic problem-solving skills for resolving personal and parenting difficulties along with group-based parent education (Wasik, 1984a, 1984b; Wasik et al., 1990a).The programme spanned three years. In development centres staff:pupil ratios ranged from 1:3 to 1:4. Transport to and from the development centre was provided to all participating families.

The LBW and VLBW children from mixed SES families in the intervention group who made use of home visits, child development centre visits and parental support meetings over the child's first three years of life benefited from the programme but the benefits diminished over time. At three years, compared with controls, low birth weight children's mean IQs on the Stanford Binet Intelligence Scale (Terman & Merrill, 1972) were thirteen points higher and very low birth weight children's IQs were seven points higher (Infant Health and Development Program, 1990). At five and eight years the low birth weight children's mean IQs on the revised Wechsler Preschool and Primary Scale of Intelligence (Wechsler, 1989) and the third revision of the Wechsler Intelligence Scale for Children (Wechsler, 1991) was four points higher than controls but the VLBW children's IQs did not differ from controls (Brooks-Gunn et al., 1994; McCarton et al., 1997). Compared with controls at three years, infants in the intervention group showed better psychosocial adjustment on the Child Behaviour Checklist (Achenbach, 1991), but no intergroup differences occurred in psychosocial adjustment at five years. Heavier infants (over 2,000 g) and children from poorer families made the greatest and longest lasting gains in IQ and psychosocial development (Berlin et al., 1998). Very low birth weight and low levels of programme participation were associated with poorest outcome (Ramey et al., 1992). At three years, very low birth weight infants who participated in the programme had IQs that were seven points higher than very low birth weight children from the control group (McCormick et al., 1993). At three years, children with failure to thrive whose families were highly involved in the programme and showed good compliance had higher IQs than families of failure-to-thrive children who showed low compliance (Casey et al., 1994).

From the results of the six studies summarized above and in Tables 2.4 and 2.5, the following conclusions may be drawn. First, complex multisystemic programmes for preventing developmental delay in low birth weight infants in which behavioural parent training is combined with child stimulation have a positive effect on infant development and parenting.

Second, multisystemic programmes had a positive effect on weight gain in only one of the two studies in which this was evaluated. The effect size for weight gain in this study was 0.7, indicating that the average infant whose family participated in the multisystemic programme was heavier afterwards than 76% of controls.

Third, multisystemic programmes had a positive effect on infant motor development in only one of the three studies in which this was evaluated. The effect size for weight gain in this study was 0.6, indicating that the average infant whose family participated in the multisystemic programme fared better afterwards than 73% of controls.

Fourth, multisystemic programmes had a positive effect on cognitive or mental development and in all six studies where cognitive development was assessed. Averaging across four studies for which there are one-year follow-up data, the average effect size was 0.6. Thus, at one year of age the average child whose family participated in a multisystemic programme fared better than 73% of controls. After age three the effects of intervention are less marked. Heavier infants, without neurological impairments, from poorer families who participated fully in multisystemic programmes made greatest gains. Lower biological vulnerability and greater environmental disadvantage coupled with high level of programme compliance are a recipe for success.

Fifth, multisystemic programmes had a positive effect on psychosocial adjustment during the first three years, with effect sizes ranging from 0.2 to 2.6 with a mean of 1.0 indicating that the average infant whose family participated in a multisystemic programme fared better afterwards than only 84% of controls. Greatest advances in psychosocial adjustment were made by neurologically impaired infants during the first year.

Sixth, multisystemic programmes had a positive impact on parenting knowledge and attitudes, and parenting skills. Effect sizes in these areas ranged from 0.6 to 0.8 with a mean of 0.7, indicating that the average mother who participated in a parent training programme fared better than 76% of controls afterwards.

Seventh, there was wide variability in drop-out rates. One three-year programme with an impressively low 7% drop-out rate provided participants with transport to and from the centres where the day programme was conducted.

Conclusions

Low birth weight is a problem that places infants at risk for developmental delay. About 7% of all births in industrialized countries have low birth weights and 1% of children at birth meet the criterion for very low birth weight. Social disadvantage and preterm birth are the main risk factors for low birth weight. Three broad types of early intervention programmes have been developed for low birth weight infants: programmes which focus exclusively on the needs and requirements of infants for an optimal level of stimulation; programmes which aim to help socially disadvantaged parents understand and meet the needs of their biologically vulnerable children; and multisystemic programmes which aim to focus on the child's needs for stimulation, the parents' needs for training and support and the dyad's needs for developing a secure attachment.

From this review of twelve controlled studies, it may be concluded that all three types of programmes can have a positive impact on child development in general and cognitive development in particular. All three types of

programme may also have a positive effect on infants' psychosocial adjustment. Parent training and multisystemic programmes lead to improvements
in parenting knowledge, attitudes and skills.

Long-term data are only available from two studies and so deserve cautious
interpretation. These data show that brief parent training programmes which
begin in hospital and are continued in the home may lead to increasingly
positive gains in cognitive development over the long term (up to nine years
of age). In contrast, complex multisystemic programmes, which include home
visiting and a day programme, may be less effective in the long term, with
diminishing improvement as children reach eight years of age. However, these
counterintuitive results require replication.

Lower biological vulnerability (as indexed by lack of neurological impairment and absence of very low birth weight) and greater environmental disadvantage (indexed by lower SES) coupled with high levels of participation in
programme activities are the main factors predictive of a positive response to
early intervention and a good outcome.

Implications for policy and practice

The implications of these conclusions for policy and practice are clear.
Families in which low birth weight infants are born should be engaged in
programmes which begin in neonatal intensive care units and involve home
visiting, community-based outpatient and preschool follow-up sessions. Such
programmes should include child stimulation, parent training and support,
and conjoint parent–child sessions to promote secure attachment. Such programmes should be continued throughout the preschool and early school
going years until a comprehensive multidisciplinary assessment indicates that
the child's development falls within normal limits. Children with a high level
of biological vulnerability as indexed by very low birth weights and neurological impairment may require more intensive programmes. Special efforts
should be made to help parents stay engaged with these programmes. Home
visiting and the provision of transport to day centres may facilitate this.

Implications for research

There is a need to evaluate not only immediate post-programme improvements on indices of child development and parenting knowledge, attitudes
and skills, but also the long-term impact of such programmes.

There is considerable evidence that father involvement in family therapy
can have a significant impact on outcome (Carr, 2001c). Despite this, programmes for low birth weight infants, such as those evaluated in the studies
reviewed in this chapter, have rarely involved fathers. Future research should
evaluate the impact of programmes that target both fathers and mothers as
programme participants.

Future research should evaluate manualized intervention programmes in which checks for programme integrity are made (which were a rarity in the studies reviewed here). In such studies, training sessions are recorded and blind raters use programme integrity checklists to evaluate the degree to which sessions approximate manualized training curricula. Such integrity checks allow researchers to say with confidence the degree to which a pure and potent version of their programme has been evaluated.

Studies that examine the impact of design features that may make programmes more effective are also required. Specifically research is needed on the effects of including different components in multisystemic programmes (child stimulation and behavioural parent training), of different sites for programme delivery (hospital-based intervention, home visiting, day programmes), and of programmes of differing durations.

Studies are required which investigate the mechanisms and processes that underpin programme effectiveness. Improvements probably occur through a variety of complex mechanisms including enhancing infant development directly through stimulation; enhancing infant development through supporting the development of secure parent–child attachments; and enhancing general child care taking by improving parental child care knowledge and skills.

There is a need to design and evaluate programmes for families that have particular difficulties in engaging in prevention programmes for low birth weight infants, because we know that a high level of participation is one of the most important factors influencing outcome.

Assessment resources

Achenbach, T. (1991). *Integrated Guide for the 1991 CBCL/4–18, YSR and TRF profiles*. Burlington: University of Vermont Department of Psychiatry.

Bayley, N. (1969). *Bayley Scales of Infant Development*. New York: Psychological Corporation.

Brazelton, T.B. (1973). Neonatal Behavioural Assessment Scale. *Clinics in Developmental Medicine*, 50. Philadelphia: Lippincott Company.

Caldwell, B. & Bradley, R. (1979). *Home Observation for Measurement of the Environment (HOME)*. Little Rock, AK: University of Arkansas.

Kaufman, A. & Kaufman, N. (1983). *Kaufman Assessment Battery for Children*. Circle Pines, MN: American Guidance Service.

McCarthy, D. (1972). *Manual for the McCarthy Scales of Children's Abilities*. New York: Psychological Corporation.

McConaughay, S.H. & Achenbach, T.M. (1988). *Practical Guide for the Child Behavior Checklist and related materials*. Burlington: University of Vermont Department of Psychiatry.

Terman L.M. & Merrill, M.A. (1972). *Stanford Binet Intelligence Scale: Manual for the third revision, Form L-M*. Boston: Houghton-Mifflin.

Thorndike, R., Hagen, E. & Sattler, J. (1986). *Stanford-Binet Intelligence Scale: Fourth Edition*. San Antonio: Psychological Corporation.

Wechsler, D. (1989). *Wechsler Preschool and Primary Scale of Intelligence – Revised (WPPSI-R)*. San Antonio: Psychological Corporation.

Wechsler, D. (1991). *Wechsler Intelligence Scale for Children. Third Edition (WISC-111)*. San Antonio: Psychological Corporation.

Programme resources

Bereiter, C. & Engleman, S. (1966). *Teaching Disadvantaged Children in the Preschool*. Englewood Cliffs: Prentice Hall.

Gordon, I. & Lally, R. (1967). *Intellectual Stimulation for Infants and Toddlers*. Gainsville, FA: Institute of Development of Human Resources.

Resnick, M. & Packer, A. (1990). *Infant Development Activities for Parents*. New York: St Martins Press.

Sparling, J. & Lewis, I. (1984). *Partners for Learning*. Lewisville, NC: Kaplan Press.

Sparling, J., Lewis, I. & Neuwirth, S. (1988). *Early Partners Curriculum Kit*. Lewisville, NC: Kaplan Press.

Sparling, J., Lewis, I., Ramey, C., Wasik, B., Bryant, D. & LaVange, L. (1991). Partners: A curriculum to help premature, low birth weight infants get off to a good start. *Top Early Child Special Education*, 11, 36–55.

Wasik, B. (1984a). *Problem Solving for Parents*. Chapel Hill, NC: Frank Porter Graham Child Development Centre.

Wasik, B. (1984b). *Coping with Parenting Through Effective Problem Solving: A Handbook for Professionals*. Chapel Hill, NC: Frank Porter Graham Child Development Centre.

Wasik, B., Bryant, D. & Lyons, D. (1990). *Home Visiting*. Newbury Park: Sage.

3 Prevention of cognitive delay in socially disadvantaged children

Gregor Lange and Alan Carr

Children from socially disadvantaged backgrounds show delayed development of cognitive abilities. They obtain lower scores on tests of intelligence, cognitive skills, language development and academic attainment, compared with children who are not reared in poverty (Guralnick, 1998; Neisser et al., 1996). The link between social disadvantage and cognitive delay – between poverty and intelligence – has traditionally been the premise from which hereditarians have argued for the innate superiority of the upper classes and environmentalists have argued for the provision of early intervention programmes to help poor children avoid the cognitive delays associated with poverty. According to the environmentalist position, the provision of an intellectually stimulating early environment for poor children should prevent cognitive delay. In contrast hereditarians would argue that no amount of environmental enrichment can improve intelligence. The validity of each of these conflicting viewpoints may be resolved by an empirical test. That is by conducting controlled research on the effectiveness of early intervention. The aim of this chapter is to review a number of methodologically robust research studies on the effectiveness of early intervention programmes in preventing cognitive delay in socially disadvantaged children; to draw reliable conclusions about the effectiveness of these; and to outline the implications of these conclusions for policy and practice.

Epidemiology

In both US and UK studies, rates of mild intellectual disability or cognitive delay are about 10% in lower socioeconomic groups compared with 2–3% in higher socioeconomic groups and cases of mild intellectual disability predominate in lower socioeconomic groups (Guralnick, 1998; Neisser et al., 1996; Scott, 1994; Simonoff et al., 1996). Language delay and academic attainment problems are also more common in lower socioeconomic groups.

Aetiology

While up to 75% of cases of severe or profound intellectual disability are due to identifiable organic causes, as few as 10% of cases of mild intellectual disability are due to discrete organic factors (Guralnick, 1998; Neisser et al., 1996; Scott, 1994; Simonoff et al., 1996). Polygenetic and sociocultural factors play a far greater role in the aetiology of mild compared with severe intellectual disability. Current evidence from twin, adoption and pedigree studies suggests that about 50% of the variation in intelligence is (poly)genetically transmitted and 50% is environmentally determined.

Risk factors for mild intellectual disability or cognitive delay include low income, limited parental education, high family stress, low family support, family disorganization with unclear rules and chaotic supervision, lack of warm parent–child attachment, and limited intellectual stimulation of the child by parents. In contrast socially disadvantaged children from families in which there is warm, positive parent–child attachment, clear rules and consistent supervision, and considerable opportunities for children to engage in intellectually stimulating activities with parents and family members do not develop cognitive delays (Scott, 1994).

Intervention

In light of these risk factors, four broad types of early intervention programmes have been developed for socially disadvantaged children: home-visiting programmes; preschool programmes; combined home-visiting and preschool programmes; and multisystemic programmes. Home-visiting programmes aim to help socially disadvantaged parents understand and meet their children's needs for intellectual stimulation, secure attachment and consistent supervision. Preschool programmes aim to directly provide disadvantaged children with a stimulating preschool environment to compensate for their intellectually impoverished home environment. Combined home-visiting and preschool programmes aim both to enhance the quality of disadvantaged children's home environments and to give them access to stimulating preschool environments. Multisystemic programmes also have these aims but they attempt in addition to extend the direct support given to disadvantaged children by continuing to offer additional educational placement and support services into middle childhood and provide long-term support to parents so that they can maintain the quality of the home environment for their children.

Previous reviews

Previous reviews of early intervention studies for socially disadvantaged children have reached a number of important conclusions (Bryant & Maxwell, 1997; Bryant & Ramey, 1987; Guralnick, 1998; White et al., 1985). First, early intervention programmes can have significant and positive effects on the development of socially disadvantaged children. Second, effective programmes have been delivered on a home-visiting basis, in preschools, and in special centres. Third, effective early intervention programmes have involved home visiting, preschool placement, combinations of these components, and multisystemic interventions. Fourth, there has been considerable variability in the intensity and duration with which programmes have been offered. Some programmes last no more than a few months while others span a number of years. Fifth, there is some evidence to show that multisystemic programmes of longer duration and greater intensity may be the most effective. Sixth, effective programmes lead to improvements in IQ, language development and attainment. Seventh, the mechanisms underpinning effective early intervention programmes are not fully understood, but programme effectiveness may be moderated by certain features of the child, family and wider social context within which the intervention programme is offered. Eighth, there has been considerable variability in scientific rigour with which evaluation studies of early intervention programmes for socially disadvantaged children have been conducted.

Method

The aim of the present review was to identify effective early intervention programmes for disadvantaged children at risk of cognitive delay. A PsychLit database search of English language journals for the years 1977 to 2000 was conducted to identify studies in which such programmes were evaluated. Keywords used in the search included: *early intervention*, *early education*, and *treatment programme* combined with such terms as *cognitive delay*, *developmental delay*, *social disadvantage*, *environmental disadvantage*, *poverty* and *low SES*. In addition, a search of relevant journals was also conducted. Studies were selected for review if they had a group design with more than five participants in each group; if groups of participants were relatively homogeneous; if a control group or baseline comparison was involved; if data for at least one post-treatment outcome measure were reported. In total 15 studies were selected for inclusion in this review.

Characteristics of the reviewed studies

The characteristics of the fifteen studies reviewed are outlined in Table 3.1. In seven studies home-visiting programmes were evaluated (Levenstein & Sunley, 1968; Karnes et al., 1970; Slaughter, 1983; Powell & Grantham-McGregor, 1989; Gutelius et al., 1972; Jester & Guinagh, 1983; Ramey & Campbell, 1991). Three studies assessed preschool programmes (Karnes et al., 1970; Lee et al., 1988, 1990; Jester & Guinagh, 1983). Six studies investigated the effectiveness of combined home-visiting and preschool programmes (Jester & Guinagh, 1983; Schweinhart et al., 1985;

Table 3.1 Characteristics of studies of programmes to prevent cognitive delay in socially disadvantaged children

Study no.		Authors	Year	Country	N per group	Mean age and range	Gender	Ethnicity	Programme setting	Programme duration
1	HV	Levenstein & Sunley	1968	USA	1. HV = 6 2. C = 5	24 m		A-A 100%	Home	4 m
2	HV	Karnes et al.	1970	USA	1. HV(total) = 15 2. C(total) = 15 3. HV(sibling) = 6 4. C(sibling) = 6	20 m 12–24,	M 70% F 30%	A-A 93%	Home and centre	15 m
3	HV	Slaughter	1983	USA	1. HV = 26 2. PE = 26 3. C = 31	18 m		A-A 100%	Home	2 y
4	HV	Powell & Grantham-McGregor	1989	Jamaica	Study 1: 1. HV (biweekly) = 26 2. HV (monthly) = 20 3. C1 = 21 Study 2: 4. HV(weekly) = 29 5. C2 = 29	20 m 6–30 m	M 50% F 50%	A-A 100%	Home	3 y
5	HV	Gutelius et al.	1972	USA	1. HV = 46 2. C = 46	Term		A-A 100%	Home	3 y
6	PS	Karnes et al.	1970	USA	1. PS-T = 28 2. PS-CI = 16 3. PS-M = 16 4. PS-E = 27	49–52 m	M 50% F 50%	A-A 67% Caucasian 33%	Preschool	7–8 m
7	PS	Lee et al.	1988 1990	USA	1. PS-HS = 414 2. PS-T = 390 3. C = 165	4–5 y	—	A-A 71%	Preschool	9 m
8	HV + PS	Jester & Guinagh	1983	USA	1. HV + PS (EEE) = 49 2. HV (EEC) = 28 3. HV + PS (CEE) = 19 4. HV + PS (ECE) = 18 5. HV (ECC) = 11 6. HV(CEC) = 24 7. PS (CCE) = 32 8. C (CCC) = 58	3 m	M 80% F 20%	A-A 80% Caucasian 20%	Home and preschool	3 y

9	HV + PS	Schweinhart et al.	1985	USA	1. HV + PS = 58 2. C = 65	3–4 y	—	A-A. 100%	Home and preschool	2 y
10	HV + PS	Andrews et al. Johnson and Walker	1982 1991	USA	1. HV + PS = 97 2. C = 119	12 m	—	Mexican-American 100%	Home, centre and preschool	2 y
11	HV + PS	Gray & Klaus	1965 1970	USA	1. HV + SS (×3) = 19 2. HV + SS (×2) = 19 3. C1 = 18 4. C2 = 27	3–4 y	—	A-A 100%	Summer school, home	2 or 3 y
12	HV + PS	Deutsch et al.	1983	USA	1. HV + PS-E = 275 2. C1 = 129 3. C2 = 180	4 y	—	A-A 100%	Home and preschool	5 y
13	HV + PS	Wasik et al.	1990b	USA	1. HV + PS-E = 15 2. HV = 24 3. C = 23	2 m	M 61% F 39%	A-A 91%	Home and preschool	5 y
14	MC	Ramey & Campbell Campbell & Ramey	1991 1994 1995	USA	1. HV + PS + S + ET = 25 2. HV = 24 3. PE + S + ET = 24 4. C = 23	3 m	M 50% F 50%	A-A 98%	Home, preschool and school	3, 5, or 8 y
15	MC	Garber	1988	USA	1. HV + PS-E + FS + DS + SS = 17 2. C1 = 11 3. C2 (low-risk) = 6	3 m		—	Home, preschool and school	10 y

Notes

HV = Home visiting programme involving child stimulation and parent education. PE = parent education. PS = preschool. PS-T = traditional preschool. PS-CI = community integrated preschool. PS-M = Montessori preschool. PS-E = experimental preschool. PS-HS = Head Start preschool. SS = summer school; S = school. ET = extra tuition. FS = family support. DS = differential school placement. MC = multisystemic programme. C = control group. E = experimental intervention for a year. EEE = experimental intervention was received for each of three consecutive years. EEC = experimental intervention was received for each of two consecutive years followed by a control year of routine intervention. A-A = African-American. m = month. y = year.

Andrews et al., 1982; Johnson & Walker, 1991; Gray & Klaus, 1965, 1970; Deutsch et al., 1983; Wasik et al., 1990b). Multisystemic programmes were evaluated in two studies (Ramey & Campbell, 1991; Garber, 1988). In some studies more than one type of programme was investigated (Jester & Guinagh, 1983; Ramey & Campbell, 1991; Campbell & Ramey, 1994, 1995).

The fifteen studies were published between 1965 and 1991. Fourteen studies were conducted in the USA and one study was from Jamaica. The minimum number of cases in a study group was six, with range from 6 to 275 across all intervention programmes. In total, these studies contained 1,419 children in early intervention programmes and 1,427 children in control or comparison groups. Participants ranged in age from birth to fourteen years. The duration of intervention ranged from four months to eight years. In thirteen studies participants were predominantly African-American. In one study participants were Mexican-Americans, and in one study participants were Jamaican. All participating families came from impoverished socio-economic backgrounds and were at risk for development of cognitive delay.

Methodological features

Methodological features of the fifteen studies are summarized in Table 3.2. Random assignment to groups occurred in twelve studies. In fourteen studies demographically similar participants were assigned to treatment and control groups. In thirteen studies a pre-treatment assessment was included and all studies had at least one post-treatment assessment. Psychometric evaluation of intelligence or cognitive abilities occurred in all studies. In thirteen studies intelligence was assessed, in five language development was assessed, in three reading and maths attainment were evaluated. In all studies evaluations were made during children's first five years. In six studies follow-up evaluations were conducted when children were between six and eleven years. In two studies children were followed up when they were between twelve and seventeen years of age. Deterioration was assessed in twelve studies, drop-out in thirteen studies, and all fifteen studies examined clinical significance of the results. Experienced therapists or trainers were used in thirteen studies interventions and supervision was provided for therapists or trainers in ten programmes. Four studies included an evaluation of programmes that were equally valued, and four studies were manualized. Programme integrity was checked in only two studies. Overall this group of studies was fairly methodologically robust. Consequently considerable confidence may be placed in the conclusions drawn from them about the effectiveness of different types of early intervention programmes.

Substantive findings

Results of the fifteen studies are summarized in Tables 3.3 and 3.4. There was considerable variation in the range of assessments made across these fifteen

Table 3.2 Methodological features from studies of programmes to prevent cognitive delay in socially disadvantaged children

Feature	Study number														
	S1	S2	S3	S4	S5	S6	S7	S8	S9	S10	S11	S12	S13	S14	S15
Control or comparison group	1	1	1	1	1	1	1	1	1	1	1	1	1	1	1
Random assignment	1	0	0	1	1	1	0	1	1	1	1	1	1	1	1
Demographic similarity	1	1	1	1	1	1	0	1	1	1	1	1	1	1	1
Pre-treatment assessment	1	1	1	1	1	1	1	0	1	1	1	0	0	1	1
Post-treatment assessment	1	1	1	1	1	1	1	1	1	1	1	1	1	1	1
Assessment at 0–5 years	1	1	1	1	1	1	1	1	1	1	1	1	1	1	1
Assessment at 6–11 years	0	0	0	0	0	0	0	1	1	0	0	0	0	1	1
Assessment at 12–17 years	0	0	0	0	0	0	0	0	1	0	0	0	0	1	0
Intelligence assessed	0	1	1	1	1	1	0	1	1	1	1	1	1	1	0
Language development assessed	1	1	1	0	1	0	1	0	1	0	0	1	0	0	0
Reading attainment assessed	0	0	0	0	0	0	0	0	1	0	0	0	0	1	0
Maths attainment assessed	0	0	0	0	0	0	0	0	1	0	0	0	0	1	0
Deterioration assessed	0	1	1	1	1	1	1	1	1	1	1	1	1	1	1
Drop-out assessed	1	1	1	1	1	1	0	1	1	0	0	1	1	0	1
Clinical significance of change assessed	1	1	1	1	1	1	1	1	1	1	1	1	1	1	1
Experienced therapists or trainers used	1	0	1	0	0	1	1	0	1	1	1	1	1	1	1
Programmes were equally valued	0	0	1	0	0	1	1	0	0	0	1	0	0	0	0
Programmes were manualized	0	0	0	1	0	0	0	1	0	0	0	1	0	1	1
Supervision was provided	0	0	1	1	0	1	0	1	1	1	0	1	1	1	1
Programme integrity checked	0	0	0	0	0	0	0	1	0	0	0	1	0	0	0
Data on concurrent treatment given	0	0	0	0	0	0	0	0	0	0	0	0	0	0	0
Data on subsequent treatment given	0	0	0	0	0	0	0	0	0	0	0	0	0	0	0
Total	10	10	13	12	11	13	9	13	17	11	11	14	11	16	13

Notes

S = study. 1 = design feature was present. 0 = design feature was absent.

Table 3.3 Effect sizes from studies of programmes to prevent cognitive delay in socially disadvantaged children

Age	Measures	Home-visiting programmes							Preschool programmes			Home-visiting + preschool programmes						Multisystemic programmes	
		S1 HV v C	S2 HV v C (total)	S3 HV v C	S4 HV (Weekly) v BL	S5 HV v C	S8 HV (0–2 y) VC	S14 HV v C	S6 PS-E v PS-T PS-CI PS-M	S7 PS-HS v C	S8 PS v C	S8 HV+PS (0–3 y) v C	S9 HV+PS v C	S10 HV+PS v C	S11 HV+SS (×2) H+SS (×3) v C	S12 HV+PS-E v C	S13 HV+PS-E v C	S14 HV+PS+S+ET v C	S15 HV+PS+FS+SS v C
0–5 y	Intelligence	—	1.6	0.7	1.0	0.7	0.3	0.6	0.7	—	0.2	0.3	0.9	0.6	0.6	0.6	0.6	0.9	2.1
	Language	0.6	—	0.2	—	—	—	—	—	—	—	—	0.9	—	—	0.4	—	—	—
6–11 y	Intelligence	—	—	—	—	—	0.8	0.2	—	0.4	0.5	0.9	0.2	—	—	0.4	—	0.2	2.2
	Language	—	—	—	—	—	—	—	—	—	—	—	0.2	—	—	—	—	—	—
	Reading	—	—	—	—	—	—	0.6	—	—	—	—	0.3	—	—	—	—	1.0	—
	Mathematics	—	—	—	—	—	—	0.6	—	—	—	—	0.0	—	—	—	—	0.7	—
12–17 y	Intelligence	—	—	—	—	—	—	—	—	—	—	—	0.0	—	—	—	—	0.4	—
	Language	—	—	—	—	—	—	—	—	—	—	—	0.8	—	—	—	—	—	—
	Reading	—	—	—	—	—	—	0.7	—	—	—	—	0.5	—	—	—	—	0.9	—
	Mathematics	—	—	—	—	—	—	0.6	—	—	—	—	0.5	—	—	—	—	0.5	—

Notes

HV = home visiting programme involving child stimulation and parent education. PE = parent education. PS = preschool. PS-T = traditional preschool. PS-CI = community integrated preschool. PS-M = Montessori preschool. PS-E = experimental preschool. PS-HS = Head Start preschool. SS = summer school. S = school. ET = extra tuition. FS = family support. DS = differential school placement. C = control group

Table 3.4 Summary of key findings from studies of programmes to prevent cognitive delay in socially disadvantaged children

Study no.	Authors	Year	N per group	Duration	Intensity	Group differences	Key findings
1	Levenstein & Sunley	1968	1. HV = 6 2. C = 5	4m	Weekly HV sessions	PPVT @ 2 y 1 > 2	• Compared with controls, 2-year-old children from families who participated in a 4-month home-visiting infant stimulation and parent education programme (Project Verbal Interaction) showed greater verbal intelligence
2	Karnes et al.	1970	1. HV(total) = 15 2. C(total) = 15 3. HV(sibling) = 6 4. C(sibling) = 6	15 m	Weekly HV sessions	S-B @ 3 y 1 > 2 3 > 4	• Compared with controls, 20-month-old children and their siblings from families who participated in a 15-month home-visiting infant stimulation and parent education programme (Mother Training Intervention Programme) showed greater intelligence at three years of age on the Stanford Binet Intelligence test
3	Slaughter	1983	1. HV = 26 2. PE = 26 3. C = 31	2 y	1. Biweekly HV sessions 2. Weekly discussion groups	Catell @ 3.5 y 1 > 2 > 3 McCarthy & PPVT@ 3.5 y 1 = 2 > 3	• Compared with controls, 18-month-old children from families who participated in a 2-year home-visiting infant stimulation and parent education programme (Levenstein Toy Demonstration Programme) or families in which mothers participated in a support and discussion group (Auerbach–Badger Mother Discussion Group Programme), showed greater intelligence at 3 years of age • The home-visiting programme led to greater gains as measured by the Cattell Infant Intelligence scale but not the McCarthy Children's Abilities Scale
4	Powell & Grantham-McGregor	1989	Study 1: 1. HV (biweekly) = 26 2. HV (monthly) = 20 3. C1 = 21 Study 2: 4. HV(weekly) = 29 5. C2 = 29	3 y	1. Biweekly HV sessions 2. Monthly HV sessions 4. Weekly HV sessions	Griffiths @ 3 y 4 > 1 > 2 = 3 = 5	• Compared with controls and infants from families who received monthly home visits, infants from families who participated in a 3-year weekly or fortnightly home-visiting infant stimulation and parent education programme (Jamaica Home Visit Programme) showed better cognitive functioning on the Griffiths test of abilities at 3 years. • Weekly visiting led to greater benefits than fortnightly visiting both in degree of development and in the number of different areas of development affected
5	Gutelius et al.	1972	1. HV = 46 2. C = 46	3 y	9 HV sessions in year 1 7 HV session in year 2 5HV sessions in year 3 1.5 hpm PE in years 1&2	Bayley @ 2 y S-B @ 3 y 1 > 2	• Compared with controls, children from families who participated in a 3-year home-visiting infant stimulation and parent education programme (Cognitive Stimulation Programme) showed better cognitive development on the Bayley scales of Infant Development at 2 years and on the Stanford Binet Intelligence Test at 3 years
6	Karnes et al.	1970	1. PS-T = 28 2. PS-CI = 16 3. PS-M = 16 4. PS-E = 27	7-8 m	Daily preschool for 2 h	S-B @ 5 y 4 > 1 = 2 = 3	• Children of 2.5 years who were enrolled in an experimental preschool programme for 8 months showed greater gains on the Stanford Binet Intelligence Test, than children who participated in traditional, Montessori or community integrated preschools
7	Lee et al.	1988 1990	1. PS-HS = 414 2. PS-T = 390 3. C = 165	9 m	—	PPVT & CPI @ 5 y 1 > 2 = 3	• Children in the Head Start preschool performed significantly better than children in other types of preschool and better than children who were not enrolled in preschool

Table 3.4 continued

Study no.	Authors	Year	N per group	Duration	Intensity	Group differences	Key findings
8	Jester & Guinagh	1983	1. HV + PS (EEE) = 49 2. HV (EEC) = 28 3. HV + PS (CEE) = 19 4. HV + PS (ECE) = 18 5. HV (ECC) = 11 6. HV(CEC) = 24 7. PS (CCE) = 32 8. C (CCC) = 58	3 y	Weekly HV sessions Biweekly preschool	S-B @ 4&6 y 1 = 2 = 3 > 8 S-B @ 4 y 5 = 7 > 8 S-B @ 6 y 4 > 8 WISC @ 10 y 1 = 2 = 3 > 8	• On the Stanford Binet Intelligence Test at 4 and 6 years and on the WISC at 10 years children who participated in a combined 2 or 3 year home-visiting and preschool programme (Gordon Parent Education Programme) showed greater gains than controls. • On the Stanford Binet Intelligence Test at 4 and 6 years and on the WISC at 10 years children who participated in a home-visiting programme during the child's first 2 years showed similar gains to those of children in the 2- and 3-year combined home-visiting and preschool programmes. • On the Stanford Binet Intelligence Test at 6 years children who participated in a programme where a year home-visiting was offered at 1 year and a year of preschool was offered at 3 years showed greater gains than controls. • Compared with controls, on the Stanford Binet Intelligence Test at 4 years children who participated in a programme which involved 2 years home-visiting when the child was 2 and 3 year old and children who participated in one year preschool programme offered at 3 years showed similar gains • Children whose families participated in a combined home-visiting and preschool programme in which intervention was offered in the child's first and third year only but not the second year fared no better than controls • Children who participated in a one-year preschool programme at age 3 fared no better than controls
9	Schweinhart et al.	1985	1. HV + PS = 58 2. C = 65	2 y	Weekly HV sessions Daily preschool for 3 h	Leiter @ 5 y PPVT @ 5 y CAT @ 14 y 1 > 2 PPVT @ 9 y SB @ 10 y WISC @ 9 &14 y1 = 2	• On the Leiter Performance test, the PPVT and the CAT at 5 and 14 years children who participated in a combined 2-year home-visiting and preschool programme (High/Scope Perry Preschool Programme) showed greater gains than controls • On the PPVT at 9 years, the Stanford Binet Intelligence Test at 10 years and the WISC at 9 and 14 years, children who participated in the programme fared no better than controls
10	Andrews et al. Johnson & Walker	1982 1991	1. HV + PS = 97 2. C = 119	2 y	Three weekly HV sessions Preschool 4 dpw for 3h	Bayley @ 2 y S-B @ 3 y 1 > 2	• On the Bayley Scales of Infant Development at 2 years and on the Stanford Binet Intelligence Test at 3 years children who participated in a combined 2-year home-visiting and preschool programme (Houston Parent–Child Development Centre Project) showed greater gains than controls
11	Gray & Klaus	1965 1970	1. HV + SS (× 3) = 19 2. HV + SS (× 2) = 19 3. C1 = 18 4. C2 = 27	2 or 3 y	10 w of summer school per year	S-B @ 6 y 1 = 2 > 3 = 4	• On the Stanford Binet Intelligence Test at 6 years children who participated in a combined 1- or 2-year home-visiting and summer school programme (Early Training Project) showed greater gains than controls • Their post-intervention IQ scores did not differ from those of non-deprived children

			Groups (N)	Age	Intervention	Measures	Results
12	Deutsch et al.	1983	1. HV + PS-E = 275 2. C1 = 129 3. C2 = 180	5 y	—	S-B & PPVT @ 6&9 y 1 > 2 = 3	• On the Stanford Binet Intelligence Test and the PPVT at 6 and 9 years children who participated in a combined 5-year home-visiting and experimental preschool programme (Institute of Development Studies Programme) showed greater gains than controls
13	Wasik et al.	1990b	1. HV + PS-E = 15 2. HV = 24 3. C = 23	5 y	Daily preschool Biweekly HV sessions Monthly HV during follow-up	Bayley @ 1.5 y S-B @ 4 y McCarthy @ 4.5 y 1 > 3 > 2	• On the Bayley Scales of Infant Development at 1.5 years, on the Stanford Binet Intelligence Test at 4 years, and on the McCarthy scales at 4.5 years children who participated in a combined 5-year home-visiting and experimental preschool programme (Project CARE) showed greater gains than children who participated in a home-visiting programme and controls
14	Ramey & Cambell Campbell & Ramey	1991 1994 1995	1. HV + PS + S + ET = 25 2. HV = 24 3. PE + S + ET = 24 4. C = 23	3, 5, or 8 y	Daily preschool for 7 h 15 HV sessions 6 w of extra tuition	WPPSI @ 5 y WISC & maths @ 8 y 1 = 2 > 3 > 4 Reading @ 8 y 1 > 2 > 3 > 4	• On the WPPSI at 5 years and on the WISC and a maths attainment test at 8 years children whose families participated in an 8-year multisystemic programme (Carolina Abecedarian Project) involving home visiting, preschool and school placement and extra tuition or an intensive home-visiting programme fared better than controls of children who attended a programme that involved preschool and school placement and extra tuition only • At 8 years children who participated in the multisystemic programme showed better reading attainment than children from other programmes and controls
15	Garber	1988	1. HV + PS-E + FS + DS + SS = 17 2. C1 = 11 3. C2 (low-risk) = 6	10 y	Daily preschool for 7h	Gesell @ 22m S-B @ 5&6 y WISC @ 10 y 1 > 2 = 3	• On the Gesell developmental schedules at 22 months, on the Stanford Binet Intelligence Test at 5 and 6 years and on the WISC at 10 years, children whose families participated in a multisystemic programme (The MilwaukeeProject) fared better than matched controls and non-disadvantaged children

Notes

HV = home-visiting programme involving child stimulation and parent education. PE = parent education. PS = preschool. PS-T = traditional preschool. PS-CI = community integrated preschool. PS-M = Montessori preschool. PS-E = experimental preschool. PS-HS = Head Start preschool. DS = differential school placement. EEE = Experimental intervention was received for each of three consecutive years. EEC = Experimental intervention was received for each of two consecutive years followed by a control year of routine intervention. C = control group. A-A = African-American. h = hour. dpw = days per week. hpm = hours per month. m = month. y = year.Leiter = Leiter International Performance Scale (Arthur, 1952). Bayley = Bayley Scales of Infant Development (Bayley, 1969). CPI = Cooperative Preschool Inventory (Caldwell, 1970). Catell = Cattell (1960). PPVT = Peabody Picture Vocabulary Test (Dunn, 1965). Gesell = Gesell Development Schedules (Gesell Institute of Human Development, 1985). Griffiths = (Griffiths, 1954). S-B = Stanford-Binet intelligence scale (Terman Merrill, 1972). CAT = California Achievement Tests (Tiegs & Clark, 1971). WPPSI = Wechsler preschool and primary scale of intelligence (Wechsler, 1967). WISC = Wechsler intelligence scale for children (Wechsler, 1974). WJ = Woodcock-Johnson Psycho-Educational Battery (Woodcock & Johnson, 1977). McCarthy = McCarthy (1972) McCarthy Scales of Children's Abilities studies. The focus in this review was on assessment of cognitive functioning and only results of tests of cognitive ability, language development and scholastic attainment were considered. There was also considerable variation in the frequency with which assessments were made within the three age bands outlined in Table 3.3 (0–5 years; 6–11 years; 12–17 years). If data were reported for yearly assessments at different ages on a specific test within an age band, only the results of the latest assessment within that age band were reported. For example, if participants in a study were assessed on the Wechsler Intelligence Scale for Children (WISC) at ages 1, 2 and 3 years only data for the assessments conducted at three years for that age band were included in Table 3.3.

Home-visiting programmes

In seven studies home-visiting programmes were evaluated (Levenstein & Sunley, 1968; Karnes et al., 1970; Slaughter, 1983; Powell & Grantham-McGregor, 1989; Gutelius et al., 1972; Jester & Guinagh, 1983; Ramey & Campbell, 1991; Campbell & Ramey, 1994, 1995). In two of these studies the home-visiting programme was a comparative condition in a multigroup study where the effectiveness of a variety of types of programmes was being investigated (Jester & Guinagh, 1983; Ramey & Campbell, 1991; Campbell & Ramey, 1994, 1995).

Compared with controls, Levenstein and Sunley (1968) found that two-year-old children from families who participated in in Project Verbal Interaction, a four-month home-visiting infant stimulation and parent education programme, showed greater verbal intelligence on the Peabody Picture Vocabulary Test after the programme (Dunn, 1965).

Compared with controls, Karnes et al. (1970) found that 20-month-old children and their siblings from families who participated in the Mother Training Intervention Programme, a fifteen-month home-visiting infant stimulation and parent education programme, showed greater intelligence at three years of age on the Stanford Binet intelligence scale after the programme (Terman & Merrill, 1972). Materials from manuals such as the Frostig Program for the Development of Visual Perception (Frostig & Horne, 1964) were used in this programme as a basis for designing activities that mothers could do with their children to stimulate them intellectually.

In the Chicago Housing Project programme, Slaughter (1983) compared the effectiveness of a home-visiting programme and a parent education programme. There was also a control group included in the design of the study. Compared with controls, Slaughter (1983) found that 18-month-old children from families who participated in the Levenstein (1970) Toy Demonstration Programme, a two-year home-visiting infant stimulation and parent education programme, or families in which mothers participated in Auerbach–Badger Mother Discussion Group Programme (Auerbach, 1968, 1971; Badger, 1968, 1971, 1973) showed greater intelligence at three years of age.

The home-visiting programme led to greater gains as measured by the Cattell (1960) Infant Intelligence scale but not the McCarthy (1972) Scales of Children's Abilities.

Compared with controls and infants from families who received monthly home visits, Powell & Grantham-McGregor (1989) found that infants from families who participated in the Jamaica Home Visit Programme, a three-year weekly or fortnightly home-visiting infant stimulation and parent education programme showed better cognitive functioning on the Griffiths (1954) Test of Abilities at three years. Weekly visiting led to greater benefits than fort-nightly visiting both in degree of development and in the number of different areas of development affected. Within this home-visiting programme mothers were taught to engage their infants in intellectually stimulating activ-ities, such as learning Piagetian concepts using the work of Uzgiris and Hunt (1978) as the basis of the curriculum. For older children, the curriculum was based on a manual by Palmer (1971) which outlined various activities that promote the learning of concepts such as shape, size, quantity, position, motion and colour. The manual classified these concepts age-appropriately and in order of difficulty.

Compared with controls, Gutelius et al. (1972) found that children from families who participated in the Cognitive Stimulation Programme, a three-year home-visiting infant stimulation and parent education programme, showed better cognitive development on the Bayley (1969) Scales of Infant Development at two years and on the Stanford Binet intelligence scale (Terman & Merrill, 1972) at three years.

Jester and Guinagh (1983) in a complex study compared the effectiveness of seven different programmes: (1) a three-year combined home-visiting and preschool programme which began at the child's birth; (2) a two-year com-bined home-visiting and preschool programme which began when the child was a year old; (3) a two-year combined home-visiting and preschool pro-gramme which began at the child's birth, stopped when the child reached one year and recommenced when the child was two years old; (4) a two-year home-visiting programme which began at the child's birth; (5) a one-year home-visiting programme conducted during the child's first year; (6) a one-year home-visiting programme conducted during the child's second year; and (7) a preschool programme conducted during the child's third year. A control group containing cases who received no intervention was also included in this study. The Gordon Parent Education Programme was central to all of the intervention groups. Manuals outlining aspects of this approach include *Baby Learning Through Baby Play* (Gordon, 1970) and *Child Learning Through Play* (Gordon et al., 1972). All children who participated in home-visiting programmes fared better than controls except those who received only a year of home visiting in their second year of life. The most effective home-visiting programme was that which spanned the child's first two years of life. On the Stanford Binet Intelligence Test at four and six years and on the WISC at ten years children who participated in a home-visiting programme during their first two years showed similar gains to those of children in the two- and three-year combined home-visiting and preschool programmes.

Ramey & Campbell (1991; Campbell & Ramey, 1994, 1995) in a complex study compared the effectiveness of three different programmes: (1) a multi-systemic programme involving home-visiting, preschool, school placement and extra tuition; (2) a home-visiting programme; and (3) a programme involving preschool, school placement and extra tuition. On the Wechsler Preschool and Primary scale of Intelligence (WPPSI) at five years and on the WISC and a maths attainment test at eight years, children whose families participated in the intensive home-visiting programme fared as well as those who participated in a multisystemic programme and better than those who participated in the programme which involved preschool, school placement and extra tuition.

From the results of the seven studies summarized here and in Tables 3.3 and 3.4 a number of conclusions may be drawn. First, programmes of intensive home visiting involving parent education and infant stimulation during children's early years may prevent cognitive delay and lead to significant gains in intelligence, language development, and scholastic attainment. Second, particularly effective programmes spanned the infants' first two years of life and involved at least weekly home visiting. Third, all home-visiting programmes led to gains in cognitive abilities during the first five years and in the small number of studies where data were available for middle childhood and adolescence, these gains persisted into adolescence.

Fourth, effect sizes based on intelligence test scores during the first five years ranged from 0.3 to 1.6 with a mean of 0.8. During the six- to eleven-year period they ranged from 0.2 to 0.8 with a mean of 0.5. In the only study for which data were available for adolescence the intelligence test score effect size was 0.5. Thus, the average child whose family participated in home-visiting programmes obtained higher intelligence test scores than 79% of control groups during the first five years, and this figure only dropped to 69% during childhood and adolescence.

Fifth, effect sizes based on language test scores during the first five years ranged from 0.2 to 0.6 with a mean of 0.4. Thus, the average child whose family participated in home-visiting programmes obtained higher language test scores than 66% of children from control groups who did not participate in such programmes.

Sixth, effect sizes from the only study in which reading and arithmetic attainment test scores were available averaged 0.6 in the six- to eleven-year period and 0.7 in the twelve- to seventeen-year period. Thus, the average child whose family participated in home-visiting programmes obtained higher attainment test scores than 73% of controls in childhood and 76% of controls in adolescence.

Preschool programmes

In three studies preschool programmes were evaluated (Karnes et al., 1970; Lee et al., 1988, 1990; Jester & Guinagh, 1983). One of these was a multiprogramme comparison study mentioned in the previous section (Jester & Guinagh, 1983). Karnes et al. (1970) in a comparative study of four preschool programmes found that two and a half year old children whose families were enrolled in an experimental preschool programme for eight months showed greater gains on the Stanford Binet intelligence scale (Terman & Merrill, 1972) than children who participated in traditional, Montessori or community integrated preschools. In the experimental preschool programme pupil–teacher ratios were 5:1, whereas in the other preschool programmes they were considerably higher. The experimental preschool programme differed from the other programmes in the extremely high level of structure involved and the breadth of the curriculum. The curriculum had social studies and science modules as well as units on topics such as body awareness, the family, mathematics, reading, and visual-motor coordination. Manipulative and multisensory materials, outdoor play equipment and traditional preschool toys were used. Content to be learned was presented to the children using a game format.

Lee et al. (1988, 1990) found that children in the Head Start preschool performed significantly better than children in other types of preschool and better than children who were not enrolled in pre-school on the Stanford Binet Intelligence Test (Terman & Merrill, 1972) at four and six years and on the WISC-R (Wechsler, 1974) at eight years.

Jester and Guinagh (1983) in a comparative study of seven programmes mentioned in the previous section found that on the Stanford Binet Intelligence Test (Terman & Merrill, 1972) at four years children who participated in a one-year preschool programme offered when they were three years of age fared as well as children who participated in a programme which involved two years of home visiting when children were two and three years old and both fared better than controls. However, children who participated in a one-year preschool programme at three years of age fared no better than controls.

From the results of the three studies summarized here and in Tables 3.3 and 3.4 a number of conclusions may be drawn. First, preschool programmes may prevent cognitive delay and lead to significant gains in intelligence and language development. Second, these programmes ranged in duration from eight months to three years and participants ranged in age from two to five years. Third, effect sizes based on intelligence test scores during the first five years ranged from 0.2 to 0.7 with a mean of 0.5. In the only study for which data were available for the six- to eleven-year period the intelligence test score effect size was also 0.5. Thus, the average child who participated in a preschool programme obtained higher intelligence test scores than 69% of controls during the first five years and these gains persisted into middle childhood.

Combined home-visiting and preschool programmes

Six studies investigated the effectiveness of combined home-visiting and pre-school programmes (Jester & Guinagh, 1983; Schweinhart et al., 1985; Andrews et al., 1982; Johnson & Walker, 1991; Gray & Klaus, 1965, 1970; Deutsch et al., 1983; Wasik et al., 1990b).

Jester and Guinagh (1983) in a comparative study of seven programmes mentioned in previous sections found that on the Stanford Binet Intelligence Scale (Terman & Merrill, 1972) at four and six years and on the WISC-R (Wechsler, 1974) at eight years children who participated in a combined two- or three-year home-visiting and preschool programme, the Gordon Parent Education Programme, showed greater gains than controls. On the Stanford Binet Intelligence Test at four and six years and on the WISC-R at eight years children who participated in a two-year home-visiting programme showed similar gains to those of children in the two- and three-year combined home-visiting and preschool programmes. On the Stanford Binet Intelligence Test at six years children who participated in a programme where a year of home-visiting programme was offered during infants' first year of life and a year of preschool was offered when children were in their third year showed greater gains than controls. Children whose families participated in a combined home-visiting and preschool programme in which intervention was offered in the child's first and third year only, but not the second year, fared no better than controls.

Schweinhart et al. (1985) found that on the Leiter International Perform-ance Scale (Arthur, 1952), the Peabody Picture Vocabulary Test (Dunn, 1965) and the California Achievement Tests (Tiegs & Clark, 1971) at five and four-teen years children who participated in the High/Scope Perry Preschool Pro-gram, a combined two-year home-visiting and preschool programme, showed greater gains than controls.

However, on the Peabody Picture Vocabulary Test at nine years, the Stan-ford Binet Intelligence Test (Terman & Merrill, 1972) at ten years and the WISC-R (Wechsler, 1974) at nine and fourteen years, children who partici-pated in the programme fared no better than controls.

Andrews et al. (1982) found that on the Bayley (1969) Scales of Infant Development at two years and on the Stanford Binet Intelligence Scale (Terman & Merrill, 1972) at three years children who participated in the Houston Parent–Child Development Centre Project, a combined two-year home-visiting and preschool programme, showed greater gains than controls.

Gray and Klaus (1965, 1970) found that on the Stanford Binet Intelligence Scale (Terman & Merrill, 1972) at six years children who participated in the Early Training Project, a combined one- or two-year home-visiting and summer school programme, showed greater gains than controls. Further-more, their post-intervention IQ scores did not differ from those of non-deprived children.

On the Stanford Binet Intelligence Scale (Terman & Merrill, 1972) and the

Peabody Picture Vocabulary Test (Dunn, 1965) at six and nine years, Deutsch et al. (1983) found that children who participated in the Institute for Developmental Studies Project, a combined five-year home-visiting and experimental preschool programme, showed greater gains than controls.

Wasik et al. (1990b) found that on the Bayley (1969) Scales of Infant Development at one and a half years, on the Stanford Binet Intelligence Test (Terman & Merrill, 1972) at four years, and on the McCarthy (1972) Scales of Children's Abilities at four and a half years, children who participated in Project CARE, a combined five-year home-visiting and experimental pre-school programme, showed greater gains than children who participated in a home-visiting programme and controls. Manuals such as *Learning Games for the First Three Years* (Sparling & Lewis, 1979) and *Learning Games for Threes and Fours* (Sparling & Lewis, 1984b) formed the basis of the curriculum for this programme.

From the results of the six studies summarized here and in Tables 3.3 and 3.4 a number of conclusions may be drawn. First, combined programmes of intensive home visiting involving parent education and infant stimulation and preschool education during children's early and toddler years may prevent cognitive delay and lead to significant gains in intelligence, language development and scholastic attainment. Second, these programmes were of two to five years' duration, involved regular weekly or fortnightly home visiting, and regular preschool attendance three to five days per week. Third, all combined home-visiting and preschool programmes led to gains in cognitive abilities during the first five years and in the small number of studies where data were available for middle childhood and adolescence, it was clear that some of these gains persisted into adolescence

Fourth, effect sizes based on intelligence test scores during the first five years ranged from 0.3 to 0.9 with a mean of 0.6. During the six- to eleven-year period they ranged from 0.2 to 0.9 with a mean of 0.5. In the only study for which data were available for adolescence the intelligence test score effect size was 0. Thus, the average child whose family participated in home-visiting programmes obtained higher intelligence test scores than 73% of control groups during the first five years. This figure only dropped to 69% during middle childhood. In adolescence there were no differences in IQ between cases who participated in early intervention programmes and controls.

Fifth, effect sizes based on language test scores during the first five years ranged from 0.4 to 0.9 with a mean of 0.7. During the six- to eleven-year period they ranged from 0.2 to 0.4 with a mean of 0.3. In the only study for which data were available for adolescence the language test score effect size was 0.8. Thus, the average child whose family participated in combined home-visiting and preschool programmes obtained higher language test scores than 76% of control groups during the first five years. This figure dropped to 62% during middle childhood but increased to 79% in adolescence.

Sixth, effect sizes from the only study in which reading and arithmetic attainment test scores were available averaged 0.2 in the six- to eleven-year period and 0.5 in the twelve- to seventeen-year period. Thus, the average child whose family participated in combined home-visiting and preschool programmes obtained higher attainment test scores than 58% of controls in childhood and 69% of controls in adolescence.

Multisystemic programmes

In two studies multisystemic programmes were evaluated (Ramey & Campbell, 1991; Campbell & Ramey, 1994, 1995; Garber, 1988). Ramey and Campbell's (1991) comparative study of the effectiveness of three different programmes has been mentioned above. On the WPPSI (Wechsler, 1967) at five years and on the WISC-R (Wechsler, 1974) and a maths attainment test at eight years children whose families participated in the Carolina Abecedarian Project, an eight-year multisystemic programme involving home visiting, preschool and school placement and extra tuition, or children whose families participated in an intensive home-visiting programme fared better than controls or children who attended a programme that involved preschool and school placement and extra tuition only. At eight years children who participated in the multisystemic programme showed better reading attainment than children from other programmes and controls. The infant curriculum *Learningames for the First Three Years* (Sparling & Lewis, 1979) was used as the basis for the early part of this programme. The *Peabody Early Experience Kit* (Dunn et al., 1976) and *Bridges to Reading* (Greenberg & Epstein, 1973) manual were used during the toddler years phase of the programme.

   Garber (1988) found that on the Gesell (1985) developmental schedules at twenty-two months, on the Stanford Binet Intelligence Scale (Terman & Merrill, 1972) at five and six years and on the WISC-R (Wechsler, 1974) at ten years, children whose families participated in the Milwaukee Project, a multisystemic programme, fared better than matched controls and non-disadvantaged children.

   From the results of these two studies, which are summarized in Tables 3.3 and 3.4, a number of conclusions may be drawn. First, multisystemic programmes that include intensive home visiting involving parent education and infant stimulation, preschool enrolment, primary school placement, and other elements such as extra tuition, summer school and family support during children's early years may prevent cognitive delay and lead to significant gains in intelligence, language development and scholastic attainment. Second, these effective multisystemic programmes were long-term interventions spanning eight to ten years and involved weekly or fortnightly home visiting in the early years, regular daily preschool attendance during the toddler years, regular daily school placement in middle childhood, and intensive additional service. Third, both multisystemic programmes led to gains in cognitive abilities during the first five years and these persisted into middle childhood. In the single study where long-term follow-up data were available, the benefits persisted into late adolescence.

Fourth, effect sizes based on intelligence test scores during the first five years ranged from 0.9 to 2.1 with a mean of 1.5. During the six- to eleven-year period they ranged from 0.2 to 2.2 with a mean of 1.2. In the study for which data were available for adolescence the intelligence test score effect size was 0.4. Thus, the average child whose family participated in a multisystemic programme obtained higher intelligence test scores than 93% of control groups during the first five years. This figure only dropped to 88% during childhood and to 66% in adolescence.

Fifth, effect sizes from the single study in which reading and arithmetic attainment test scores were available averaged 0.9 in the six- to eleven-year period and 0.7 in the twelve- to seventeen-year period. Thus, the average child whose family participated in a multisystemic programme obtained higher attainment test scores than 82% of controls in childhood and 76% of controls in adolescence.

Conclusion

Children from socially disadvantaged backgrounds show delayed development of cognitive abilities. They obtain lower scores on tests of intelligence, cognitive skills, language development and academic attainment, compared with children who are not reared in poverty. Rates of cognitive delay are about 10% in lower socioeconomic groups compared with 2–3% in higher socioeconomic groups. Four broad types of early intervention programmes have been developed for socially disadvantaged children. Home-visiting programmes aim to help socially disadvantaged parents understand and meet their children's needs for intellectual stimulation, secure attachment and consistent supervision. Preschool programmes aim to directly provide disadvantaged children with a stimulating preschool environment to compensate for their intellectually impoverished home environment. Combined home-visiting and preschool programmes aim both to enhance the quality of disadvantaged children's home environments and to give them access to enriched preschool environments. Multisystemic programmes attempt in addition to extend support services for children and families into middle childhood.

From Table 3.5, it may be seen that multisystemic programmes are the most effective. Overall, the average child who participates in a multisystemic early intervention programme fares better than 93% of children whose families do not participate in this type of programme. In rank order of effectiveness after multisystemic programmes are: home-visiting programmes; combined home-visiting and preschool programmes; and programmes that involve preschool enrolment only. From Table 3.5 it may also be seen that overall, longer programmes are more effective than shorter programmes and the most effective programmes extend beyond five years.

Table 3.5 Mean effect sizes for early intervention programmes differing in type and duration

	Intervention programme	N	Average effect size
Type of programme	Multisystemic	2	1.5
	Home visiting only	7	0.8
	Home visiting and preschool	6	0.6
	Preschool only	3	0.5
Duration of programme	>5 year	4	1.1
	2–3 years	4	0.8
	1–2 years	4	0.8
	<1 years	3	0.5

Note
Mean effect sizes were calculated using effect sizes outlined in Table 3.3. Effect sizes were averaged within each programme first and then across programmes.

Implications for policy and practice

The main implications for policy and practice arising from this review are that disadvantaged children at risk for cognitive delay should be offered effective early intervention programmes to prevent such delays occurring. From Table 3.6, it may be seen that effective programmes have distinctive key features. The list in Table 3.6 is based on careful analysis of descriptions of particularly effective programmes reviewed in this chapter. Effective programmes involve a comprehensive range of components delivered by a multidisciplinary team who receive continuous training and supervision. Effective programmes are intensive, involving frequent and long-term contact. They involve children's families fully and build upon their cultural beliefs, traditions and practices. Preschools in effective programmes have small child–teacher ratios and modify the curriculum to meet the unique needs of individual children. Effective programmes use manualized curricula to ensure that all staff involved in implementation provide the intervention as intended. Effective programmes also evaluate participants with appropriate assessment instruments before, during and after the intervention and at follow-up to monitor progress and respond to children who are having difficulties benefiting from participation. Effective programmes also include additional supports to maintain initial positive effects.

Implications for research

Future studies should evaluate manualized intervention programmes in which checks for programme integrity are made. In such studies, home visits, preschool classes, and other intervention sessions are recorded and blind raters use programme integrity checklists to evaluate the degree to which sessions approximate manualized training curricula. Such integrity checks

Table 3.6 Key features of effective early intervention programmes

Timing and duration	• Interventions that begin earlier and continue longer produce better effects than short-term programmes
Intensity	• More intensive intervention programmes produce larger positive effects • Programmes with small child–teacher ratios produce better outcomes
Breadth	• Interventions that provide more comprehensive services and use multiple complex components to enhance children's development generally are more effective than less comprehensive programmes
Individual difference	• Effective programmes modify their curriculum and design to meet the unique needs of individual children
Environmental maintenance	• Effective programmes include additional supports to maintain initial positive effects
Cultural appropriateness and relevance	• Effective programmes build upon participants' cultural beliefs, traditions, and practices
Family involvement	• Effective programmes involve children's families as part of the intervention
Experienced staff	• Effective programmes are implemented by experienced multidisciplinary staff • Staff receive continuous training and supervision
Manualized curricula	• Effective programmes use manualized curricula to ensure that all people involved in the implementation of the programmes provide the treatment as intended. Furthermore, this allows for replication, and cross-study comparison
Systematic evaluation and monitoring	• Effective programmes evaluate participants with appropriate assessment instruments before, during and after the intervention and at follow-up

allow researchers to say with confidence the degree to which a pure and potent version of their programme has been evaluated.

Studies are required which investigate the mechanisms and processes which underpin programme effectiveness. Improvements probably occur through a variety of complex mechanisms including enhancing child development directly through stimulation, preschool and school-based education; enhancing child development through supporting the development of secure parent–child attachments; and enhancing general child care-taking by improving parental child care knowledge and skills.

There is a need to design and evaluate programmes for socially disadvantaged families that have particular difficulties in engaging in early intervention programmes. There is also a need to design programmes that maximize the involvement of both parents. There is considerable evidence that father involvement in family therapy can have a significant impact on outcome (Carr, 2001c). Despite this, programmes for socially disadvantaged children, such as those evaluated in the studies reviewed in this chapter, have rarely involved fathers. Future research should evaluate the impact of programmes that target both fathers and mothers as programme participants.

Assessment resources

Arthur, G. (1952). *The Arthur Adaptation of the Leiter International Performance Scale*. Beverly Hills, CA: Psychological Service Center Press.

Bayley, N. (1969). *Bayley Scales of Infant Development*. New York: Psychological Corporation.

Caldwell, B.M. (1970). *Cooperative Preschool Inventory: Revised edition*. Menlo Park, CA: Addison-Wesley.

Cattell, P. (1960). *The Measurement of Intelligence of Infants and Young Children (Revised Edition)*. New York: Johnson Reprint.

Dunn, L.M. (1965). *Peabody Picture Vocabulary Test Manual*. Minneapolis, MN: American Guidance Service.

Gesell Institute of Human Development (1985). *Gesell Development Schedules*. New Haven, CT: Author.

Griffiths, R. (1954). *The Abilities of Babies*. London: University of London Press.

McCarthy, D. (1972). *Manual: McCarthy Scales of Children's Abilities*. New York: Psychological Corporation.

Ramey, C.T. & Smith, B.J. (1977). Assessing the intellectual consequences of early intervention with high-risk infants. *American Journal of Mental Deficiency*, *81*, 318–324.

Terman, L. & Merrill, M. (1972). *Stanford Binet Intelligence Scale: Manual for the Third Revision, Form L-M*. Boston: Houghton Mifflin.

Tiegs, E.W. & Clark, W.W. (1971). *California Achievement Tests*. Monterey Park, CA: California Test Bureau (McGraw-Hill).

Wechsler, D. (1955). *Wechsler Adult Intelligence Scale*. New York: The Psychological Corporation.

Wechsler, D. (1967). *Wechsler Pre-school and Primary Scale of Intelligence*. New York: The Psychological Coporation.

Wechsler, D. (1974). *Manual for the Wechsler Intelligence Scale for Children (Rev. ed.)*. New York: The Psychological Corporation.

Woodcock, R.W. & Johnson, M.B. (1977). *Woodcock–Johnson Psycho-Educational Battery*. Hingham, MA: Teaching Resources Corporation.

Intervention resources

Dunn, L.M., Chun, L.T., Crowell, D.C., Dunn, L.M., Alexy, L.G. & Yachel, E.R. (1976). *Peabody Early Experience Kit*. Circle Pines, MN: American Guidance Services.

Frostig, M. & Horne, D. (1964). *The Frostig Program for the Development of Visual Perception*. Chicago: Follett.

Gordon, I.J. (1970). *Baby Learning Through Baby Play*. New York: St Martin's Press.

Gordon, I.J., Guinagh, B.J. & Jester, R.E. (1972). *Child Learning Through Play*. New York: St Martin's Press.

Greenberg, P. & Epstein, B. (1973). *Bridges to Reading*. Morristown, NJ: General Learning Corp.

Palmer, F. (1971). *Concept Training Curriculum For Children Ages Two to Five*. Stony Brook, NY: State University of New York, Stony Brook.

Sparling, J. & Lewis, I. (1979). *Learningames for the First Three Years: A Program for Parent/Center Partnership*. New York: Walker Educational Book Corp.

Sparling, J. & Lewis, I. (1984). *Learningames for Threes and Fours: A Guide To Parent-Child Play*. New York: Walker.

Uzgiris, I.G. & Hunt, J.McV. (1978). *Assessment in Infancy: Ordinal Scales of Psychological Development*. Chicago, IL: University of Illinois Press.

4   Prevention of adjustment problems in children with cerebral palsy

Brian Waldron and Alan Carr

Cerebral palsy is a disorder of movement and posture that results from an insult to, or anomaly of, the immature central nervous system in centres which govern motor activity (Shapiro & Capute, 1999). Symptoms of cerebral palsy include extreme muscular tension and muscular rigidity with a partial paralysis or a loss of voluntary movement together with spasm of the affected muscles. Cerebral palsy may not become apparent until after six months when the infant develops to the stage where reflex action is largely replaced by purposive movements and motor skills for which an intact central nervous system is essential. Motor delay is the basis for diagnosis of cerebral palsy and may vary from minimal to severe-profound (Capute & Shapiro, 1985). Insults to, or anomalies of, the central nervous system which cause cerebral palsy in some cases may also cause other co-morbid disabilities including intellectual disability, seizure disorders, visual and auditory impairments, learning difficulties and behaviour problems. The more profound the motor impairments and the more extensive the co-morbid disabilities, the greater the adjustment difficulties youngsters with cerebral palsy face (Pellegrino, 1997). A variety of early intervention programmes have been developed for children with cerebral palsy to prevent or minimize such adjustment problems. The effectiveness of many of these remains untested (Harris, 1997). The aim of this chapter is to review methodologically robust research studies on the effectiveness of such early intervention programmes, draw reliable conclusions about the effectiveness of these, and outline the implications of these conclusions for policy and practice.

Aetiology

Cerebral palsy is a non-progressive condition caused by cerebral lesions, which interrupt motor function and can have diverse causes occurring at the prenatal, perinatal and postnatal stages (Boyce et al., 1999; Pellegrino, 1997; Shapiro & Capute, 1999). These include blood rhesus factor incompatibility, anoxia, cerebral vascular accident, trauma and bacterial or viral infection. Low birth weight and associated cerebral ischaemia are significant risk factors. There are different subtypes of cerebral palsy and these are associated with different types of cerebral lesions.

Cerebral palsy may be classified according to the type of motor impairment that predominates. Distinctions are made between spastic, dyskinetic and ataxic conditions. Spastic cerebral palsy is further subclassified according to the distribution of limbs involved. Distinctions are made between hemiplegia (affecting one side of the body), quadriplegia (affecting all four limbs), and diplegia (affecting the lower limbs). Spastic hemiplegia is associated with unilateral brain damage whereas diplegia and quadriplegia are associated with bilateral brain damage.

Dyskinetic conditions include athetoid cerebral palsy involving fluctuating muscle tone and dystonic cerebral palsy involving rigid muscle tone. Ataxic cases are characterized by poor muscle tone, balance and co-ordination problems.

Damage to the corticospinal tracts, basal ganglia, brainstem and cerebellum is responsible for the differing types of motor symptoms. Corticospinal damage is associated with spasticity, basal ganglial damage with dyskinesia, and cerebellar damage with ataxia.

Cases of cerebral palsy may be classified as mild, moderate or severe depending upon their level of overall motor functioning as indexed by observations and scales based on motor development quotients, such as the Bayley Scales of Infant Development (Bayley, 1993; Capute & Shapiro, 1985; Coolman et al., 1985).

Epidemiology

Cerebral palsy is the most common movement disorder and affects 2.3 per 1,000 live births or about 1 in 400 children (Boyce et al., 1999; Goodman, 1994; Kolb & Whishaw, 1990; Pellegrino, 1997; Shapiro & Capute, 1999). Spastic cerebral palsy is the most common subtype, accounting for 50–75% of all cases. About 25% of cases are athetoid, about 10% are dystonic, and about 10% are ataxic. Co-morbid intellectual disability occurs in about 60% of cases of cerebral palsy; co-morbid seizure disorders occur in about 50% of cases; co-morbid behavioural and psychological problems occur in about 50% of cases; co-morbid hearing, speech and language impairments occur in 30% of cases; and co-morbid visual impairments in a proportion of cases. Feeding problems may also occur in cerebral palsy due to poor control of oral muscles. About 50% of people with cerebral palsy develop functional independence in the community in adulthood and about 25% develop partial independence. Outcome in adulthood is dependent upon both the degree of initial disability and the quality of rehabilitative and preventative intervention during the preschool and school-going years.

Intervention

For people with cerebral palsy, it is widely accepted that best practice involves offering comprehensive multidisciplinary rehabilitative programmes of care specifically designed to minimize the impact of the constraints placed by the disability on the child's physical and psychosocial development and to meet the unique needs of each case (Pellegrino, 1997; Shapiro & Capute, 1999).

Such programmes may include environmental alterations to manage the musculoskeletal complications of cerebral palsy including braces, splints and casts to prevent contractures. They may involve introducing positioning devices such as sidelyers, prone wedgers, standers or mobility devices such as wheelchairs, scooters and tricycles.

Comprehensive programmes may include medication to reduce spasticity and rigidity such as diazepam, baclofen and dantrolene. Nerve blocks and motor point blocks to reduce spasticity in specific muscle groups may also be considered. Some programmes may include surgery, for example to place a pump in the abdomen to deliver antispasticity medication directly into spinal fluid. In other cases orthopaedic surgery may be required to correct deformities due to the asymmetrical distribution of muscle tone.

In addition to these essentially physical interventions comprehensive rehabilitative care programmes also include a variety of types of physio-therapy and occupational therapy the aim of which is promote optimal motor functioning, optimal communicative functioning, and optimal involvement in activities of daily living. In many respects these programmes aim to prevent secondary handicaps. It is with these aspects of comprehensive care plans that the current review is concerned. Neurodevelopmental therapy, thera-peutic electrical stimulation and conductive education deserve particular mention.

Neurodevelopmental therapy

Therapeutic exercise based on one or more of the neurofacilitation approaches is central to all major early intervention programmes for infants and children with motor disabilities. Neurodevelopmental treatment developed by Karel and Berta Bobath in the 1940s is the most widely used of these (Bobath & Bobath, 1972; Bobath, 1980). In neurodevelopmental ther-apy, the therapist uses movement and handling to alter muscle tone and to facilitate normal movement patterns and postural reactions. These exercises substitute for normal voluntary motor activity which cannot be initiated by people with cerebral palsy. However, through repetition of these exercises, new motor patterns are developed. A second aspect of neurodevelopmental therapy is the use of movement and handling exercises to inhibit abnormal muscle tone and primitive reflex activity.

A recent modification of neurodevelopmental therapy is neurobehavioural motor intervention. With this approach, rather than using therapeutic exercises to improve a wide range of movement patterns and postural reactions, there is a focus on developing specific movements and postures which are absent from the child's repertoire but are essential for the completion of specific developmentally appropriate functional tasks (such as moving from a chair to a wheelchair or dressing). Behavioural methods including shaping and reinforcement are combined with neurodevelopmental therapeutic exercises in this approach (Horn et al., 1995).

Therapeutic electrical stimulation

In cerebral palsy the absence of continual neuromuscular activity prevents normal muscle development. Therapeutic electrical stimulation aims to compensate for this absence of muscular activity. In therapeutic electrical stimulation muscles are continuously activated by electrical pulses passed through electrodes on the skin (Barry, 1996). Therapeutic electrical stimulation has been used with children who have cerebral palsy to maintain or improve range of motion, to facilitate voluntary muscle control, and to reduce spasticity.

Conductive education

Conductive education, which was developed in Hungary by András Petö during the 1940s and 1950s, is a system for promoting motor, cognitive and social development so that children with cerebral palsy can enter mainstream schooling and participate in normal community activities (Bairstow et al, 1993, Hari & Tillemans, 1984; Hari & Akos, 1988; Sutton, 1988). Conductive education, as practised at the András Petö Institute for Motor Disorders in Budapest, is an intensive residential programme facilitated by specialized staff (conductors) with four years of training. Conductors work in teams with the groups of children to help them learn motor skills, cognitive skills and social skills. The work is functional and goal directed. The focus is on learning skills necessary to fulfil functions essential for independent living such as mobility and self-care. Achievable goals are set by analysing large tasks into their component parts. In working towards goals compensatory strategies may be used such as using rhyme, song and rhythmic self-instruction (referred to as rhythmic intention) to initiate, guide and refine motor actions. Use is made of two pieces of equipment – the plinth and ladder-back chair – within the programme. The process of conductive education depends upon a close working relationship between conductors and youngsters and upon the motivation and achievement orientation generated by group cohesion. So each child's progress assists the progress of others within the group. Conductive education is holistic insofar as the focus is on the overall development of the child and it is child-centred insofar as the process of learning is shaped by each child's unique capabilities. In the UK, since the 1980s the process is practised at the Birmingham Institute for

Conductive Education. There are also centres in Ireland and Australia where conductive education is practised.

Previous reviews

From previous reviews of studies of early intervention programmes for children with cerebral palsy a number of conclusions may be drawn (Barry, 1996; Harris, 1987, 1997; Piper, 1990; Tirosh & Rabino, 1989; Turnbull, 1993). First, early intervention programmes involving physiotherapy, particularly neurodevelopmental therapy, lead to only small improvements in motor functioning. In contrast, recent single case design studies support the effectiveness of neuromotor behavioural intervention programmes which aim to help youngsters develop functional skills (rather than reach motor milestones as is the case with neurodevelopmental therapy). Second, improvements in cognitive and social functioning arising from traditional neurodevelopmental physiotherapy programmes are greater than those for motor functioning. Third, the outcome of physiotherapy is better for cases with milder disabilities. Fourth, earlier intervention is associated with better outcome. Fifth, to derive benefit from physiotherapy youngsters must participate in at least one session per week over an extended time period. Sixth, youngsters who receive more structured and intensive physiotherapy involving frequent sessions over longer time periods make better progress. Seventh, both routine special education and conductive education are equally effective in promoting motor, cognitive and social development. Eighth, some environmental manipulations such as the use of tone-reducing casts can improve motor functioning. Previous reviews have cast a wide net and based their conclusions on both uncontrolled and controlled studies and on single case designs as well as group studies. In the present review the focus was exclusively on controlled group outcome studies.

Method

The aim of the present review was to identify effective programmes for preventing adjustment problems in children with cerebral palsy. PsychLit and Medline database searches of English language journals for the years 1977 to 2000 were conducted to identify studies in which such prevention programmes were evaluated. The terms *cerebral palsy* and *spastic paresis* were combined with such terms as *programme*, *study*, *evaluation*, *treatment*, *group outcome*, *conductive education*, *therapeutic electrical stimulation* and *neurodevelopmental therapy*. A manual search through the bibliographies of all recent reviews, and relevant journals on prevention was also conducted. Studies were selected for review if they had a group design which included a treatment and control or comparison group; if at least ten cases were included in each group; and if reliable pre- and post-treatment measures were included. Using these criteria thirteen studies were selected for review.

Characteristics of the studies

The characteristics of the thirteen studies are given in Table 4.1. Five focus on the evaluation of neurodevelopmental therapy (Goodman et al., 1985; Weindling et al., 1996; Mayo, 1991; Palmer et al., 1988, 1990; Law et al., 1991). Two compared the effectiveness of physiotherapy programmes which varied in intensity and the specificity with which goals were set (Bower et al., 1996, 2001). Two studies evaluated the effects of therapeutic electrical stimulation (Hazelwood et al., 1994; Steinbok et al., 1997). Four studies compared the effectiveness of conductive education with that of traditional special education (Bairstow et al., 1993; Hur, 1997; Coleman et al., 1995; Catanese et al., 1995; Reddihough et al., 1998). Five were conducted in the UK, three in Australia, three in Canada, one in the USA and one in South Africa. All of the studies were conducted between 1985 and 2001. There were a total of 601 children in various treatment and control groups over the fifteen studies. Treatment and control group sizes ranged from 9 to 44. Children's ages ranged from birth to twelve years. However, most children were in the two- to eight-year age range. Fifty-six per cent of cases were male and 44% were female. All participants in the studies had a diagnosis of cerebral palsy although there was considerable heterogeneity in the subtypes of the disorder shown by children within these studies. The settings in which programmes were offered varied from study to study. Neurodevelopmental therapy and routine physiotherapy programmes involved regular attendance at hospital clinics and home practice. The therapeutic electrical stimulation programmes were largely home-based. Conductive education programmes were offered in school or preschool settings. Programmes ranged in duration from ten hours over a couple of weeks to five days per week over a couple of years.

Methodological features

The methodological features of studies are given in Table 4.2. In all thirteen studies, cases were assigned to treatment and control or comparison groups and in ten studies such assignment was random. Matching was used in four studies. With respect to subtyping of cerebral palsy, in six studies relatively homogeneous groups of cases were used and in nine studies cases were demographically similar. In eleven studies cases were assessed before treatment and in all studies blind or independent post-intervention evaluations were conducted. In nine studies follow-up assessments were carried out at six months. In seven, one-year follow-up evaluations were conducted and in two studies follow-up was conducted after two years. In all studies gross motor functioning was assessed. Other outcome variables were also assessed in some studies. Fine motor functioning and play skills were evaluated in seven studies, cognitive functioning in six, communication and parental satisfaction in five, activities of daily living in four, parent–child relationships in three, and parental well-being in two. In all studies deterioration and drop-out were assessed.

Table 4.1 Characteristics of prevention studies for children with cerebral palsy

Study no.	Authors	Year	Country	N per group	Mean age and range	Gender	Primary diagnosis	Programme setting	Programme duration
1	Goodman et al.	1985	South Africa	1. NDT = 40 2. C = 40	34 wGA	M 49% F 51%	At risk	Clinic and home	45 minpm for 1 y
2	Weindling et al.	1996	UK	1. Early NDT = 44 2. Standard NDT = 43	At term	M 56% F 44%	At risk	Clinic and home	1 hpw physiotherapy.
3	Mayo	1991	Canada	1. Intense NDT = 17 2. Regular NDT = 12	< 18 m 11 m	—	Mixed types	Clinic and home	1. NDT 1 pw for 6 m 2. NDT 1 pm for 6 m
4	Palmer et al.	1988 1990	USA	1. NDT + CS = 23 2. NDT = 25	12–19 m 15 m	M 75% F 25%	Spastic diplegia	Clinic and home	1. IS 2 × m for 6 m and NDT for 6 m 2. NDT 2 × m for 12 m
5	Law et al.	1991	Canada	1. Intense NDT/C = 19 2. Regular NDT/C = 17 3. Intense NDT = 18 4. Regular NDT = 18	1–8 y	M 39% F 61%	Hemiplegic and quadriplegic spastic CP	Clinic and home	1&3. NDT 2 × 45 minpw + 30-H for 1 y 2&4. NDT 1 × 45minpw + 15-H for 1 y
6	Bower et al.	1996	UK	1. Intense PT/G = 11 2. Regular PT/G = 11 3. Intense PT/A = 11 4. Regular PT/A = 11	3–11 y	—	Quadriplegic CP	Clinic	1&3. 5 hpw for 2 w 2&4. 1 hpw for 2 w
7	Bower et al.	2001	UK	1. Intense PT/G = 15 2. Regular PT/G = 13 3. Intense PT/A = 13 4. Regular PT/A = 15	3–12 y 5 y	M 55% F 45%	Bilateral CP	Clinic	1&3. 5 hpw for 6 m 2&4. 1 hpw for 6 m
8	Hazlewood et al.	1994	UK	1. TES = 10 2. C = 10	5–12 y 8 y	M 75% F 25%	Hemiplegic CP	Home	1. 1 hpd for 5 w
9	Steinbok et al.	1997	Canada	1. TES = 20 2. C = 21	4–10 y 7 y	—	Spastic diplegia	Home	1. 8–12 hpn for 1 y
10	Bairstow et al. Hur	1993 1997	UK	1. CE = 19 2. SE = 17	3–5 y	M 42% F 58%	Mixed types	School	5 dpw for 2 y

11	Coleman et al.	1995	Australia	1. CE = 11 2. SE = 9	19–69 m 45 m	M 50% F 50%	Mixed types	Preschool	3 d minpw for 26 w
12	Catanese et al.	1995	Australia	1. CE = 17 2. SE = 17	4–7 y	M 53% F 47%	Mixed types	Preschool	3 d minpw for 26 w
13	Reddihough et al.	1998	Australia	1. CE = 17 2. SE = 17	12–36 m 23 m	M 63% F 37%	Mixed types	Preschool	3 d minpw for 27 w

Notes
NDT = neurodevelopmental therapy. NDT/C = neurodevelopmental therapy and casting. CS = child stimulation programme. PT/G = physical therapy based on general aims. PT/A = Physical therapy based on specified goals. PT/A = Physical therapy based on general aims. TES = therapeutic electrical stimulation. CE = conductive education. C = control. CP = cerebral palsy. min = minutes. wGA = weeks gestational age. h = hour. d = day. w = week. m = month. y = year. hpw = hours per week. hpd = hours per day. hpn = hours per night. minpm = minutes per month. minpw = minutes per week.

Table 4.2 Methodological features of studies of children with cerebral palsy

Feature	Study number												
	S1	S2	S3	S4	S5	S6	S7	S8	S9	S10	S11	S12	S13
Control or comparison group	1	1	1	1	1	1	1	1	1	1	1	1	1
Random assignment	1	1	1	1	1	1	1	1	1	0	0	0	1
Matched groups	0	0	0	0	0	0	0	1	0	1	0	1	1
Diagnostic homogeneity	0	0	0	1	1	1	1	1	1	0	0	0	0
Demographic similarity	0	1	0	1	1	1	1	1	0	1	0	1	1
Pre-treatment assessment	0	0	1	1	1	1	1	1	1	1	1	1	1
Up to 6 months assessment	0	0	1	1	1	1	1	0	0	0	1	1	1
1-year assessment	1	1	0	0	0	0	0	0	0	0	0	0	0
2-year assessment	0	1	0	0	0	0	0	0	0	0	0	0	0
Objective or blind assessments	1	1	1	1	1	1	1	1	1	1	1	0	1
Cognitive function assessed	1	1	0	0	0	0	0	0	0	0	0	0	1
Communication assessed	1	0	0	0	0	0	0	0	0	1	1	1	1
Gross motor function assessed	1	1	1	1	1	1	1	1	1	1	1	1	1
Fine motor functioning assessed	1	1	0	0	1	0	0	0	0	1	1	1	1
Social functioning and play assessed	1	1	0	1	0	0	0	0	0	1	1	0	1
Activities of daily living assessed	0	0	0	0	0	0	0	0	0	1	1	1	1
Parent–child relationship assessed	0	0	0	1	0	0	0	0	0	0	1	0	1
Parental satisfaction assessed	0	0	0	0	0	0	1	0	0	1	1	1	1
Parental well-being assessed	0	0	0	0	0	0	0	0	0	1	0	0	1
Deterioration assessed	1	1	1	0	1	1	1	1	1	1	1	1	1
Drop-out assessed	1	1	1	1	1	1	1	1	1	1	1	1	1
Experienced therapists or trainers used	1	1	1	1	1	0	0	0	0	1	1	1	1
Programmes were equally valued	0	0	1	0	0	0	1	1	0	1	1	0	0
Programmes were manualized	1	1	1	1	0	0	0	0	1	0	0	0	0
Supervision was provided	1	1	1	1	1	0	0	1	0	0	0	0	0
Programme integrity checked	0	0	0	0	0	0	0	0	1	0	0	0	0
Data on concurrent treatment given	0	0	0	1	1	0	1	1	0	0	0	0	0
Total	14	15	11	19	16	12	15	14	12	19	15	17	20

Notes

S = study. 1 = design feature was present. 0 = design feature was absent.

Experienced therapists were used in all studies. These professionals were all committed to their theoretical approach and programmes were equally valued in studies where two different types of programmes were compared. In six studies it was mentioned that supervision was available and this was usually in the context of parental supervision for home components of the interventions. Manualized programmes were used in seven studies. Checks on programme integrity were specifically reported in only two studies. In four studies data on concurrent treatment were given but no study gave details of subsequent treatment. These were a methodologically robust group of studies.

Substantive findings

A summary of the results of the studies is contained in Tables 4.3 and 4.4.

Neurodevelopmental therapy

In five studies neurodevelopmental therapy was evaluated (Goodman et al. 1985; Weindling et al., 1996; Mayo, 1991; Palmer et al., 1988, 1990; Law et al., 1991). Goodman et al. (1985) and Weindling et al. (1996) found that when newborn infants at high risk for a diagnosis of cerebral palsy received neurodevelopmental therapy from birth, they fared no better on any of the Griffiths (1954) cognitive, motor or social development scales than infants who received routine services or neurodevelopmental therapy offered later in the first year when clear physical signs of cerebral palsy became apparent.

However, Mayo (1991) found that with older infants who were on average eleven months, intensive neurodevelopmental therapy led to significant improvement. Compared with children who received a routine monthly neurodevelopmental therapy, those who received an intensive weekly neurodevelopmental therapy programme showed better motor development over six months. The effect size for improvement in gross motor development was 1.3, indicating that the average infant who received the intensive programme fared better after six months than 90% of infants who received routine physiotherapy.

Results of two further studies show that the efficacy of neurodevelopmental therapy may be increased by coupling it with other interventions, specifically infant stimulation (Palmer et al., 1988, 1990) and the use of inhibitive limb casting (Law et al., 1991). Palmer et al. (1988, 1990) found that, compared with infants who received a year of neurodevelopmental therapy only, infants who received a six-month programme of intensive neurodevelopmental therapy preceded by a six-month home-based programme of infant stimulation made greater gains in cognitive motor and social development on the Bayley Scales of Infant Development (Bayley, 1969) and the Vineland Social Maturity Scale (Doll, 1965) and their mothers were rated as showing greater emotional and verbal responsiveness on the Home Observation for

Table 4.3 Summary of results of treatment effects and outcome rates for studies of children with cerebral palsy

Study type and number. Column groups: **Neurodevelopmental therapy** (Study 1–5); **Goals and intensity** (Study 6–7); **TENS** (Study 8–9); **Conductive education** (Study 10–13).

Variable	Study 1 NDT v C	Study 2 Early NDT v Standard NDT	Study 3 Intense NDT v Regular NDT	Study 4 NDT+ICS v NDT	Study 5 Intense NDT/C v Regular NDT	Study 6 Goals v Aims	Study 6 Intense v Regular	Study 7 Goals v Aims	Study 7 Intense v Regular	Study 8 TES v C	Study 9 TES v C	Study 10 CE v SE	Study 11 CE v SE	Study 12 CE v SE	Study 13 CE v SE
Improvement at up to 6 months															
Cognitive function	0.0	0.0	—	0.6	—	—	—	—	—	—	—	—	—	-0.4	0.3
Communication	0.3	—	—	—	—	—	—	—	—	—	—	—	0.0	-0.1	-0.1
Gross motor function	0.0	0.0	1.3	0.8	0.8	0.9	0.6	0	0.5	1.2	—	—	-0.2	0.7	0.3
Fine motor function	-0.1	0.0	—	—	0.2	—	—	—	—	—	—	—	-0.1	0.6	-0.1
Social interaction and play	0.3	0.0	—	0.3	—	—	—	—	—	—	—	—	0.1	0.1	0.3
Activities of daily living	—	—	—	—	—	—	—	—	—	—	—	—	0.1	—	0.3
Parent–child relations	—	—	—	—	—	—	—	—	—	—	—	—	0.0	—	0.0
Parent satisfaction	—	—	—	—	—	—	0.5	-0.1	0.5	—	—	—	0.0	0.7	0.0
Parental well-being	—	—	—	—	—	—	—	—	—	—	—	—	—	—	0.0
Improvement at up to 1 year															
Cognitive function	—	0.0	—	0.5	—	—	—	—	—	—	—	0.0	—	—	—
Communication	—	—	—	—	—	—	—	—	—	—	—	0.1	—	—	—
Gross motor function	—	0.0	—	0.8	0.8	—	—	0.0	0.0	—	—	0.0	—	—	—
Fine motor function	—	0.0	—	—	0.3	—	—	—	—	—	1.2	-0.1	—	—	—
Social interaction and play	—	—	—	0.4	—	—	—	—	—	—	—	0.2	—	—	—
Activities of daily living	—	—	—	0.5	—	—	—	—	—	—	—	0.4	—	—	—
Parent–child relations	—	—	—	—	—	—	—	—	—	—	—	—	—	—	—
Parent satisfaction	—	—	—	—	—	—	—	-0.2	0.5	—	—	0.7	—	—	—
Parental well-being	—	—	—	—	—	—	—	—	—	—	—	0.0	—	—	—
Improvement at 2 years or over															
Cognitive function	—	0.0	—	—	—	—	—	—	—	—	—	0.0	—	—	—
Communication	—	—	—	—	—	—	—	—	—	—	—	0.2	—	—	—
Gross motor function	—	0.0	—	—	—	—	—	—	—	—	—	-0.3	—	—	—
Fine motor function	—	0.0	—	—	—	—	—	—	—	—	—	-0.4	—	—	—
Social interaction and play	—	0.0	—	—	—	—	—	—	—	—	—	0.4	—	—	—
Activities of daily living	—	—	—	—	—	—	—	—	—	—	—	0.1	—	—	—
Parent–child relations	—	—	—	—	—	—	—	—	—	—	—	—	—	—	—
Parent satisfaction	—	—	—	—	—	—	—	—	—	—	—	0.6	—	—	—
Parental well-being	—	—	—	—	—	—	—	—	—	—	—	0.2	—	—	—

Notes
NDT = neurodevelopmental therapy. NDT/C = neurodevelopmental therapy and casting. CS = child stimulation. TES = therapeutic electrical stimulation. CE = conductive education. SE = routine special education. C = control.

Measurement of the Environment scales (Bradley & Caldwell, 1977). The infant stimulation intervention was based on *Learningames* (Sparling & Lewis, 1979), a programme that consists of 100 explicitly defined and illustrated cognitive, sensory, language and motor activities of increasing developmental complexity appropriate for children from birth to three years of age. Average effect sizes across all domains at six months and a year were each 0.6. Thus the average infant who participated in the infant stimulation and neurodevelopmental therapy programme fared better at six months and a year later than 73% of cases who received a year of neurodevelopmental therapy only.

Law et al. (1991), in an attempt to improve motor functioning in the arms of children with cerebral palsy, combined intensive neurodevelopmental therapy with upper extremity casting to inhibit spasticity and reduce contractures. Children received two 45-minute sessions of neurodevelopmental therapy per week, and completed 30 minutes of physiotherapy exercises per day at home. In addition to this, for four hours each day they wore bivalved, fibreglass, short arm casts which extended from below the elbow to the palm of the hand to inhibit spastic contractions. Children who participated in this intensive programme with arm casting showed much greater gains in upper limb gross motor functioning than children who received a neurodevelopmental therapy programme that was about half as intense and involved no casting. Effect sizes after treatment and nine months later were 0.8, indicating that the average child who participated in the intensive neurodevelopmental therapy with upper arm inhibitive casting showed better upper limb motor functioning afterwards and at follow-up than 79% of children who received routine neurodevelopmental therapy. The combined programme had minimal effect on fine motor development.

From these five studies it may be concluded that neurodevelopmental therapy can improve motor functioning in children with cerebral palsy. However, the effectiveness of neurodevelopmental therapy depends upon the timing of the intervention, the intensity of the programme and the other therapeutic interventions that are combined with it. To be effective neurodevelopmental therapy must be offered at a high level of intensity with clinic physiotherapy sessions once or twice a week and daily home practice. Such intensive programmes should not be offered until the infant is six months and should be preceded by an infant stimulation programme. When coupled with inhibitive limb casting neurodevelopmental therapy is particularly effective in improving the motor functioning of limbs for which inhibitive casts are worn for a set period of time each day.

Goal setting and programme intensity

In two studies, the efficacy of physiotherapy programmes which varied in intensity and the specificity with which goals were set were compared (Bower et al., 1996, 2001). In each of these studies high intensity physiotherapy

Table 4.4 Summary of key findings for studies of children with cerebral palsy

No.	Authors	Year	N per group	Duration	Group differences	Key findings
1	Goodman et al.	1985	1. NDT = 40 2. C = 40	45 minpm for 1 y	1 = 2	• Children in both the neurodevelopmental therapy programme and those that received routine services made similar gains in motor functioning and cognitive development after a year of treatment
2	Weindling et al.	1996	1. Early NDT = 44 2. Standard NDT = 43	1 hpw physiotherapy	1 = 2	• Children in both the early and standard neurodevelopmental therapy made similar gains in motor functioning and cognitive development at 12 and 30 months
3	Mayo	1991	1. Intense NDT = 17 2. Regular NDT = 12	1. NDT 1 pw for 6 m 2. NDT 1 pm for 6 m	1 > 2	• Compared with children who received a routine monthly neurodevelopmental therapy programme, those who received an intensive weekly neurodevelopmental therapy programme showed better motor development over 6 months
4	Palmer et al.	1988 1990	1. NDT + CS = 23 2. NDT = 25	1. IS 2 × m for 6 m & NDT for 6 m 2. NDT 2 × m for 12 m	1 > 2	• Compared with children who received neurodevelopmental therapy, those who received a 6-month programme of child stimulation in addition to neurodevelopmental therapy showed better motor and cognitive development at 6 months and continued to show motor (but not cognitive) development at 12 months • Compared with parents of children who received neurodevelopmental therapy, those whose children received a 6-month programme of child stimulation in addition to neurodevelopmental therapy showed greater maternal emotional and verbal responsiveness at 6 months
5	Law et al.	1991	1. Intense NDT/C = 19 2. Regular NDT/C = 17 3. Intense NDT = 18 4. Regular NDT = 18	1&3. NDT 2 × 45 minpw + 30-H for 1 y 2&4. NDT 1 × 45 minpw + 15-H for 1 y	1 = 2 > 3 = 4	• Children whose arms were in casts showed better functioning on a measure of upper extremity skills • For improving hand functioning the regular and intensive neurodevelopmental therapy programmes were equally effective
6	Bower et al.	1996	1.Intense PT/G = 11 2.Regular PT/G = 11 3.Intense PT/A = 11 4.Regular PT/A = 11	1&3. 5 hpw for 2 w 2&4. 1 hpw for 2 w	1 = 2 > 3 = 4	• For motor functioning, physiotherapy programmes that involved specific goal setting led to greater improvement than those in which general aims were set when planning rehab strategies for children. • For motor functioning, there was a trend for children who received intensive physiotherapy to perform better than children who received routine services
7	Bower et al.	2001	1. Intense PT/G = 15 2. Regular PT/G = 13 3. Intense PT/A = 13 4. Regular PT/A = 15	1&3. 5 hpw for 6 m 2&4. 1 hpw for 6 m	1 = 2 = 3 = 4	• For motor functioning, intensive and regular physical therapy programmes that involved specific goal setting and general aims led to similar outcomes
8	Hazlewood et al.	1994	1. TES = 10 2. C = 10	1. 1 hpd for 5 w	1 > 2	• Compared with controls, children who received therapeutic electrical stimulation showed an increase in passive range of motion of the ankle following treatment
9	Steinbok et al.	1997	1. TES = 20 2. C = 21	1. 8–12 hpm for 1 y	1 > 2	• For gross motor functioning and parental reports of improvement, children who received therapeutic electrical stimulation made greater gains than controls. Participants in the study had undergone lubosacral rhizotomy prior to intervention.

#	Study	Year	Groups	Dosage	Outcomes	Findings
10	Bairstow et al. Hur	1993 1997	1. CE = 19 2. SE = 17	5 dpw for 2 y	1 = 2	• After more than a year of intervention and at one-year follow-up on parents rating of children's communication, physical development, social development and self-help skills both conductive education and special education were equally effective • After more than a year of intervention and at one-year follow-up teacher's ratings of children's gross motor development, interpersonal skills, engagement in play and leisure, and ADL skills both programmes were equally effective • Compared with children in special education, children in the conductive education programme developed deterioration in the mobility of the hips
11	Coleman et al.	1995	1. CE = 11 2. SE = 9	3 h minpw for 26 w	1 = 2	• After 6 months of intervention on blind researcher ratings of language, motor development and self-care both conductive education and special education were equally effective • After 6 months of intervention on parental ratings of language, self-care, social development and family stress both conductive education and special education were equally effective
12	Catanese et al.	1995	1. CE = 17 2. SE = 17	3 h minpw for 26 w	Motor functioning, ADL and parental stress 1 > 2 Social functioning and play 2 > 1	• After 6 months of intervention on objective ratings of gross and fine motor function and activities of daily living children in the conductive education programme performed better than those in traditional Australian early intervention programme • After 6 months of intervention on parental ratings of toileting behaviour and family stress cases in the conductive education programme fared better than those in traditional Australian early intervention programme • After 6 months of intervention on parental ratings of social interaction and play children in the conductive education programme improved less than those in traditional Australian early intervention • After 6 months of intervention both groups showed cognitive improvement with greater gains made by children in the traditional Australian early intervention programme
13	Reddihough et al.	1998	1. CE = 17 2. SE = 17	3 h minpw for 27 w	Cognitive function Toileting 1 > 2 Organizational behaviour 2 > 1	• After 6 months of intervention on objective ratings of cognitive functioning children in the conductive education programme performed better than those in traditional Australian early intervention programme • After 6 months of intervention on parental ratings of dressing behaviour cases in the conductive education programme fared better than those in traditional Australian early intervention programme • After 6 months of intervention on objective ratings of organizational skills children in traditional Australian early intervention programme performed better than those the conductive education programme • After 6 months of intervention on blind researcher ratings of expressive language, and on Reynell Developmental Language Scale both conductive education and special education led to significant improvements • After 6 months of intervention on parental ratings of language, self-care, social development and family stress both conductive education and special education were equally effective in leading to significant improvements • After 6 months of intervention both groups show equal improvements in gross motor functioning

Notes

NDT = neurodevelopmental therapy. NDT/C = neurodevelopmental therapy and casting. CS = child stimulation programme. PT/C = physical therapy based on specified goals. PT/A = physical therapy based on general aims. TES = therapeutic electrical stimulation. CE = conductive education. SE = routine special education. C = control. min = minutes. ADL = activities of daily living. h = hour. d = day. w = week. m = month. y = year. hpw = hours per week. hpd = hours per day. hpn = hours per night.minpm = minutes per month. minpw = minutes per week.

programmes involved one hour per day, five days per week whereas low intensity programmes involved only one hour per week. Also distinctions were made in these studies between general aims which were vaguely stated and specific goals which were measurable and operationally defined behavioural targets. An example of an aim would be to increase mobility. In contrast, an example of goal would be to be able to move independently from a static chair to a wheelchair within a two-minute period without assistance. Thus in these studies goals were formulated in such a way that there was no doubt as to the extent to which they had been achieved when performance was reviewed. In the first of these two studies the treatment lasted for two weeks and in the second treatment duration was six months.

When high and low intensity programmes were compared, after-treatment effect sizes for gross motor functioning ranged from 0.5 to 0.6 with a mean of 0.6 (rounded to one decimal place) but in the second study the effect size at six-month follow-up was 0. Thus the average child who participated in an intensive daily physiotherapy programme showed better gross motor functioning after treatment than 73% of children who received routine once weekly physiotherapy, but these gains did not persist over the long term. Also, in the second study the effect size for parental satisfaction was 0.5 after treatment and at follow-up, indicating that the average parent of a child who received intensive therapy reported greater satisfaction with treatment afterwards and at follow-up than 69% of parents of children who received routine treatment.

When programmes with specific goals and general aims were compared, after-treatment effect sizes for gross motor functioning ranged from 0 in the six-month programme to 0.9 in the two-week programme. It is not meaningful to average these effect sizes since it is clear that using specific goals (rather than general aims) has an immediate short-term benefit over two weeks of therapy, but no such benefit after six months of therapy.

From these two studies it may be concluded that intensive daily treatment (rather than routine weekly therapy) and the use of specific goals (rather than general aims) may lead to immediate improvements in motor functioning but do not confer long-term benefits.

Therapeutic electrical stimulation

In two studies the effects of therapeutic electrical stimulation were evaluated (Hazlewood et al., 1994; Steinbok et al., 1997). In the programme evaluated by Steinbok et al. (1997) children received therapeutic electrical stimulation for eight hours a night over a period of a year following posterior rhizotomy. The muscles stimulated included the abdominal and gluteal muscles, the quadriceps femoris and the tibialis anterior. The anterior tibial and extensor digitorum muscles were stimulated for an hour per day for five weeks in the programme evaluated by Hazlewood et al. (1994). Parents administering the home treatments had written and illustrated instructions and supervision. In both studies effect sizes of 1.2 occurred for gross motor functioning, indicating that the average child treated with therapeutic electrical stimulation fared better afterwards than 88% of untreated children. From these studies it may be concluded that therapeutic electrical stimulation is an effective treatment for improving gross motor functioning in children with cerebral palsy.

Conductive education

In four studies the effectiveness of conductive education was compared with that of traditional special education (Bairstow et al., 1993; Hur, 1997; Coleman et al., 1995; Catanese et al., 1995; Reddihough et al., 1998). In the three Australian studies children received at least three mornings per week of conductive education for a six-month period, but in many instances they received considerably more. In the UK study, participants received five days per week of conductive education over a period of about two years. In all four studies comprehensive, reliable and valid assessment protocols were used to evaluate children's functioning in a range of domains including cognitive, communicative, motor and social development. Ratings of parent–child relationships, parental satisfaction with treatment and parental well-being were also made in some of the studies. Effect sizes obtained at six months from the three Australian studies and those obtained after one year from the UK study across all assessment domains ranged from -0.2 to +0.2 with a mean of less than 0.1. In the UK study effect sizes at two years ranged from 0 to 0.6 with a mean of 0.1. These results show that conductive education and routine UK and Australian special education led to broadly similar outcomes for children with cerebral palsy. However, an important question is whether these studies represent fair trials of conductive education. The programmes evaluated in these studies were non-residential whereas conductive education as practised at the András Petö Institute for Motor Disorders in Budapest is an intensive residential programme. On the other hand, in the UK study conductive education involved far more hours of treatment than routine special education.

Conclusions

Cerebral palsy is a disorder of movement and posture that results from an insult to, or anomaly of, the immature central nervous system in centres which govern motor activity and affects about 1 in 400 children. Children with cerebral palsy often have other co-morbid disabilities including intellectual disability, seizure disorders, visual and auditory impairments, learning difficulties and behaviour problems. Best practice involves offering comprehensive multidisciplinary rehabilitative programmes of care specifically designed to minimize the impact of the constraints placed by cerebral palsy and co-morbid conditions on the child's physical and psychosocial development. Such programmes may include environmental alterations to manage the musculoskeletal complications of cerebral palsy; the use of carefully designed devices to aid posture and mobility; medication, nerve blocks and motor point blocks and neurosurgery to reduce spasticity; and orthopaedic surgery. In addition to these essentially physical interventions, studies reviewed in this chapter suggest that neurodevelopmental therapy, infant stimulation, therapeutic electrical stimulation, special education and conductive education may be effective components within overall multidisciplinary care plans.

Clinical implications

To be effective neurodevelopmental therapy must be offered at a high level of intensity with clinic physiotherapy sessions once or twice a week and daily home practice. Such intensive programmes should not be offered until the infant is six months and the effectiveness of this type of treatment for infants is enhanced if it is preceded by an infant stimulation programme during the child's first six months. In toddlers and young children, when coupled with inhibitive limb casting, neurodevelopmental therapy is particularly effective in improving the motor functioning of limbs for which inhibitive casts are worn for a set period of time each day.

Therapeutic electrical stimulation may be offered as a parent-administered manualized home-based programme to improve gross motor functioning in specific muscles or muscle groups.

Special education and conductive education when offered as day programmes are equally effective in promoting cognitive, motor and social development in young children. As yet there are no outcome data for the effectiveness of conductive education offered on a residential basis.

Implications for research

Studies that evaluate the effectiveness of comprehensive multidisciplinary programmes and the contribution of their constituent elements to their overall effectiveness are required in this area. The benefits of evaluating multicomponent programmes is particularly evident from the studies of neurodevelopmental therapy reviewed here. These showed that when combined with other interventions such as infant stimulation or inhibitive casting, the effectiveness of neurodevelopmental therapy is greatly enhanced.

There is also a need for evaluation studies of popular and high profile single component programmes, particularly conductive education. A fair treatment trial of intensive residential conductive education as it is practised at the András Pető Institute for Motor Disorders in Budapest is needed.

Future evaluation studies should include assessments of the integrity of programmes that have been manualized and are protocol based. In such studies, training sessions are recorded and blind raters use programme integrity checklists to evaluate the degree to which sessions approximate manualized training curricula. Such integrity checks allow researchers to say with confidence the degree to which a pure and potent version of their programme has been evaluated.

Studies are required which investigate the psychological and physiological processes which underpin programme effectiveness. Neurobehavioural motor intervention offers a good model for this type of research. The focus in neurobehavioural programmes is on developing specific movements and postures which are absent from the child's repertoire but are essential for the completion of specific developmentally appropriate functional tasks. The degree to which functional goals are achieved may be correlated with the degree to which the specific movements and postures initially absent from the child's repertoire are acquired (Horn et al., 1995). In studies of interventions where the putative mechanism of change is physiological, changes on appropriate physiological variables may be correlated with the attainment of specific treatment goals. There is also a need to replicate studies of the effects of infant stimulation and identify the neuropsychological processes involved.

There is a need to use homogeneous groups of cases in programme evaluation studies in this area because children with different types of cerebral palsy and different disability profiles clearly have differing treatment needs.

Assessment resources

Abidin, R.R. (1983). *The Parenting Stress Index*. University of Virginia, USA: Paediatric Psychology Press.

Alpern, G., Ball, T. & Shearer, M. (1986). *Developmental Profile 2*. Los Angeles: Western Psychological Services.

Bayley, N. (1969). *Bayley Scales of Infant Development*. New York: Psychological Corporation.

Bayley, N. (1993). *Bayley Scales of Infant Development* (Second Edition). New York: Psychological Corporation.

Bradley, R.H. & Caldwell, B.M. (1977). Home Observation for Measurement of the Environment: A validation study of screening efficiency. *American Journal of Mental Deficiency*, 81, 417–420.

Capute, A. & Shapiro, B. (1985). The motor quotient: A method for the early detection of motor delay. *American Journal of Disability in Children*, 139, 940–941.

Coolman, R., Bennett, F., Sells, C., Sweanson, M., Andrews, M. & Robinson, N. (1985). Neuromotor development of graduates of the neonatal intensive care unit. Patterns encountered in the first two years of life. *Journal of Developmental and Behavioural Pediatrics*, 6, 327–333.

Doll, E. (1965). *Vineland Social Maturity Scale*. Circle Pines, MN: American Guidance Service.

Evans, P.M. & Alberman, E. (1985). Recording motor defects of children with cerebral palsy. *Developmental Medicine and Child Neurology*, 27, 401–406.

Folio, R., Fewell, R. & Dubose, R.F. (1983). *Peabody Developmental Motor Scales*. Toronto: Teaching Resources Co.

French, J.L. (1964). *The Pictorial Test of Intelligence*. Boston: Houghton Mifflin.

Friedrich, W.N., Greenberg, M.T. & Crnic, K. (1983). A short form of the Question-naire on Resources and Stress. *American Journal of Mental Deficiency*, 88, 41–48.

Griffiths, R. (1954). *The Abilities of Babies: A Study in Mental Measurement*. Thet-ford, Norfolk: Lowe and Brydone for the Association For Research in Infant and Child Development.

Holroyd, J. (1974). The Questionnaire on Resources and Stress: An instrument to measure family response to a handicapped family member. *American Journal of Community Psychology*, 2, 92–94.

King, S., Rosenbaum, P. & King, G. (1995). *The Measure of Process of Care: A Means to Assess Family Centred Behaviours of Healthcare Providers*. Hamilton, Ontario: Neurodevelopmental Research Unit, McMaster University.

Knobloch, H. & Pasamanick, B. (1974*). Gesell and Amatruda's Developmental Diag-nosis*. Hagerstown, MD: Harper & Row.

Knobloch, H., Stevens, F. & Malone, A. (1980). Manual of Developmental Diagnosis: The Administration and Interpretation of the Revised *Gesell and Amatruda's Developmental and Neurologic Examinations*. Hagerstown, MD: Harper & Row.

Russell, D.J., Rosenbaum, P.L., Cadman, D.T., Gowland, C., Hardy, S. & Jarvis, S. (1989). The Gross Motor Function Measure: A means to evaluate the effects of physical therapy. *Developmental Medicine and Child Neurology*, 31, 341–352.

Sparrow, S.D., Bella, D.A. & Cicchetti, D.V. (1985). *The Vineland Adaptive Behaviour Scales*. Circle Pines, MN: American Guidance Services.

Vulpe, S.G. (1982). *Vulpe Assessment Battery*. Toronto: National Institute on Mental Retardation.

Therapy resources

Basmajian, J. & Wolf, S. (1990). *Therapeutic Exercise* (Fifth Edition). Baltimore, MD: Williams & Wilkins.

Bobath, K. (1980). *A Neurophysiological Basis for the Treatment of Physiotherapy. Clinics in Developmental Medicine No 75* (Second Edition). Philadelphia, PA: Lippincott.

Hari, M. & Akos, K. (1988). *Conductive Education*. London: Routledge.

Scrutton, D. (1984). *Management of the Motor Disorders of Children with Cerebral Palsy*. London: Spastics International Medical Publications.

Sparling, J. & Lewis, I. (1979). *Learningames for the First Three Years*. New York: Walker.

5 Prevention of adjustment difficulties in children with sensory impairments

Aine Fahey and Alan Carr

Children born with sensory impairments such as hearing or visual impairment – deafness or blindness – or multisensory impairment can develop serious adjustment problems (Hindley & Brown, 1994). The more profound the impairments, and the earlier the onset, the greater the effect. Sensory impairments can prevent children from developing adequate cognitive, communication and social skills and this in turn can lead to emotional and behavioural problems, relationship difficulties and a restricted lifestyle. A variety of early intervention programmes have been developed to prevent such adjustment problems developing in children with sensory impairments. The effectiveness of many of these remains untested (Calderon & Greenberg, 1997; Davidson & Harrison, 1997). The aim of this chapter is to review methodologically robust research studies on the effectiveness of such early intervention programmes, draw reliable conclusions about the effectiveness of these, and outline the implications of these conclusions for policy and practice.

Hearing impairment

Normal hearing refers to the ability to detect sounds of within 0 to 15–20 dB HL at a variety of frequencies (e.g. 500 Hz, 1000 Hz etc.) and hearing loss refers to deficits in this sensory ability, with such deficits being classified as mild (15–30 dB HL), moderate (31–60 dB HL), severe (61–90 dB HL) and profound (90 dB HL or greater) (American National Standards Institute, 1989; Bess & Humes, 1995). Distinctions are made between congenital deafness, which is present from birth, and deafness which occurs postnatally. Further distinction exists between the deterioration of hearing loss over time, termed progressive hearing loss, and acquired hearing loss, which occurs following a period of normal development.

Aetiology

Sensorineural and conductive hearing loss constitute the main types of hearing loss (Carney & Moeller, 1998). The former is associated with defects of the auditory nerve, the cochlea, the organ of Corti, or the central nervous system and is indicative of more severe hearing loss than the conductive form, which involves the middle ear. Both types of hearing loss can occur simultaneously. Heredity and meningitis are the main causes of hearing loss. Maternal rubella, birth trauma, complications of pregnancy, prematurity, Rh incompatibility, postnatal infections and viruses such as mumps and measles, high fever and otitis media are also cited as potential precursors of hearing impairment.

Epidemiology

One in every 1,000 children is born with severe to profound hearing loss and the prevalence of deafness, if acquired cases are included, is about 4 per 1,000 (Hindley & Brown, 1994). Hearing loss presents in the majority of these cases before the age of three years and mostly during the first year of life. Eighty per cent of hearing loss involves sensorineural defects, 25% of deaf children have multiple disabilities, while 90% of deaf children have hearing parents (Strong et al., 1992).

Impact of deafness on development

Regardless of type, time of onset, severity or cause, language, cognitive, social and emotional development is invariably more problematic for the hearing impaired child (Carney & Moeller, 1998; Hindley & Brown, 1994). Impoverished linguistic input associated with hearing impairment compromises the ability of the child with hearing loss to extract linguistic cues from the environment and leads to delays in all aspects of language development. Since language is indispensable to the development of appropriate strategies for reading and writing, literacy skills are also compromised. Children with moderate and severe degrees of hearing loss also have difficulties in discriminating and labelling speech sounds. These phonetic deficiencies make speech production difficult. With respect to social and emotional development, a higher level of impulsiveness, more limited problem-solving skills and a greater difficulty in labelling and identifying emotions make deaf children more vulnerable to developing psychological problems than their hearing peers.

Visual impairment

Visual impairment refers to corrected visual acuity (in the better eye) of less than 6/18 metres and no more than 6/60 metres, or a central visual field of less than 10 degrees (Davidson & Harrison, 1997; World Health Organization, 1984). A distinction is made between severe visual impairment (corrected acuity of between 6/60 and 3/60 metres) and blindness (corrected visual acuity worse than 3/60 metres).

Aetiology

Central nervous system damage due to maternal infections during pregnancy, alterations of embryonic development, genetic factors and birth complications are the main pre- and perinatal factors associated with visual impairment (Palumba et al., 1995). Children rendered blind after birth are termed adventitiously blind. Adventitious blindness is rare and is usually caused by traumatic brain injury and neoplasms affecting the visual system (Robinson & Jan, 1993).

Epidemiology

About 1 in every 3,000 children has severe visual impairment (Olson, 1987; Hindley & Brown, 1994). Hereditary retinopathy accounts for 25–50% of cases. Congenital rubella accounts for a further 10% of cases. Up to 50% of children with blindness have additional disabilities including intellectual disability, cerebral palsy, epilepsy and hearing impairment.

Impact of blindness on development

Variations in blind children in terms of aetiology, time of onset, severity and type of visual impairment create an idiosyncratic developmental trajectory for each blind child. However, broad conclusions about the impact of blindness on development can be drawn from available developmental studies (Fraiberg, 1977; Norris et al., 1957). The development of motor activities, particularly those which involve visual-motor integration, are delayed in blind children. Motor limitations diminish the availability of sensory stimulation for the blind child which inhibits the integration of sensorimotor experiences. Hearing becomes the dominant sense with which to organize the world into a coherent and meaningful framework. The acquisition of object concept, object permanence, spatial conservation and understanding of causality is delayed as a result of blindness. Consequently, higher order cognitive skills such as classification and conservation are inhibited. A limited experiential base hinders the development of language, symbolic play and non-verbal communication such as facial expressions. Lack of reciprocity in blind child–caregiver interactions interferes with the development of attachments. In later years, blind children may have difficulty initiating and maintaining peer relations due to their lack of awareness of non-verbal social cues and strategies which facilitate social relations such as smiling, nodding and using eye contact.

Previous reviews

From previous reviews of the literature on the effectiveness of early intervention programmes for children with sensory impairments a number of conclusions may be drawn (Calderon & Greenberg, 1997; Carney & Moeller, 1998; Davidson & Harrison, 1997; Meadow-Orlans, 1987; Olson, 1987; Vergara et al., 1993). First, children with sensory impairments (both deafness and blindness) can probably benefit from early intervention programmes. Second, for blind children, the relative effectiveness of one programme over another or the effectiveness of specific programme variables has not yet been demonstrated. Third, for deaf children, programmes that involve teaching manual or signing forms of communication, such as Rochester fingerspelling, American Sign Language (ASL) and manual English, are probably more effective in promoting language development and academic achievement than those based on oral communication only. Fourth, the setting (home or preschool) in which programmes are offered has little impact on outcome.

Fifth, research in this area has been primarily concerned with the impact of specific early intervention curricula on the development of cognitive, linguistic and communication skills. There is a need to expand this focus and investigate the impact not only of curricula but of factors within the child's social system, such as parental and family factors, that may influence the impact of the curriculum, on a wider range of outcome variables which tap psychosocial development in addition to cognitive and linguistic development. Sixth, multisystemic early intervention programmes for deaf and blind children which involve both parents and children and which are staffed by multidisciplinary teams hold considerable promise and deserve evaluation.

Seventh, hearing aids and FM systems can improve speech and language acquisition in young children and their effectiveness can be enhanced if coupled with tactile aids. FM systems improve speech perception in noisy environments by reducing the amount of background noise. FM systems include a microphone and pocket-sized transmitter worn by the speaker. Listeners wear pocket-sized receivers connected to their hearing aids through which they hear the voice of the speaker as he or she speaks into the microphone. The tactile aids alone have minimal effect on speech and language development. Eighth, while there is good evidence that cochlear implants can facilitate the development of speech and language in older children, there is insufficient evidence to show that they are effective with young children. Ninth, there is no evidence to support the effectiveness of sensory aids such as the Sonic Guide or the Lobster Pot in facilitating development in young children and what evidence there is suggests that these aids will not make a major contribution to future effective early intervention programmes.

Tenth, there are numerous obstacles to conducting rigorously controlled outcome research in this field including the low incidence of children with sensory impairment in the general population; the heterogeneous nature of blindness and deafness; the unavailability of outcome measures standardized on deaf and blind children; difficulties in child–evaluator communication; and ethical problems associated with withholding potentially beneficial intervention programmes from control groups. It is therefore not surprising that most studies which evaluate early intervention programmes for children with sensory impairments have methodological shortcomings including the study of aetiologically heterogeneous groups of cases, the absence of control groups, lack of random assignment of cases to groups, and the use of outcome measures standardized on children without sensory impairments.

The degree of confidence that can be placed in the conclusions drawn from the reviews mentioned above is limited by the quality of the studies included in the reviews. All of these reviews contained some studies that were poorly designed. In this chapter our aim was to draw conclusions from the better-designed studies in this area.

Method

The aim of the present review was to identify effective early intervention programmes for children with sensory impairments. PsychLit, ERIC and Medline database searches of English language journals for the years 1977 to 2000 were conducted using the terms *deaf, blind, hearing impairment, visual impairment*, combined with terms such as *early intervention, early childhood education, intervention programmes, treatment*. These were complemented by a manual search of the bibliographies of recent review papers. Prominent researchers in the field were also contacted by telephone or email in order to establish whether they had conducted any recent studies in the area. Over 30 studies in which quantitative methods were used to examine the effectiveness of a particular early intervention programme for children with sensory disabilities were identified. Studies which examined the effectiveness of sensory aids were excluded, because our focus was primarily on educational and psychological intervention programmes. Initially, only studies involving prospective group designs with more than five participants in the intervention and control group and reliable pre- and post-intervention measures were selected. However, only eight studies met these stringent methodological criteria. Because such a small number of studies was identified, five other studies, which did not meet our initial stringent methodological criteria, but which were fairly methodologically robust, were selected for review also. Three of these studies lacked control groups and two had control groups but involved retrospective designs. In two of the three studies that lacked control groups, statistical procedures were used to control for maturational processes and the third study lacking a control group was included because it was the only quantitative evaluation of an early intervention programme for children with multiple sensory impairments (deaf-blind children) identified. In one of the studies with a retrospective design, a comprehensive procedure was used to match intervention and control groups and in the other statistical procedures were used to control for the effects of possible confounding variables on which groups were not matched.

Characteristics of the studies

Characteristics of the thirteen selected studies are set out in Table 5.1. All studies were conducted between 1985 and 1998. In eight studies programmes for deaf children were evaluated. In two studies programmes for blind children were evaluated and in three studies the children were both deaf and blind. Of the thirteen studies six evaluated exclusively school-based programmes, six assessed exclusively home-based programmes and in the remaining two studies the programmes were conducted partially or wholly in special day centres. In the case of the home-based interventions, home visits took place either on a daily or weekly basis or a few times per month, over time periods ranging from fifteen months to three years. The principles learnt during these visits were implemented during the week by parents. School-based programmes were implemented during the school term over time periods ranging from seven months to three years. Aggregated across all studies, a total of 2,919 deaf children, 36 deaf-blind children and 45 blind children received intervention, while 115 deaf children, 15 deaf-blind and 63 blind children acted as controls. Of the deaf children who received intervention, 2,768 received the SKI*HI service. This is a family-centred, home-based, early intervention programme for enhancing language and communicative development in deaf children. Children's ages ranged from six months to twelve years. Of the studies in which gender details were given, 54% of cases were male and 46% female.

Methodological features

Methodological features of each study are outlined in Table 5.2. In ten out of thirteen studies, a control or comparison group was used but in only one study were cases randomly assigned to treatment and control groups. Diagnostic homogeneity was established in all thirteen studies to the extent that children in all studies were diagnosed as having hearing or visual impairment or both. Demographic similarity between intervention and control groups was present in nine of the studies. With the exception of the two retrospective studies, both pre- and post-programme measures were incorporated into the experimental design. No studies included controlled follow-up assessments, although uncontrolled one- and two-year follow-up assessments were carried out in one study, and qualitative data were reported on the maintenance of post-intervention gains in another study. Both retrospective studies provided follow-up data only. Children's self-report measures were not used to evaluate outcomes in any of the studies, while teacher ratings were used in four studies and parent ratings in eight studies. Ratings by early interventionists or by researchers were used in seven studies while psychometric tests of language, speech and academic attainments and tests of general and visual development were used in all but one of the studies. In five studies treatment drop-out was reported; in the case of deaf-blind children, drop-outs were replaced on a

Table 5.1 Characteristics of prevention studies for children with sensory impairments

Study no.	Dis-ability	Authors	Year	N per group	Mean age and range	Gender	Family characteristics	Programme setting	Programme duration
1	Deaf	Greenberg & Kusche	1998	SBP-S = 29 C = 28	9 y 5–12 y	M 47% F 53%	Caucasian 83% DP 0% DS 7% DR 9%	Special class Mainstream school	54 × 20–40 min less for 22 w
2	Deaf	Greenberg & Kusche	1993	SBP-S = 7 C = 8	—	—	—	Special class Mainstream school	54 × 20–40 min less
3	Deaf	Hindley & Reed	1999	SBP-S = 24 C = 31	9 y 7–11 y	M 62% F 38%	HP 100%	Special school	4 × 30 min less pw for 1 y or 2 × 60 min less pw for y
4	Deaf	Moog & Geers	1985	SBP-L = 15 C = 18	7 y 6 y–9 y	—	—	School	3 y during school term
5	Deaf	Strong et al.	1994	FCP-L = 2,768.	2 y	—	Caucasian 73%	Home	1 hpw PA visit over 15 m
6	Deaf	Watkins	1987	FCP-L = 46 C = 46	10 y	—	Mid SES	Home	1 hpw PA visit
7	Deaf	Watkins et al.	1998	FCP-L-DM = 18 FCP-L = 18	2 y 0–5 y	—	—	Home	11 hpw PA DIP-P 6.5 hpm DM over 18 m
8	Deaf	Greenberg Greenberg et al.	1983 1984	FCP-L = 12 C = 12	2 y	—	DP 8%	Home Centre	1 hpw PA 6.5 hpm DM for 18 m
9	Blind	Beelman & Brambring	1998	FCP-L-S = 10 C = 40	1–3 y	M 58% F 42%	Mixed SES	Home	2 spm over 3 y
10	Blind	Sonksen et al.	1991	FCP-S-L-V = 35 FCP-S-L = 23	27 < 6 m 31 > 6 m	M 62% F 38%	—	Centre	CrBS DIP-P for 12 m
11	Deaf-blind	Watkins et al.	1993	FCP = 24	—	M 46% F 54%	SPF 14% Low SES 10% Caucasian 82%	Home	1 hpw PA 10 hpw 1 for 3 y
12	Deaf-blind	Watkins et al.	1993	FCP-S-L = 15 FCP = 15	—	M 43% F 57%	—	Home	1 hpw PA 10 hpw 1 for 2 y
13	Deaf-blind	Rowland & Schweigert	2000	SBP-C = 12	4 y 3–5 y	M 58% F 42%	—	School	During school-term for 3 y

Notes

SBP-S = school-based programme focusing on social-emotional development. SBP-L = school-based programme promoting cognitive and communicative development. FCP- L = family-centred home-based programme focusing mainly on language development, using signed or spoken English. FCP-L-DM = family-centred and child-centred home-based programme focusing on language and communication development, using a deaf mentor. FCP-S-L = family-centred programme focusing on social and language development. FCP-S-L-V = family-centred programme focusing on social, language and visual development. C = control group. SES = socioeconomic status. SPF = single parent family. DP = deaf parents. DS = deaf siblings. DR = deaf relative. HP = hearing parent. PA = parent adviser. DM = deaf mentor. I = intervener. min = minutes. h = hour. d = day. w = week. pw = per week. m = month. y = year. less = lessons. hpm = hours per month. hpw = hours per week. Cr = centre. CrBS = centre-based sessions. DIP-P = daily implementation of programme by parents.

Table 5.2 Methodological features of studies for children with sensory impairments

Feature	S1	S2	S3	S4	S5	S6	S7	S8	S9	S10	S11	S12	S13
Control or comparison group	1	1	1	1	0	1	1	1	1	1	0	1	0
Random assignment	1	0	0	0	0	0	0	0	0	0	0	0	0
Diagnostic homogeneity	1	1	1	1	1	1	1	1	1	1	1	1	1
Demographic similarity	1	0	1	1	1	0	1	0	0	0	1	1	1
Pre-treatment assessment	1	1	1	1	1	0	1	1	1	1	1	1	1
Post-treatment assessment	1	1	1	1	1	1	0	0	1	1	1	1	1
Follow-up assessment	1*	0	0	0	0	0	0	1	0	1‡	0	0	1†
Children's self-report	0	0	0	0	0	0	0	0	0	0	0	0	0
Parent ratings	1	1	1	0	0	0	0	0	1	0	0	0	0
Teacher ratings	1	1	1	0	0	0	0	0	0	0	0	0	0
Researcher/Early interventionist ratings	1	1	1	0	1	1	0	1	1	1	1	1	1
Measures of general/visual development	0	0	0	1	0	0	1	1	1	0	1	1	0
Tests of language/speech/academic attainment	1	1	1	1	1	1	1	1	0	1	0	1	0
Deterioration assessed	1	0	1	0	0	0	0	0	1	1	0	0	0
Drop-out assessed	1	0	1	0	0	0	0	0	0	1‡	1†	1†	1†
Clinical significance of change assessed	0	0	0	0	0	0	0	0	0	1‡	0	0	0
Experienced therapists or trainers used	1	1	1	1	1	1	1	0	1	0	1	1	1
Programmes were manualized	1	1	1	0	1	1	1	0	0	0	1	1	1
Supervision was provided	1	1	1	0	1	1	1	0	0	0	1	1	1
Programme integrity checked	1	1	1	0	0	1	0	1	1	0	1	0	0
Data on concurrent treatment given	0	0	0	0	0	0	0	0	0	1	0	0	0
Data on subsequent treatment given	0	0	0	0	0	0	0	0	0	0	0	0	0
Total	17	12	15	8	9	9	9	8	10	11	11	12	10

Notes
S = study. 1 = design feature was present. 0 = design feature was absent. *uncontrolled follow-up, ‡qualitative data only, †drop-outs replaced on a continual basis.

continuous basis. Four studies provided qualitative data regarding deterioration on specific outcome variables, while the clinical significance of post-intervention change was analysed descriptively in one study. In all studies but one, in which the absence of trained counsellors was acknowledged, early interventionists received training prior to intervention. In seven studies programmes were manualized. Supervision was provided in ten programmes and programme integrity was verified in all but four studies, either by completion of progress reports or by direct observation of intervention procedures by a supervisor. Data on concurrent treatment were reported in one study, while no study reported data on subsequent intervention or treatment.

Substantive findings

Substantive findings from the thirteen studies selected for review are summarized in Tables 5.3 and 5.4. The early intervention programmes evaluated in these studies may be broadly classified as school- as opposed to home-based interventions; and interventions which focus on enhancing social development as opposed to those which focus mainly on improving cognitive, linguistic and communicative functioning. Within the home-based programmes a further distinction can be made between programmes that are family centred and those that are child centred. Family-centred interventions focus on teaching parents strategies to promote their children's cognitive and communicative development and on providing emotional support and advice to the family within a collaborative framework. In contrast, in child-centred programmes, a professional works directly with the child to enhance language, speech and communicative development. Programmes can also be distinguished by their primary method of communication and programmes reviewed here entail signed English, spoken English, simultaneous communication (signed plus spoken English), total communication (a variety of communications, both auditory–oral and manual), and American Sign Language.

Programmes for deaf children

Of the eight studies of programmes for deaf children, three evaluated a programme designed to enhance social development (Greenberg & Kusche, 1993, 1998; Hindley & Reed, 1999) and five evaluated programmes where the enhancement of communicative skills and cognitive development were the main goals (Moog & Geers, 1985; Strong et al., 1994; Watkins, 1987; Watkins et al., 1998; Greenberg, 1983; Greenberg et al., 1984).

School-based programmes for promoting social development in deaf children

The PATHS (Promoting Alternative Thinking Strategies) programme, which aims to promote effective interpersonal problem-solving in deaf children, was

Table 5.3 Summary of results of treatment effects and outcome rates for studies of children with sensory disabilities

	Study number and condition												
	Deaf								Blind		Deaf-Blind		
Variable	Study 1	Study 2	Study 3	Study 4	Study 5	Study 6	Study 7	Study 8	Study 9	Study 10	Study 11	Study 12	Study 13
	SBP-S v C	SBP-S v C	SBP-S v C	SBP-L v C	FCP-L	FCP-L v C	FCP-L-DM v FCP-L	FCP-L v C	FCP-S-L v C	FCP-S-L-V v C	FCP	FCP-S-L v FCP	SBP-C
Child's communication													
Speech and language test performance	—	—	—	1.0	0.4	0.5	0.7	—	—	—	—	—	—
Researcher ratings of communication	—	—	—	—	—	—	—	1.0	—	—	—	—	—
Parent ratings of communication	—	—	—	—	—	0.5	—	1.9	—	—	0.4	0.7	—
Child's behavioural adjustment													
Teacher ratings	0.3	—	0.9	—	—	—	—	1.2	—	—	0.7	0.9	—
Parent ratings	0.7	—	—	—	—	0.5	—	1.5	—	—	—	—	—
Researcher ratings	—	—	—	—	—	—	—	—	—	—	—	—	—
General development													
Academic attainments	0.6	1.5	0.3	1.0	—	0.5	—	—	1.0*	—	—	—	—
Social-emotional understanding	1.3	1.8	0.9	—	—	—	—	—	—	—	—	—	—
Visual development	—	—	—	—	—	—	—	—	—	0.7	0.8	0.6	—
Parental stress and well-being	—	—	—	—	—	—	—	1.3	—	—	—	—	—
% Drop-out	5%	—	14%	—	—	—	—	—	—	40%	—	—	—

Notes

SBP-S = school-based programme focusing on social-emotional development. SBP-L = school-based programme focusing on language. SBP-C = school-based programme promoting cognitive and communicative development. FCP-L = family-centred home-based programme focusing mainly on language development, using signed or spoken English. FCP-L-DM = family-centred and child-centred home-based programme focusing on language and communication development, using a deaf mentor. FCP-S-L = family-centred programme focusing on social and language development. FCP-S-L-V = family-centred programme focusing on social, language and visual development. C = control group. *This effect size is for full-term infants at 30 months.

Table 5.4 Summary of key findings from studies of children with sensory disabilities

Study no.	Disability	Authors	Year	N per group	No. of sessions	Group differences	Key findings
1	Deaf	Greenberg & Kusche	1998	SBP-S = 29 C = 28	54 20–40 min sess for 22 school w	1 > 2	• Compared with controls, deaf children who completed the PATHS programme (a school-based programme to improve social adjustment) in a US school where spoken and signed language were used showed improved social-emotional understanding, social competence, and teacher-rated behavioural adjustment
2	Deaf	Greenberg & Kusche	1993	SBP-S = 7 C = 8	54 20–40 min sess	1 > 2	• Compared with controls, deaf children who completed the PATHS programme (a school-based programme to improve social adjustment) in a US school where only spoken language was used showed improved social-emotional understanding
3	Deaf	Hindley & Reed	1999	SBP-S = 24 C = 31	4 30 min pw or 2 h less pw for 1 y	1 > 2	• Compared with controls, deaf children who completed a UK adapted version of the PATHS programme (a school-based programme to improve social adjustment) in a UK school showed improved social-emotional understanding and teacher-rated behavioural adjustment
4	Deaf	Moog & Geers	1985	SBP-L = 15 C = 18	3 y during school term	1 > 2	• Compared with controls, deaf children who participated in a school-based language-focused programme showed improved speech and language development and higher academic attainment
5	Deaf	Strong et al.	1994	FCP-L = 2,768.	1 hpw PA visit over 15 m DIP-P	Language improvement	• Deaf children who participated in the SKI*HI programme (a home-based language-focused programme) showed greater rates of language development following intervention than that predicted by pre-programme test scores
6	Deaf	Watkins	1987	FCP-L = 46 C = 46	1 hpw PA visit DIP-P	1 > 2	• Compared with controls, deaf children who had participated in the SKI*HI programme (a home-based language-focused programme) as preschoolers showed better language, academic and social functioning at 6–13 y
7	Deaf	Watkins et al.	1998	FCP-S-L = 18 FCP-L = 18	1 1 hpw PA DIP-P 6.5 hpm DM over 18 m	1 > 2	• Compared with deaf children in the routine SKI*HI programme, those exposed to a bi-lingual, bi-cultural learning environment who received regular contact with a deaf mentor in addition to participation in the SKI*HI programme showed better language development
8	Deaf	Greenberg Greenberg et al.	1983 1984	FCP-L-B = 12 FCP-L = 12	HV 2 spw C 1 spw for 1 year Occasional PGA	1 > 2	• Compared with controls, deaf preschool children who participated in a home- and centre-based multisystemic programme which focused on both family adjustment and communication showed better language development and behavioural adjustment • Compared with controls, mothers of deaf children who participated in a home- and centre-based multisystemic programme which focused on both family adjustment and communication showed lower levels of stress

Table 5.4 continued

Study no.	Disability	Authors	Year	N per group	No. of sessions	Group differences	Key findings
9	Blind	Beelman & Brambring	1998	FCP-L-S = 10 C = 40	2 spm over 3 y	1 > 2	• At 2.5 y and 3 y, compared with matched controls, blind full-term infants whose families participated in a home-based parent training programme showed a significantly greater level of overall development • From 2.5 y to 3 y the differences between full-term infants intervention and control groups decreased • Among pre-term children, the control group showed significantly greater developmental progress than intervention groups at both age levels.
10	Blind	Sonksen et al.	1991	FCP-S-L-V = 35 FCP-S-L = 23	CrBS for 12 m DIP-P	1 > 2	• Compared with infants whose families participated in a routine family education programme, blind infants who participated in a multisystemic programme including a special component to enhance visual development made greater developmental progress.
11	Deaf Blind	Watkins et al.	1993	FCP = 24	1 hpw PA DIP-P 10 hpw I for 3 y	Accelerated development	• Following a multisystemic family-based programme, focusing on both children and parents, deaf-blind children made significantly greater general developmental progress than that predicted due to maturational factors alone
12	Deaf Blind	Watkins et al.	1993	FCP-S-L = 15 FCP = 15	1 hpw PA DIP-P 10 hpw I for 2 y	1 > 2	• Following a multisystemic home-based programme, focusing on both children and parents, deaf-blind children made significantly greater general developmental progress than children from families who participated in programme which focused largely on training parents • Children in the multisystemic programme spent a greater number of hours interacting with other family members
13	Deaf Blind	Rowland & Schweigert	2000	SBP-C = 12	During school-term for 3 years	Greater cognitive and communicative development	• Deaf-blind children who participated in a school-based language and communication-focused programme showed significant improvement in cognitive and communicative functioning

Notes

SBP-S = school-based programme focusing on social-emotional development. SBP-L = school-based programme focusing on language, academic and speech development. SBP-C = school-based programme promoting cognitive and communicative development. FCP-L = family-centred home-based programme focusing mainly on language development, using signed or spoken English. FCP-L-DM = family-centred and child-centred home-based programme focusing on language and communication development, using a deaf mentor. FCP-S-L = family-centred programme focusing on social and language development. FCP-S-L-V = family-centred programme focusing on social, language and visual development. C = control group. PA = parent adviser. DM = deaf mentor. I = Intervener, min = minutes. h = hour. d = day. w = week. pw = per week. sess = sessions. less = lessons. y = year. m = month. hpm = hours per month. hpw = hours per week. spw = sessions per week. spm = sessions per month. Cr = centre. CrBS = centre-based sessions. DIP-P = daily implementation of programme by parents.

evaluated in three studies (Kusche & Greenberg, 1994). The PATHS programme includes three units, each of which focuses on teaching a specific set of skills. In the first unit children learn to 'stop and think' and control impulsivity when faced with new or challenging situations. The metaphor of a turtle who 'stops to think' is used in this unit. Developing a vocabulary to label emotional states is the focus of the second unit. In the third unit, children learn interpersonal problem-solving skills, with an emphasis on identifying problems, examining alternative solutions and planning implementation of preferred solutions. In the third unit, children use their 'stop and think' skills to create a context for interpersonal problem-solving. They also use their emotion labelling skills when considering the impact of possible solutions to interpersonal problems on the emotional state of others. Thus the programme is progressive and cumulative in that skills learned in the first two units are the bedrock upon which skills in the final unit are acquired.

Greenberg and Kusche (1998, 1993) and Hindley and Reed (1999) evaluated the impact of the PATHS programme in a series of three waiting list control design studies. In the first study, elementary school children selected from eleven special classes for the deaf in six mainstream schools were randomly assigned to intervention and control groups in which normal teaching methods were used (Greenberg & Kusche, 1998). Uncontrolled follow-up assessments were conducted at one and two years. This study involved children educated in a total communication setting in which both signed and spoken English were used. In the second study Greenberg and Kusche (1993) evaluated the effectiveness of the PATHS programme in a school where only oral English was used. Hindley and Reed (1999) evaluated the effectiveness of a version of the PATHS curriculum adapted for use in the UK. In addition to the units described above, children learnt how to use role-play and give and receive compliments as a prelude to joint social problem-solving. Participants in this study used signed English as their main communication modality.

After one year effect sizes for academic attainment from these three studies ranged from 0.3 to 1.5 with a mean of 0.8, indicating that the average child who participated in the PATHS programme was reading better than 79% of controls. Reading ability was assessed in the US studies with the Special Edition for Hearing Impaired Students of the Stanford Achievement Test (Madden et al., 1972) and in the UK with the Edinburgh Reading Test (University of Edinburgh, 1981).

After one year effect sizes for social-emotional understanding from these three studies ranged from 0.9 to 1.8 with a mean of 1.3, indicating that the average child who participated in the paths programme showed better social-emotional adjustment than 90% of controls. In the US studies the Social Problem Solving Assessment Measure-Revised (Elias et al., 1978) was used and in both the US and UK studies the Kusche Emotional Inventory (Kusche, 1984) was used to evaluate social-emotional understanding. For the US studies effect sizes were aggregated across both instruments.

After one year effect sizes for teacher-rated behavioural adjustment, from these three studies, ranged from 0.0 to 0.9 with a mean of 0.4, indicating that the average child who participated in the PATHS programme showed better social-emotional adjustment than 66% of controls. In the US studies behavioural adjustment was evaluated by teachers using the Meadow/Kendall Social-Emotional Assessment Inventory for Deaf Children (Meadow, 1983), the Health Resource Inventory (Gersten, 1976) and the Walker Behaviour Problem Identification Checklist (Walker, 1976); in the UK study only the first of these three instruments was used.

After one year there were no intergroup differences in the two US studies on parent-rated behaviour problems as assessed by the Child Behaviour Checklist (Achenbach, 1991) and the Eyeberg Child Behaviour Inventory (Robinson et al., 1980). A floor effect due to the absence of serious behaviour problems in the sample at pre-test may have accounted for the negligible effect sizes for parent- and teacher-rated behaviour problems.

In an uncontrolled follow-up carried out a year after the programme had finished Greenberg and Kusche (1998) obtained effect sizes of 0.7 and 0.5 for measures of social understanding and reading achievement respectively, suggesting that one year following intervention, the average child who participated in the programme was still functioning better than between 69% and 76% of non-intervention children in these domains.

School-based programme for enhancing communication and cognitive development in deaf children

Compared with a control group, Moog and Geers (1985) found that children who participated in the Experimental Project in Instructional Concentration (EPIC) showed a significantly greater level of language development, superior speech production and higher academic attainment levels than the control group. Programme features included homogeneous grouping based on ability level in each subject area; instructional groups of variable size; hierarchical organization of instructional objectives in each skill area so that proficiency was needed on one level before a child could proceed to the next objective; flexible length of teaching blocks in each area to accommodate the variable rates of progress of each child; and a team approach to teaching which aimed to enhance programme flexibility and to facilitate co-operation between teachers.

Language was assessed using the Peabody Picture Vocabulary Test (Dunn, 1965); the Auditory Association and Grammatical Closure subtests of the Illinois Tests of Psycholinguistic Abilities (Kirk et al., 1968); the Northwestern Syntax Screening Test (Lee, 1971); the Test of Syntactic Abilities (Quigley et al., 1978) and the Grammatical Analysis of Written Language (Geers et al., 1981). Speech production was evaluated using a procedure described by Monsen (1983) in which the child's speech was taped and rated in terms of degree of intelligibility. The American School Achievement Test (Pratt et al., 1975) was used as a measure of academic performance. An effect size of

1.0 was obtained across all language measures, on the measure of speech production and on the word and sentence meaning subtest of the American School Achievement Test, indicating that following intervention, children who participated in the EPIC programme were functioning better in these domains than 84% of children who received routine instructional programmes.

Home-based programmes for enhancing language and communicative development in deaf children

In three studies the SKI*HI (Watkins & Clark, 1992) family-centred, home-based, early intervention programme for enhancing language and communicative development in deaf children was assessed (Strong et al., 1994; Watkins, 1987; Watkins et al., 1998). Central components of the model are procedures for screening and identifying infants early in life; home visits; and provision of family support services. Families in the SKI*HI programme receive weekly home visits from a parent adviser who assesses the needs of the child and advises parents on topics such as hearing aid use, parent–child communication, the use of American Sign Language, cognitive and language development, and the development of warm and stimulating parent–child relationships. Strategies for promoting optimal child development are modelled by the parent adviser and practised by the parents in the sessions. In addition, the parent adviser helps the family access other social, health and educational services.

Strong et al. (1994) in a single group outcome predictive design evaluated the rate of progress beyond that attributable to maturational factors after 15 months of 2,768 deaf children (mean age of two years) who participated in the SKI*HI programme. Predicted post-test scores were calculated by dividing pre-programme developmental age by pre-programme chronological age and multiplying by post-programme chronological age (Sheehan, 1979). Using predicted post-programme scores as controls, an effect size of 0.4 was obtained for both expressive and receptive language on the Language Development Scale for deaf children (Tonelson & Watkins, 1979). This indicates that following the SKI*HI programme the average participant showed better language development than would be expected from 66% of cases, if they had not participated in the programme.

In a retrospective study, Watkins (1987) found that, compared with matched controls, children who participated in the SKI*HI programme during their preschool years showed better language development, greater academic achievement, and better social-emotional adjustment at age eight to eleven years. An effect size of 0.6 was obtained on measures of communication, language, academic attainments, and teacher-rated behavioural adjustment, indicating that following intervention, the average child who participated in the programme was functioning better in these domains than 73% of controls.

Watkins et al. (1998) evaluated the impact of augmenting the routine SKI*HI programme with a deaf mentor home-based programme. This deaf mentor programme involved the introduction of children to a bi-lingual, bi-cultural environment in which American Sign Language (ASL) was taught in regular home visits by deaf mentors concurrently with signed and spoken English (Total Communication). Deaf mentors also acted as advocates for the deaf culture, promoting a deeper understanding in parents of the culture and facilitating the development of a positive sense of identity and pride in the child as a member of the deaf community. An effect size of 0.7 was obtained on the Language Development Scale (Tonelson & Watkins, 1979), which indicates that following intervention, the average child in the SKI*HI and Deaf Mentor programme had better language abilities than 76% of children who participated in the routine SKI*HI programme.

Greenberg evaluated the effectiveness of a Counselling and Home Training Programme for deaf children (Greenberg, 1983; Greenberg et al., 1984). The programme comprised six specific components: an initial parent counselling service; weekly home visits by a teacher of the deaf to facilitate communicative development (both signed and oral/aural); weekly home sign language instruction by a deaf adult who also promoted a deeper understanding and appreciation among parents and children of the deaf culture; weekly sign language group-based classes at a centre for the deaf; and occasional parent group activities at the centre for the deaf such as lectures and counselling sessions to stimulate relations among families, staff and members of the deaf community.

Evaluation was carried out one to four months post intervention by an outside evaluation team. Parent and family stress and parental knowledge of deaf issues were evaluated using the Questionnaire on Resources and Stress (Holroyd, 1973); a modified version of the Parental Information and Attitudes Scale for Parents of Hearing-Impaired Children (Brown, 1972); and Parent Knowledge of Audiological Matters (Schlesinger & Meadow, 1976). Developmental level was assessed with the Leiter Performance Scale (Levine, 1986) and the Alpern–Ball Developmental Profile (Alpern et al., 1986). Interviewer ratings of child and family adjustment were also documented during two family interviews. Parent–child communication was assessed by video-taping the children in a naturalistic setting for 30 minutes while they interacted with their mothers.

Four months after enrolment in the programme effect sizes of 1.0 and 1.9 were obtained for researcher and parent ratings of communication skills respectively. Effect sizes for researcher and parent ratings of behavioural adjustment were 1.5 and 1.2 respectively. Averaging parent and researcher effect sizes in each of these domains, it may be concluded that the average child in the programme had better developed communication skills and showed better behavioural adjustment than 92% of controls. Researcher ratings were based on direct observation of parent–child interaction and parents gave their ratings on the Alpern–Ball Developmental Profile (Alpern et al.,

1986). An effect size of 1.3 was obtained for maternal well-being as assessed by the total score on the Questionnaire on Resources and Stress (Holroyd, 1973). Thus, the average mother who participated in the programme was less stressed than 90% of mothers from the control group.

The studies reviewed in this section on hearing impairment show that both school- and home-based early intervention programmes for deaf children with the goals of enhancing social and communicative skills and preventing adjustment problems in these domains can be highly effective in the short and long term.

Programmes for children with visual impairment

In two studies, family-centred programmes for blind children were evaluated (Beelman & Brambring, 1998; Sonksen et al., 1991). Beelman and Brambring, (1998) assessed the effectiveness of a home-based programme for congenitally blind children. The programme included a child-focused component to facilitate children's cognitive, motor and visual development and a parent-focused component involving problem-focused counselling in a family context. Throughout the programme particular emphasis was placed on blindness-specific domains of development, especially tactile and auditory perception, spatial orientation, mobility, and daily living skills. Parents were trained in skills required to promote optimal development in blind children and information was provided on how to optimally structure children's environments by using orientation aids within the home and appropriate play materials. For full-term children, an overall effect size of 1.0 was obtained at 30 months on the Bielefeld Developmental Test for Blind Infants and Preschoolers (Brambring, 1989). This indicates that the average child who participated in the programme was functioning better than 84% of controls. However, six months later, the effect size had fallen to 0.5, indicating that the impact of the programme diminished over time. Preterm children did not benefit from the programme.

Sonsken et al. (1991) examined the incremental effectiveness of adding a special module which aimed to promote visual development in preschoolers to a centre-based parent-oriented intervention programme which focused on general development. The programme for general development covered language, non-verbal concept formation, localization skills (sound and touch), manipulative and tactile discrimination ability, and gross motor skills. Strategies to promote development in these domains and which could be incorporated into daily play and routine activities were modelled for parents. The additional module on visual development involved training parents to identify visually arresting objects or events to which their infants reacted and coaching parents in reinforcing infants for responding to these objects and events. Parents were also trained in how to help their children increase the range of visually arresting objects and events to which they responded. After a year, compared with controls who completed the general development programme only, children who completed the general development pro-gramme and the additional module on visual development showed superior performance on measures of visual progress including near acuity, distance acuity, near following, distance tracking and sphere of attention. The effect size after a year was 0.7, indicating that the average child in the more com-prehensive programme showed better progress in visual functioning than 76% of those who participated in the routine programme.

The results of the two studies reviewed in this section show that family-focused early intervention programmes can enhance general and visual func-tioning in visually impaired preschool children and so prevent adjustment problems.

Programmes for children with multisensory impairments

In three studies programmes for children with multisensory impairments were evaluated (Watkins et al., 1993; Rowland & Schweigert, 2000). In two of these, Watkins et al. (1993), examined the effectiveness of the Intervenor Service Model for deaf-blind children and their families. Based on the one-to-one service provided by Annie Sullivan to Helen Keller, within this pro-gramme the intervener becomes the 'eyes and ears of the child'. Interveners implement a 10-hour weekly individualized programme of tactile, visual and auditory sensory stimulation in order to facilitate learning and interaction and minimize self-stimulating and injurious behaviours. Alongside this child-focused intervention, parents receive weekly home visits from parent advisers who follow the SKI*HI curriculum mentioned earlier in the section on programmes for deaf children.

In the first study a single group predictive design was used in which the rate of progress made by children in the programme over and above that expected due to maturation was assessed on the Callier-Azusa Developmental Scale (Stillman & Battle, 1985) and the Insite Developmental Scale (Morgan & Watkins, 1989). Predicted post-programme scores were calculated by dividing pre-programme developmental age by pre-programme chronological age and multiplying by post-programme chronological age (Sheehan, 1979). Using predicted post-test scores as controls, effect sizes of 0.8, 0.4 and 0.7 were obtained for visual development, communication development and behavioural adjustment respectively. This indicates that following the inter-vention programme, the average participant showed better development in these domains than would be expected from between 66% and 79% cases, if they had not participated in the programme.

In the second study families participating in the intervener programme were compared with matched controls who participated in a parent adviser home-visiting programme. Effect sizes of 0.6, 0.7 and 0.9 were obtained for visual development, communication development and behavioural adjust-ment respectively on these same instruments as were used in the first study. This indicates that following the intervention programme, the average participant showed better development in these domains than between 73% and 82% of controls.

Rowland and Schweigert (2000) evaluated the effectiveness of a school-based programme for children with multisensory impairments. The goal of the programme was to enhance the communicative and cognitive functioning of deaf-blind children by organizing all classroom activities so as to maximize the child's opportunities to interact with people and objects. Individualized programmes were collaboratively formulated by teachers, parents and project staff, based on a thorough assessment of the functional level of each child. Target skills were reinforced and generalized throughout the school day. Participants in this single group outcome study made modest gains in cognitive and communication skills, but the design of the study precluded the calculation of effect sizes.

The results of the three studies reviewed in this section show that family-focused early intervention programmes which include a child-centred intervener and a parent adviser, and individually tailored school-based programmes for young children can enhance functioning of children with multisensory impairments and so prevent adjustment problems.

Conclusions

From this review, a number of conclusions may be drawn. First, both home- and school-based early intervention programmes for children with sensory impairments can prevent adjustment difficulties and promote psychological development in a range of domains including communication, behavioural adjustment, social-emotional understanding and academic attainment. Home-based programmes may be most appropriate for infants and preschool children. School-based programmes are more appropriate for children over the age of five.

Second, the SKI*HI (Watkins & Clark, 1992) programme for families with preschool deaf children is a particularly well-researched and effective programme. The SKI*HI programme is a multisystemic family-oriented approach which actively promotes early identification of hearing loss, provides weekly instruction and advice to parents and family regarding strategies to enhance the deaf child's cognitive and language development, uses an auditory-oral and signed English approach, and helps the family access a wide range of support services from other disciplines. The effectiveness of this programme, and other similar multisystemic programmes, is enhanced if children in addition have direct child-centred input from a deaf mentor as well as family support from a home-visiting parent adviser. Furthermore, early preschool gains made by children in the SKI*HI programme are sustained right up until late childhood.

Third, maternal stress may be reduced by participating in multisystemic family-based programmes, with both child-focused and parent-focused components.

Fourth, for school-aged children, the PATHS programme (Kusche & Greenberg, 1994), which consists of a series of daily school lessons to teach children interpersonal problem-solving skills, is effective in promoting social-emotional understanding and behavioural adjustment in deaf primary school children.

Fifth, an intensive school-based curriculum which adopts a systematic approach to teaching based on the individual needs and abilities of each child appears to be more effective than normal teaching methods in enhancing speech and language and academic attainment in primary school children with hearing loss.

Sixth, for visually impaired infants, multisystemic child- and parent-focused programmes in which direct intervention with children in blind-specific areas such as motor co-ordination and orientation, combined with parent training in strategies to promote child development, and the provision of a family-counselling service, are particularly effective. Visual development in visually impaired youngsters is enhanced if parents are taught strategies to maximize their child's opportunities to engage in active looking as opposed to passive 'seeing'.

Seventh, for deaf-blind children, multisystemic programmes in which children are assigned an intervener to provide intensive weekly individualized programmes of sensory stimulation and communicative interaction for the child, in conjunction with parent training and education, are effective in promoting development in most domains of functioning. Effective school-based interventions for deaf-blind children maximize children's opportunities to interact with their peers, teachers and with the physical environment throughout the school day.

Implications for policy and practice

The evidence reviewed in this chapter has implications for the development of prevention programmes for children with sensory impairments. Developmental screening procedures should be implemented to facilitate early identification. Multisystemic family-based early intervention programmes should be offered to families with children who are detected through screening procedures as having sensory impairments. These multisystemic family-based early intervention programmes should include child-focused and parent-focused components and these components should be offered flexibly on a home-visiting basis and at local health, social or educational centres for families of children with sensory impairments. The SKI*HI curriculum is a good example of this type of intervention. Child-centred interventions should focus on promoting the use of all senses including the impaired sense, especially in the case of visually impaired children. In addition child-centred interventions should focus on training the child in communication skills including oral speech and sign language. Child-centred interventions may be taught by an adult with a sensory impairment who acts as an advocate and role model for the child, introducing them to the deaf and blind minority cultures. Parent-centred interventions should provide information on sensory impairment, and coaching in techniques that parents can use to help their children learn communication and social skills. Parent-centred interventions should also provide parents with ongoing personal support and advice on how to access health, social and educational services. For school-aged children, school-based programmes should follow on from home-based child-centred programmes. In school-based programmes, systematic and intensive instruction, tailored to children's unique learning profiles, should be used to promote language development. Social problem-solving skills should also be taught to promote social understanding and behavioural adjustment, as in the PATHS programme. Long-term parent-centred programmes should run in parallel with the child-centred school-based programmes, to provide a forum within which parents can address the various problems that occur as their sensorily impaired children make various life-cycle transitions such as entering puberty and leaving secondary school.

Implications for research

The studies reviewed in this chapter have implications for future research. There is a need to evaluate the long-term impact of multisystemic programmes that begin in infancy and carry on into the school-going years.

There is considerable evidence that father involvement in family-based intervention can have a significant impact on outcome (Carr, 2001c). Despite this, programmes, such as those evaluated in the studies reviewed in this chapter, have rarely involved fathers. Future research should evaluate the impact of programmes that target both fathers and mothers as programme participants.

Future research should evaluate manualized intervention programmes in which checks for programme integrity are made. In such studies, training sessions are recorded and blind raters use programme integrity checklists to evaluate the degree to which sessions approximate manualized training curricula. Such integrity checks allow researchers to say with confidence the degree to which a pure and potent version of their programme has been evaluated.

Studies that examine the impact of design features that may make programmes more effective are required. Specifically research is needed on the effects of including different components in multisystemic programmes and the effects of programmes of differing durations.

Studies are required which investigate the mechanisms and processes which underpin programme effectiveness. Improvements probably occur through a variety of complex mechanisms including increasing support to parents; enhancing parenting skills; improving infants' and children's sensory, communicative and social skills; and supporting the development of good parent–child relationships.

Not all children and families respond equally to early intervention programmes. There is a need to design and evaluate programmes for children and families that have particular difficulties in responding to routine prevention programmes. For example, low birth weight infants with visual impairments have difficulties responding to programmes to promote visual development. Further research is needed to identify programmes that can be effective with this vulnerable group of children.

Assessment resources for deaf children

Brown, P. (1972). *Parental Information and Attitude Scale For Parents of Hearing-Impaired Children*. Washington, DC: Gallaudet College.

Kusche, C.A. (1984). *The Understanding of Emotion Concepts by Deaf Children: An Assessment of an Effective Education Curriculum*. Unpublished doctoral dissertation, University of Washington.

Levine, M. (1986). *Leiter International Performance Scale: A Handbook*. Los Angeles, CA: Western Psychological Services.

Madden, R., Gardner, E., Rudman, H., Karlsen, B. & Merwin, J. (1972). *Stanford Achievement Test for Hearing Impaired Students*. New York: Harcourt Brace Jovanovich.

Meadow, K.P. (1983). *Revised Manual. Meadow/Kendall Social-Emotional Assessment Inventory for Deaf and Hearing-Impaired Children*. Washington, DC: Pre-College Programs, Gallaudet Research Institute.

Monsen, R.B. (1983). Towards measuring how well hearing-impaired children speak. *Journal of Speech and Hearing Research*, 21(2), 197–219.

Moog, J.S., Kozak, V.J. & Geers, A.E. (1983). *Grammatical Analysis of Elicited Language: Pre-sentence Level (GAEP-P)*. St Louis, MO: Central Institute for the Deaf.

Schlesinger, H. & Meadow, K.P. (1976). *Studies of Family Interaction, Language Acquisition and Deafness*. Washington, DC: Office of Maternal and Child Health.

Tonelson, S. & Watkins, S. (1979). *Instruction Manual for the SKI*HI Language Development Scale: Assessment of Language Skills for Hearing Impaired Children from Infancy to Five Years of Age*. Logan, UT: SKI*HI institute, Utah State University.

Winton, P. (1998). The family focused interview: An assessment measure and goal setting mechanism. In D. Bailey & R. Simeounson (Eds.), *Family Assessment in Early Intervention* (pp. 195–205). Columbus, OH: Merrill.

Assesment resources for blind children

Brambring, M. (1989). Methodological and conceptual issues in the construction of a developmental test for blind infants and preschoolers. In M. Brambring, F. Losel & H. Skowronek (Eds.), *Children at Risk: Assessment, Longitudinal Research, and Intervention* (pp. 136–154), Berlin, NY: de Gruyter.

Davis, C. (1980). *Perkins–Binet Tests of Intelligence for the Blind*. Watertown, MA: Perkins School for the Blind.

Newland, T. (1971). *Blind Learning Aptitude Test*. Champaign, IL: University of Illinois Press.

Reynell, J. (1979). *Manual for the Reynell–Zinkin Scales, Developmental Scales for*

Visually Handicapped Children. Part 1: Mental Development. Windsor, Berks: NFER.

Assessment resources for children with multisensory impairment

Morgan, E. & Watkins, S. (1989). *Assessment of Developmental Skills for Young Multi-handicapped Sensory-impaired Children.* Logan, UT: HOPE.

Rowland, C. (1990, 1996). *Communication Matrix.* Portland, OR: Oregon Health Sciences University.

Rowland, C. & Schweigert, P. (1997). *Hands-on Problem-Solving for Children with Deafblindness (SIPPS, HIPSS, TAPPS and Guide to Assessment and Teaching Strategies).* Portland, OR: Oregon Health Sciences University.

Rowland, C. & Schweigert, P. (2000). *Time to Learn.* Portland, OR: Oregon Health Sciences University.

Stillman, R. & Battle, C. (1985). *Callier-Azusa Scale (H): Scales for the Assessment of Communicative Abilities.* Dallas: University of Texas at Dallas, Callier Centre for Communication Disorders.

Programme resources for deaf children

Kusche, C.A. & Greenberg, M.T. (1994). *The PATHS Curriculum.* Seattle, WA: Developmental Research and Programs.

Moores, D. (1978). *Educating the Deaf. Psychology Principles and Practices.* Boston, MA: Houghton Mifflin.

Quigley, S. & Kretschmer, R. (1982). *The Education of Deaf Children.* Baltimore, MD: University Park Press.

Schneider, M. & Robin, S. (1978). *Manual for the Turtle Technique.* Unpublished manual, Department of Psychology, State University of New York at Stony Brook.

Watkins, S. & Clark, T.C. (1992). *The SKI*HI model: A Resource Manual for Family-Centred, Home-based Programming for Infants, Toddlers, and Pre-school-aged Children with Hearing Impairment.* Logan, UT: HOPE.

Weissberg, R.P., Gesten, E.L., Liebenstein, N.L., Doherty-Schmid, K.D. & Sutton, H. (1980). *The Rochester Social Problem-Solving (SPS) Program.* Rochester, NY: University of Rochester.

Programme resources for blind children

Anderson, S., Boignon, S. & Davis, K. (1991). *The Oregon Project for Visually Impaired and Blind Preschool Children.* Medford, OR: Jackson Education Service District.

Barraga, N. (1980). *Program to Develop Efficiency in Visual Functioning.* Louisville, KY: American Printing House for the Blind.

Blind Children Centre (1993). *First Steps: A Handbook for Teaching Young Children who are Visually Impaired.* Los Angeles, CA: Blind Children's Centre.

Programme resources for deaf-blind children

Condon, R. (1979). Pre-language Development: Communication training for the deaf–blind. In O. Peak (Ed.), *Educational Methods for Deaf-blind and Severely Handicapped Students*, Volume 1 (pp. 125–134). Austin, TX: Texas Education Agency, Department of Special Education, Special Education Developmental Services Centre for Deaf-Blind.

Freeman, N.B.E. (1985). *The Deaf-blind Baby: A Programme of Care*: London: William Heinemann Medical Books.

Resources for parents

Chen, D., Friedman, C.T. & Calvello, G. (1991). *Learning Together: A Parent Guide to Socially-based Routines for Visually Impaired Infants*. Unpublished guide of the PAVII-project.

Ferrell, K. (1985). *Reach out and Teach. Materials for Parents of Visually Handicapped and Multihandicapped Young Children*. New York: American Foundation for the Blind.

Freeman, R., Carbin, C. & Boese, R. (1981). *Can't your Child Hear?: A Guide for those who Care about Deaf Children*. Baltimore, MD: University Park Press.

Garretson, M. (1994). *Deafness: Life and Culture*. Silver Spring, MD: National Association of the Deaf.

Kates, L. & Schein, J.D. (1980). *A Complete Guide to Communication with Deaf-blind Persons*. Silver Spring, MD: National Association of the Deaf.

Luterman, D. & Ross, M. (1991). *When your Child is Deaf. A Guide for Parents*. Parkton, MD: New York Press.

6　Prevention of adjustment problems in children with autism

Linda Finnegan and Alan Carr

Autism is a pervasive developmental disorder characterized by profound cognitive, social and communication deficits and by repetitive behaviours (Howlin, 1998; Cohen & Volkmar, 1997). Autism, first described by Leo Kanner in 1943, is now classified within ICD 10 and DSM IV as one of a group of pervasive developmental disorders.

Diagnostic criteria for autism, from both ICD 10 and DSM IV, are presented in Table 6.1. A triad of deficits typify most autistic children (Cohen & Volkmar, 1997). These are often called Wing's triad, after the eminent researcher Lorna Wing. These deficits occur in social development, language and behaviour, particularly imaginative or make-believe play. Abnormalities in social behaviour, which first appear in infancy, include the absence of eye-to-eye signalling; the absence of the use of social or emotional gestures; a lack of reciprocity in social relationships; attachment problems such as an inability to use parents as a secure base; little interest in peer relationships; lack of empathy; and little interest in sharing positive emotions such as pride or pleasure with others. Language development in autistic children is usually delayed and the language of autistic children is characterized by a variety of pragmatic abnormalities including pronominal reversal, echolalia, neologisms and speech idiosyncrasies. With pronominal reversal, the child uses the pronoun *you* in place of the pronoun *I*. With echolalia the child repeats the exact words that someone has said to them with the same intonation. Autistic children rarely engage in extended conversations focusing on social or affective topics and display little creativity in language use. The behaviour of autistic children is characterized by stereotyped repetitive patterns and confined in its range by the restricted interests that most autistic children display. There is also a strong desire to maintain routines and sameness and a resistance to change. Imaginative or make-believe play is virtually absent.

Epidemiology

The prevalence rate for autism based on studies conducted from the 1960s to the 1970 was 2–5 per 10,000 (Howlin, 1998; Cohen & Volkmar, 1997). However, Gillberg and Coleman (2000) in a review of more recent epidemiological

Table 6.1 Diagnostic criteria for autism in the *Diagnostic and Statistical Manual of Mental Disorders*, Fourth Edition (DSM IV) and the International Classification of Diseases, 10th revision (ICD 10)

DSM IV	ICD 10
A. At least six of the following with at least two items from 1 and one each from 2 and 3	A pervasive developmental disorder defined by the presence of abnormal and/or impaired development that is manifest before the age of 3 years, and by the characteristic type of abnormal functioning in three areas of social interaction, communication and restricted repetitive behaviour.
1. Qualitative impairment of social interaction as manifested by at least two of the following: (a) Marked impairments in the use of multiple non-verbal behaviours such as eye-to-eye gaze, facial expression, body postures, and gestures to regulate social interaction (b) Failure to develop peer relationships appropriate to developmental level (c) A lack of spontaneous seeking to share enjoyment, interests, or achievements with other people (d) lack of social or emotional reciprocity	Usually there is no prior period of unequivocally normal development but, if there is, abnormality becomes apparent before the age of 3 years. There are always qualitative impairments in reciprocal social interaction. These take the form of an inadequate appreciation of socio-emotional cues, as shown by a lack of responses to other people's emotions and/or a lack of modulation of behaviour according to social context; poor use of social signals and a weak integration of social, emotional, and communicative behaviours; and, especially, a lack of socio-emotional reciprocity.
2. Qualitative impairments in communication as manifested by at least one of the following: (a) Delay in, or total lack of, the development of spoken language (b) In individuals with adequate speech, marked impairment in the ability to initiate or sustain a conversation with others (c) Stereotyped and repetitive use of language or idiosyncratic language (d) Lack of varied, spontaneous make-believe play or social imitative play appropriate to developmental level	Similarly qualitative impairments in communication are universal. These take the form of a lack of social usage of whatever language skills are present; impairment of make-believe and social imitative play; poor synchrony and lack of reciprocity in conversational interchange; poor flexibility in language expression and a relative lack of creativity and fantasy in thought processes; lack of emotional response to other people's verbal and non-verbal overtures; impaired use of variations in cadence or emphasis to reflect communicative modulation; and a similar lack of accompanying gesture to provide emphasis or aid meaning in spoken communication.
3. Restricted repetitive and stereotyped patterns of behaviour, interests and activities as manifested by at least one of the following: (a) Encompassing preoccupation with one or more stereotyped and restricted patterns of interest that is abnormal either in intensity or focus (b) Apparently inflexible adherence to specific, non-functional routines or rituals (c) Stereotyped and repetitive motor mannerisms (d) Persistent preoccupation with parts of objects	The condition is also characterized by restricted, repetitive and stereotyped patterns of behaviour, interests and activities. These take the form of a tendency to impose rigidity and routine on wide range of aspects of day-to-day functioning; this usually applies to novel activities as well as to familiar habits and play patterns.
B. Delays or abnormal functioning in at least one of the following areas, with onset prior to age 3 years: (1) social interaction, (2) language as used in social communication, or (3) symbolic or imaginative play	In early childhood there may be attachment to unusual, typically non-soft objects. The children may insist on the performance of particular routines or rituals of a non-functional character; there may be stereotyped preoccupations with interests such as dates, routes or timetables; often there are motor stereotypies; a specific interest in non-functional elements of objects (such as their smell or feel) is common; and there may be resistance to changes in routine or details of the personal environment.
C. The disturbance is not better accounted for by Rett's disorder or childhood disintegrative disorder	

Sources: Adapted from DSM IV (APA, 1994) and ICD 10 (WH0, 1992, 1996) with permission.

studies concluded that the prevalence rate for autism is now 9.6 per 10,000. This dramatic rise in the prevalence of autism may reflect an increase in prevalence of the disorder, a change in diagnostic practices or both. The male–female ratio for autism is 3 or 4:1. Children with autism may also suffer from co-morbid cognitive and physical conditions which affect their overall adjustment (Howlin, 1998; Cohen & Volkmar, 1997).

In the cognitive domain, it is noteworthy that about 75% of children with autism have IQs below 70 and the characteristic profile is for the non-verbal or performance IQ score to be greater than the verbal IQ. An IQ above 50, especially a verbal IQ above 50, is a particularly significant protective factor associated with a better prognosis. Age-appropriate language development at five years is also a good prognostic sign. Some youngsters with autism have islets of ability. For example, they may be able to play many tunes by ear or remember a catalogue of facts. However, the most noticeable cognitive deficit in autism is an inability to solve social or interpersonal problems.

In the domain of physical development, up to a third of autistic children develop epilepsy in late adolescence. Many have elimination problems including encopresis and enuresis. Some also develop physical complications due to self-injurious behaviour such as head-banging or biting.

The outcome for children with autism is poor. Up to 60% are unable to lead an independent life and only 4% reach a stage where they are indistinguishable from normal children. Children with a non-verbal IQ in the normal range and some functional language skills at the age of five have the best prognosis. However, underestimating the potential of children with pervasive developmental disorders to develop life skills is the major pitfall to be avoided. Autistic children with severe to profound cognitive impairment rarely develop speech and commonly develop adjustment problems including self-injury.

Aetiology

Theories of autism fall into three broad categories: psychogenic, biogenic and cognitive (Cohen & Volkmar, 1997). Psychogenic theories argue that psychosocial processes are central in the aetiology of autism whereas biogenic theories look to biological factors as the basis for the condition.

Most recent research points to the neurobiological aetiology of autism and to the centrality of cognitive rather than emotional factors as underpinning the main clinical features (Bailey et al., 1996, Gillberg & Coleman, 2000). Evidence from twin and family studies shows that genetic factors contribute to the development of autism; that the mode of transmission is quite complex; and probably involves multiple genes. There is also an association between autism and a variety of genetic disorders including fragile X anomaly, tuberous sclerosis, and untreated phenylketonuria. Tuberous sclerosis is a neurocutaneous disorder characterized by skin lesions and neurological features, and both epilepsy and learning difficulties also occur in many cases.

The risk of parents having a second child with autism is between 3 and 7%. Some cases of autism are due to congenital rubella and some may be due to obstetric complications. A higher incidence of prenatal problems has been found in children with autism and those identified consistently in the literature include advanced maternal age, birth order (first- or fourth-born or later), use of medication, prematurity, postmaturity, and early or mid-trimster bleeding (Tsai, 1987). The precise biological characteristics that are genetically transmitted or that develop as a result of congenital infection or obstetric complication and which underpin the clinical features of autism are still unclear and future research will continue to investigate the neuroanatomical, neurochemical, psychophysiological, endocrinological and immunological characteristics of people with autism (Bailey et al., 1996; Gillberg & Coleman, 2000).

Cognitive theories of autism are concerned, not with identifying the primary causes of autism, but with explaining the patterning of symptoms in terms of specific underlying cognitive deficits. Cognitive theories of autism posit central cognitive deficits which may account for some or all of the clinical features and symptoms that characterize the condition. A wide variety of cognitive deficits have been proposed and these include problems with encoding, sequencing and abstraction (Hermelin & O'Connor, 1970); processing socially significant information (Sigman, 1995); processing emotive facial expressions (Hobson, 1993); developing a theory of mind (Baron-Cohen, 1995); recalling episodic autobiographical memories (Jordon & Powell, 1995); seeking central coherence (Frith & Happé, 1994); and executive functioning (Ozonoff, 1994). There is some evidence to support each of these theories and it seems quite probable that some combination of all seven of these cognitive deficits accounts for the main clinical features of autism. Future research will aim to clarify this and also the relationship between these cognitive deficits and the neurobiological correlates of autism.

Previous reviews

A wide range of intervention programmes for autism has been developed. There is no scientific evidence for the effectiveness of most of these (Green, 1996; Jordon & Jones, 1996). This does not mean that they are not effective. It simply means that we do not currently know whether they are effective or not. Some may be effective in some cases; some may be ineffective but benign in some cases; and some may be harmful in some cases. Without empirical evaluation, the only evidence available is unsubstantiated anecdotal testimonials. These are an interesting basis for hypotheses deserving scientific testing, but no substitute for empirical evidence from controlled clinical trials.

Given that autism is a neurodevelopmental disorder, whose aetiology is not yet fully understood, it is not surprising that currently there is no definitive cure for this condition (Cohen & Volkmar, 1997). Pharmacological interventions which reduce the frequency and intensity of some symptoms have been developed and evaluated (Lord & Rutter, 1994). With respect to non-pharmacological interventions, there are a number of secondary prevention programmes for autism-related adjustment difficulties which have been scientifically investigated. Two broad approaches to intervention have been taken (Rogers, 1998). On the one hand, highly specific individually tailored intervention programmes have been developed for dealing with particular adjustment problems such as challenging behaviour, sleep difficulties or lack of social skills. The impact of these programmes has been evaluated using applied behavioural analysis, controlled single case design methodologies. On the other hand, broad-based comprehensive secondary prevention programmes have been developed which aim to improve overall cognitive, linguistic and social functioning. These have been evaluated using controlled group-based treatment outcome studies. In this chapter, the focus is on these group-based treatment outcome studies which evaluated comprehensive programmes. Examples of individually tailored programmes for specific challenging behaviours, developed within an applied behavioural analysis framework, are described in Chapter 7. The programmes described in Chapter 7 were developed for children with intellectual disabilities and in some cases the children also had autism.

Previous reviews of the impact of comprehensive secondary prevention programmes for children with autism have highlighted the effectiveness of Lovas's (1987) behavioural intervention programme; Schopler's (Ozonoff & Cathcart, 1998) TEACCH programme; and intensive speech- and language-focused programmes (Dawson & Osterling, 1997; Green, 1996; Howlin, 1997, 1998; Rogers, 1998).

Method

The aim in this chapter was to review well-designed studies in which early intervention programmes for preventing adjustment problems in children with autism were evaluated. A computer-based literature search of the PsychLit database was conducted in which the term *autism* was combined with relevant secondary terms such as *early intervention*, *prevention* and *treatment*. The search was confined to English language journals and books covering the period 1977–2000. This computer-based search was complemented by a manual search of the bibliographies of recent review papers of psychological interventions for autism. Since the review was concerned primarily with the *prevention* of adjustment problems, only early intervention studies in which the programme began before children were five years of age were considered for inclusion. Studies of exclusively pharmacological interventions were not considered, since our concern was primarily with psychological prevention programmes. With respect to methodological criteria, studies were selected for inclusion in this review if all participants had a diagnosis of autism; if the study included an intervention and control group; and if both pre- and post-intervention assessments were conducted. Eight studies met these criteria.

Characteristics of the studies

The characteristics of the eight studies reviewed are outlined in Table 6.2. The eight studies included four which evaluated behavioural intervention programmes (Lovaas, 1987; McEachin et al., 1993; Birnbrauer & Leach, 1993; Sheinkopf & Siegel, 1998; Fenske et al., 1985), one study of Schopler's TEACCH programme for autistic children (Ozonoff & Cathcart, 1998), and three studies that focused on speech and language training (Harris et al., 1983, 1990; Bloch et al., 1980). Seven of the studies were conducted in the United States and one in Australia. All were published in peer-reviewed journals within the last 20 years. In all eight studies, secondary prevention programmes were evaluated (rather than primary or tertiary preventative interventions). Programmes ranged in duration from five months to six years. Six of the studies involved home-based intervention either alone or in conjunction with preschool or community-based intervention. In two of the speech and language programme studies, intervention was conducted in the school only. A total of 180 children participated in these studies and of these 82 were in intervention groups and 98 were in control groups. The mean age across the eight studies was 44 months and the age range was 23 months to 101 months. The gender balance in the six studies for which such data were available was 81% male and 19% female. For those studies in which information of family circumstances was provided, participants came from two-parent middle-class families.

Methodological features

The methodological features of the eight studies reviewed are outlined in Table 6.3. All eight studies were outcome studies in which a control or comparison group was used. A multiple baseline design across groups was used in one study. Random assignment of participants to groups did not occur in any of the studies, although in all studies groups were sufficiently similar at the outset of the studies for us to have confidence that post-intervention differences were not due to major pre-intervention inter-group differences (Baer, 1993; Gresham & MacMillan, 1998). Diagnostic homogeneity was established in all eight studies, with all cases having a diagnosis of autism. Demographic similarity of intervention and control group was established in five of the eight studies. Pre- and post-treatment assessments were carried out in all eight studies, but only one study provided long-term follow-up data by assessing subjects more than three months after treatment had finished. In six studies assessments were made from more than one perspective. In seven studies assessments were based on researcher ratings; in five studies they were based on parent ratings; in five they were based on intervention staff ratings; and in two studies they were based on teacher ratings. Drop-out was assessed in all eight studies and deterioration in two studies. The clinical significance of change was assessed in three studies. In half of the studies experienced

Table 6.2 Characteristics of secondary prevention studies of autism

Study no.	Study type	Authors	Year	N per group	Mean age and range	Gender	Family characteristics	Programme setting	Programme duration
1	BIP	Lovaas McEachin et al.	1987 1993	1. BIP = 19 2. C1 = 19 3. C2 = 21	35 m 24–46 m	NS	Mixed SES	Home + school + community	2– 6 y
2	BIP	Birnbrauer & Leach	1993	1. BIP = 9 2. C = 5	36 m 24–48 m	M 71% F 29%	majority 2-parent families	Home	24 m
3	BIP	Sheinkopf & Siegel	1998	1. BIP = 11 2. C = 11	35 m 23–47 m	NS	NS	Home	16 m
4	BIP	Fenske et al.	1985	1. BIP = 9 2. C = 9	75 m 42–156 m	M 89% F 11%	NS	Home + school	1 = 45.9 m 2 = 72.4 m
5	TEACCH	Ozonoff & Cathcart	1998	1. TEACCH = 11 2. C = 11	53 m 31–69 m	M 82% F 18%	All 2-parent families 95% Caucasian American	Home	4 m
6	SLP	Harris et al.	1983	1. SLP = 4 2. C = 5	43 m 27–56 m	M 90% F 10%	All middle class 2-parent families	Home	13 m
7	SLP	Harris et al.	1990	1. SLP = 5 2. C = 5	53 m 40–66 m	M 80% F 20%	NS	School	5–11 m
8	SLP	Bloch et al.	1980	1. SLP = 14 2. C = 12	50 m 35–74 m	M 77% F 23%	NS	School	15 – 24 m

Notes

BIP = behavioural intervention programme. TEACCH = Schopler's TEACCH programme for autistic children (TEACCH stands for Treatment and Education of Autistic and related Communication handicapped Children). SLP = speech and language programme. C = control group. SES = socioeconomic status. NS = not specified. m = months. y = years.

Table 6.3 Methodological features of secondary prevention studies of autism

Feature	Study number							
	S1	*S2*	*S3*	*S4*	*S5*	*S6*	*S7*	*S8*
Control or comparison group	1	1	1	1	1	1	1	1
Random assignment	0	0	0	0	0	0	0	0
Diagnostic homogeneity	1	1	1	1	1	1	1	1
Demographic similarity	0	0	1	0	1	1	1	1
Pre-treatment assessment	1	1	1	1	1	1	1	1
Post-treatment assessment	1	1	1	1	1	1	1	1
3-month follow-up assessment	1	0	0	0	0	0	0	0
Children's self report	0	0	0	0	0	0	0	0
Parents' ratings	1	1	1	1	0	0	0	1
Teachers' ratings	0	0	0	1	0	0	0	1
Therapists' or trainers' ratings	0	1	0	0	0	1	1	1
Researcher ratings	1	1	1	1	1	1	1	0
Deterioration assessed	1	0	0	0	0	0	1	0
Drop-out assessed	1	1	1	1	1	1	1	1
Clinical significance of change assessed	1	0	0	1	0	0	0	1
Experienced therapists or trainers used	0	0	0	1	0	1	1	1
Programmes were equally valued	0	0	0	0	0	0	1	1
Programmes were manualized	1	1	1	0	1	0	0	0
Supervision was provided	0	1	1	0	1	1	0	0
Programme integrity checked	0	0	0	0	1	1	0	0
Data on concurrent treatment given	1	0	1	0	1	0	0	0
Data on subsequent treatment given	0	0	0	0	0	0	0	0
Total	12	10	11	10	10	11	11	12

Note
S = study. 1 = design feature was present. 0 = design feature was absent.

therapists or trainers conducted the prevention programme while the other half depended on graduate students or volunteers. Only two studies compared two different treatment programmes and in both of these studies the prevention programmes compared were equally valued by the research team. In four of the studies the treatment was manualized or offered according to an explicitly stated treatment protocol. Supervision was provided in four studies and programme integrity was checked in two. In three studies data on concurrent treatment were reported and data on subsequent treatment were not provided for any of the studies. The statistical significance of treatment gains was reported in seven of the eight studies but only two studies presented data on the clinical significance of treatment effects in terms of the number of cases judged to be clinically improved following treatment. Out of a total of twenty-two design features summarized in Table 6.3, the mean number present in these eight studies was eleven. Overall from a methodological perspective it may be concluded that the studies reviewed here are sufficiently well designed to allow relatively reliable conclusions to be drawn from them about the types of psychological interventions they evaluated.

Substantive findings

Of the eight well-controlled studies identified for this review, four evaluated the effects of intensive behavioural intervention programmes (Lovaas, 1987; McEachin et al., 1993; Birnbrauer & Leach, 1993; Sheinkopf & Siegel, 1993; Fenske et al., 1985); one evaluated the TEACCH programme (Ozonoff & Cathcart, 1998) and three evaluated the impact of speech and language training (Harris et al., 1983, 1990; Bloch et al., 1980). Effect sizes and outcome results for the eight studies are outlined in Table 6.4 and a narrative account of the main conclusions is given in Table 6.5. It is noteworthy that there is considerable overlap between the group of well-controlled studies identified

Table 6.4 Summary of results of secondary prevention studies of autism

Variable	Behavioural intervention				TEACCH	Speech and language		
	Study 1	Study 2	Study 3	Study 4	Study 5	Study 6	Study 7	Study 8
	BIP v C	BIP v C	BIP v C	BIP v C	TEACCH v C	SLP v BPT	SLP-I v SLP-S	SLP v C
Improvement after programme								
IQ	1.1	1.1	1.6	—	—	—	—	—
Overall developmental change	—	—	—	—	0.4	—	—	—
Language	—	0.1	—	—	0.3	—	0.0	0.7
Adaptive behaviour	—	0.7	—	—	—	—	—	—
Symptom severity	—	—	0.8	—	—	—	—	—
Educational placement	0.5	—	—	1.5	—	—	—	—
Improvement at follow-up								
IQ	1.1	—	—	—	—	—	—	—
Maladaptive behaviour	0.8	—	—	—	—	—	—	—
Educational placement	0.6	—	—	—	—	—	—	—
Positive clinical outcomes								
% improved after treatment	47% v 2%	44% v 20%	—	67%	—	—	—	67%
% improved at follow-up	47%	—	—	—	—	—	—	58% v 14%
Negative clinical outcomes								
% Deterioration	5%	—	—	—	—	—	—	7%
% Drop-out	0%	21%	18%	0%	0%	18%	0%	0%

Notes

BIP = behavioural intervention programme. TEACCH = Schopler's TEACCH programme for autistic children. (TEACCH stands for Treatment and Education of Autistic and related Communication handicapped Children). SLP = speech and language programme. SLP-I = Speech and language programme conducted in an integrated class. SLP-S = speech and language programme conducted in a segregated class. BPT = behavioural parent training. C = control group.

Table 6.5 Summary of key findings of secondary prevention studies of autism

Study no.	Study type	Authors	Year	N per group	No. of sessions	Group differences	Key findings
1	BIP	Lovaas McEachin et al.	1987 1993	1. BIP = 19 2. C1 = 19 3. C2 = 21	1 = 40 hpw × 2 – 6 y 2 = 10 hpw × 2 – 6 y 3 = 0	1 > 2 = 3	• The group treated with the behavioural intervention programme had higher IQs and better adjustment within educational placements than controls or cases who received minimal treatment. • 47% of the treated group achieved normal intellectual and educational functioning compared with 2% of the control group. • After treatment the group treated with the behavioural intervention programme had gained an average of 30 IQ points and this was maintained at age 13 y. • The experimental group also showed more adaptive behaviours and fewer maladaptive behaviours than did the control group.
2	BIP	Birnbrauer & Leach	1993	1. BIP = 9 2. C = 5	18.72 hpw × 24 m	1 > 2	• 44% of cases treated with the behaviour intervention programme showed signs of approaching normal levels of functioning on measures of language, IQ and adaptive behaviour, compared with 20% of controls. • Improvements in the remainder of the children were moderate to minimal.
3	BIP	Sheinkopf & Siegel	1998	1. BIP = 11 2. C = 11	27hpw × 16 m	1 > 2	• After treatment the group treated with the behavioural intervention programme had gained an average of 25 IQ points compared with a matched control group who received standard school-based interventions. • The group that received the behavioural intervention programme showed a reduction in symptom severity although there was no notable difference in number of symptoms or diagnostic classification. Cases in both groups still met the criteria for autism or PDD.
4	BIP	Fenske et al.	1985	1. BIP = 9 2. C = 9	27.5 hpw × 11 m	1 > 2	• For the younger children in the study, 67% of cases treated with a behavioural intervention programme continued residence with parents and attendance at public school classes compared with 11% of the older group. • Age at programme entry was found to be strongly related to positive treatment outcome with younger cases showing a better treatment response.
5	TEACCH	Ozonoff & Cathcart	1998	1. TEACCH = 11 2. C = 11	1 hpw × 10 w	1 > 2	• Children who participated in the TEACCH programme showed greater improvement than control group on measures of imitation, fine motor, gross motor, and non-verbal conceptual skills. • Progress in the TEACCH group was three to four times greater than in the control group on all outcome tests.

6	SLP	Harris et al.	1983	1. SLP = 4 2. BPT = 5	1 hpw × 13 w	1 > 2	• Parental speech-therapy training led to greater improvements than behavioural parent training. • A substantial rise in parental speech-oriented language was noted after parental speech therapy training. • A substantial rise in child speech was obvious when their parents completed the speech therapy training. • The verbal children accounted for the changes in the two groups since the mute children made no improvements in language usage.
7	SLP	Harris et al.	1990	1. SLP-I = 5 2. SLP-S = 5	Daily preschool × 5–11 m	1 = 2	• Children treated with a speech and language programme made better than normative progress in rate of language development. • There were no significant differences in changes in language ability between the autistic children in the segregated and integrated classes.
8	SLP	Bloch et al.	1980	1. SLP = 14 2. C = 12	2 × .5 hpw × 15 – 24m	1 > 2	• At the end of the second year 58% of cases in the intensive experimental speech and language programme achieved criterion on all seven language ability measures compared with 14% of the control group.

Note

BIP = behavioural intervention programme. TEACCH = Scholper's TEACCH programme for autistic children. (TEACCH stands for Treatment and Education of Autistic and related Communication handicapped Children). SLP = speech and language programme. SLP-I = speech and language programme conducted in an integrated class. SLP-S = speech and language programme conducted in a segregated class. BPT = behavioural parent training. C = control group. hpw = hours per week. w = weeks. y = year. m = months.

in this review and those identified by other reviewers (Dawson & Osterling, 1997; Green, 1996; Howlin, 1997, 1998; Rogers, 1998).

Behavioural intervention programmes

Four studies evaluated the effects of intensive behavioural intervention programmes (Lovaas, 1987; McEachin et al., 1993; Birnbrauer & Leach, 1993; Sheinkopf & Siegel, 1993; Fenske et al., 1985). Three of the four were based on the Young Autism Programme developed by Lovaas and his colleagues which is outlined in a treatment manual (Lovaas et al., 1980) and instructional videotapes (Lovaas & Leaf, 1981). Within this model an attempt is made to maximize behavioural treatment gains by treating autistic children for most of their waking hours over many years with procedures based on the principles of operant conditioning. All significant persons in the child's social system and a roster of operant therapists are recruited to assist with the delivery of the treatment programme. The central aim of the programme is to construct an intense, comprehensive learning environment for very young autistic children based on operant conditioning principles, to help them catch up with normal peers by the time they start school.

The programme begins with a broad developmental analysis of skills and deficits and a fine-grained behavioural analysis of skill use or lack thereof in particular situations. In light of this behavioural analysis, a set of highly specific treatment goals are established and behavioural methods for achieving these specified. Parents and school staff or other involved front-line professionals such as nurses or child care workers are trained to implement these programmes.

Children with autism may have a variety of difficulties in learning self-care and academic skills (Bregman & Gerdtz, 1997). In all instances the curriculum materials are matched to the child's developmental stage. Where low IQ or limited language usage prevents or impairs the child's understanding, simplified verbal or pictorial communication methods are used. Large tasks are broken down into smaller more manageable tasks that make success more likely. Where children show lack of initiative, they are encouraged to choose the learning materials in which they are most interested, and the tasks are structured so as to maximize success. So, if the child is learning a new skill, trials of learning the new unfamiliar skill are interspersed with trials of executing related skills that have already been mastered. Where children show resistance to learning a new skill, reinforcement should be arranged so that it is delivered intermittently, on a variable interval or ratio schedule. However, when it is delivered, the child receives it immediately and naturally occurring reinforcers rather than contrived reinforcers (such as sweets or candy) are used. Generalization of skills learned in one context to multiple contexts is a major problem in the education of children with autism. In this programme children are encouraged and prompted to exercise newly learned skills in many different environments and reinforced for doing so since this maximizes the chances of generalization occurring.

In the first of the four studies of behavioural programmes (Lovaas, 1987; McEachin et al., 1993) each youngster in the intervention group was assigned several well-trained student therapists who worked with the subject in the subject's home, school and community for an average of 40 hours per week for two or more years. Parents worked as part of the treatment team throughout the intervention and were extensively trained so that treatment could continue 365 days a year. Whenever possible the children were integrated into regular preschools. The intervention programme focused primarily on developing language, increasing social behaviour, and promoting cooperative play with peers together with independent and appropriate toy play. All cases in the intervention group received two or more years of intensive intervention. Those who went on to a normal first grade had their treatment reduced from 40 hours per week to ten hours or less per week during kindergarten. After a participant had started first grade, the project maintained a minimal contact with some families. Participants who did not recover received 40 hours or more per week of one-to-one treatment for more than six years (more than 14,000 hours of one-to-one treatment). At age six after two to four years of intervention the effect size for IQ (based on comparison with a control group that received a minimal intervention of about ten hours of intervention per week) was 1.1, indicating that the average case that received intensive intervention fared better than 86% of cases in the minimal intervention control group. The effect size for placement status was 0.5, indicating that the average case that received intensive intervention fared better than 69% of cases in the minimal intervention control group in terms of being placed in a mainstream school class with classroom support.

When cases in this study were an average of thirteen years old, McEachin et al. (1993) found that gains in IQ and placement status were maintained. Effect sizes computed using data from the intensive intervention group compared with the minimal intervention control group were 1.1 for IQ and 0.6 for placement status. This indicates that the average participant who received intensive intervention fared better on IQ than 86% of the minimal intervention control group and better than 73% of the control group on placement status. McEachin et al. (1993) also found that eight of the nineteen cases (42%) in the intensive intervention group were indistinguishable from normal children on tests of intelligence and adaptive behaviour at thirteen years of age.

In the second behavioural intervention study Birnbrauer and Leach (1993) attempted to partially replicate and extend the findings of Lovaas (1987) using an approach based on Lovaas's model but departing from the programme in several key respects. Aversive physical consequences for aggressive and self-injurious behaviour were not used. Volunteers, half of whom were recruited by the parents, implemented programmes rather than graduate student therapists. Also, Birnbrauer and Leach's programme was about half as intense as the Lovaas programme (an average of 18.72 hours per week as compared to 40 hours). The control group in this study received no specialist intervention whatsoever. Individual programmes were drawn up for each child with each child allocated a treatment team which consisted of one of the researchers, a programme co-ordinator, the parents and up to 24 volunteers each of whom committed themselves to a minimum of 2.5 hour sessions per week in the child's home for a minimum of four months. After two years of intervention, as with the Lovaas et al. (1987) study, the effect size for IQ was 1.1, indicating that the average participant who received intensive intervention fared better on IQ than 86% of the control group. An effect size of 0.7 was obtained for adaptive behaviour, indicating that following two years of intensive intervention, the average participant was functioning better than 76% of control group cases. After two years of intervention, four out of nine participants (44%) were rated as highly improved across the domains of IQ, language development and adaptive behaviour compared to one child out of five (20%) in the control group. Involvement in the programme was also associated with reduced stress levels among mothers.

In the third behavioural study, Sheinkopf and Siegel (1998) reviewed the records from a database of a larger longitudinal study of eleven autistic youngsters who had received an intensive behavioural intervention programme and eleven age- and IQ-matched autistic controls who had received routine educational services. Those who participated in behavioural programmes received an average of 27 hours intervention per week over 20 months, based on Lovaas's (1987) protocol. For IQ, an effect size of 1.6 was obtained, indicating that after about two years of intervention, the average treated case was functioning better than 95% of untreated controls. An effect size of 0.4 was obtained for percentage of positive symptoms present, indicating that following treatment the average treated case was functioning better than 66% of untreated controls. An effect size of 0.8 was obtained for symptom severity, indicating that following treatment the average treated case was functioning better than 76% of untreated controls. However, both treated cases and controls all met the diagnostic criteria for autism at the conclusion of the study.

To assess the relationship between age at programme entry and treatment outcome, Fenske et al. (1985) compared the treatment outcomes of nine autistic children who began receiving intensive behavioural intervention prior to five years of age with outcomes for nine other children who entered the same intervention programme after their fifth birthday. All eighteen children involved in the study were diagnosed as autistic and enrolled in the Princeton Child Development Institute's day school and treatment programme during the period 1975–1983. An applied behaviour analysis approach to intervention was used. Participants received 27.5 hours of intervention per week, 11 months of the year. Parents were trained to become home tutors and therapists for their children. Children were provided with individualized transition programmes when observational data indicated significant developments and generalization of language skills, social skills, and behavioural self-control. Discharge occurred when children's performance data indicated that they had generalized their new skills and their control of behaviour problems to a mainstream school setting. Children who entered the intervention pro-gramme before five years received an average of four years of intervention whereas those who entered the programme after five years received six years of intervention. Of the nine younger children six (67%) were discharged compared with one older child (11%).

Conclusions for behavioural intervention programmes

From these four behavioural studies it can be concluded that intensive behavioural early intervention programmes can improve non-verbal IQ scores, educational adjustment and social adjustment. Intensive behavioural programmes can prevent educational exclusion and behavioural adjustment problems. Greatest gains are made on IQ and educational placement. Smallest gains are made in language. Moderate gains are made in adaptive behaviour and symptom severity. Greatest gains are made by cases who enter prevention programmes early (before five years). Greatest gains are made by youngsters who received 20–40 hours of intervention per week for at least two years, although children who do not improve after such intensive intervention may improve after a period of further intensive intervention. In the short term, children who receive 20 hours of intervention per week, fare as well as those who receive 40 hours per week. However, we do not know if less intensive programmes (of 20 hours per week) have as positive long-term outcomes as more intensive programmes (of 40 hours per week). In the single study where long-term follow-up data were collected, it was found that gains of up to 30 IQ points shown by children who received 40 hours of intervention per week over a period of 2–4 preschool years were maintained right into adolescence. About four out of ten children who received intensive early behavioural inter-vention (40 hours per week) may no longer meet the diagnostic criteria for autism in adolescence. Children who received behavioural intervention programmes of only 10 hours fared no better than untreated controls.

Structured teaching: Schopler's TEACCH programme

One of the eight studies in this review evaluated the TEACCH programme (Ozonoff & Cathcart, 1998). TEACCH is an acronym for Treatment and Education of Autistic and related Communication Handicapped Children. Schopler, and the group that developed the TEACCH system, place struc-tured learning at the heart of their very comprehensive approach to autism (Schopler, 1997). The TEACCH approach aims to make the world intelligible to the autistic child by acknowledging deficits (such as communication prob-lems and difficulties in social cognition) and structuring learning activities so that they capitalize upon the strengths of children with autism. Children with autism have excellent visual processing abilities and good rote memory abilities; and many have unique special interests. Thus, learning activities should be structured so that the child can visualize what is expected to achieve success. Activities should depend upon visual memory for sequences of tasks. And the content of the tasks should capitalize upon any special interests that the child has shown. So, for example, photographs of stages of task completion should be used rather than extensive verbal instructions, where language development is delayed. If the child is interested in toy cars, then these may be used to teach counting or language.

Schopler's group use a system where two clinicians work with each case: one is designated the child therapist and the other is the parent consultant (Schopler, 1997). At each clinical contact, the child therapist works directly with the child developing a written programme of home teaching activities for the parent to carry out each week. Concurrently the parent consultant works with the parent reviewing and planning future child management strategies for developing productive routines and managing challenging behaviour. Parents are invited to observe the programmes developed by the child therapist and practise these with the child at home for about 20 minutes per day. Typical programmes involve four or five activities, selected to match the child's profile of strengths and weaknesses. Schopler and his group have catalogued the types of activities that may be included in such programmes in two volumes (Schopler et al., 1979, 1980). Parents are advised to develop highly structured work routines with their children. The same time and place for work should be used each day and the environment should be free of distractions. Materials for tasks to be completed should be placed on the left and when the work is finished, the materials should be stored in a tray on the right marked *finished*. Parents are shown how to model all activities for their children and then to instruct them and give feedback in simple language. This highly structured approach capitalizes upon the affinity that children with autism have for sameness and their resistance to changes of routine.

Ozonoff and Cathcart (1998) evaluated the effectiveness of the TEACCH intervention programme in a single outcome study. The improvement shown on the Psycho Educational Profile-Revised (PEP-R, Schopler et al., 1990) by a group of eleven autistic children who received a four-month trial of the TEACCH programme was compared with that of a matched control group. Participants and controls were aged two to six years, came from two-parent families, and were simultaneously receiving services from local day treatment programmes. The groups were matched on age, severity of autism, and initial PEP-R score. The PEP-R, an instrument designed for evaluating autistic children, measures functioning in the following domains: imitation, perception, fine and gross motor skills, eye–hand coordination, and non-verbal and verbal conceptual ability. The programme was delivered by trained psychology graduate students and parents collaborated with therapists in implementing home-based aspects of the treatment programme. Post-intervention assessments were carried out four months after participants began the treatment programme

In chronological terms, over a four-month time-span, youngsters who participated in the TEACCH programme made an average overall developmental gain of 9.6 months. An effect size, based on overall PEP-R scores, of 0.4 was obtained, indicating that after the intervention programme, the average treated case was functioning better than 66% of untreated controls across the seven domains assessed by the PEP-R. There was some variability in improvement across the domains assessed by the PEP-R. An effect size of 0.6 was obtained for the cognitive performance subtest, indicating that following treatment the average treated case was functioning better than 73% of the control group in this domain. An effect size of 0.5 was obtained for the fine motor skills subtest, indicating that, in this domain, following treatment the average treated case was functioning better than 69% of the control group. An effect size of 0.4 was obtained in the imitation, perception and gross motor skills domains, indicating that following treatment the average treated case was functioning better than 66% of the control group in these areas. Finally an effect size of 0.3 was obtained for the cognitive verbal subtest, indicating that following treatment the average treated case was functioning better than 62% of the control group. Greatest improvements were made by children who had milder autistic symptoms and better language skills.

Conclusion concerning effectiveness of the TEACCH programme

This study shows that children in routine day-care placements who participate in the TEACCH programme can make significant developmental improvement over periods as short as four months. Greatest gains are made in the non-verbal cognitive domain and greatest gains are made by children with milder autism symptoms and better language skills.

Speech and language programmes

Three studies evaluated the impact of speech and language training on communicative skills of children with autism (Harris et al., 1983, 1990; Bloch et al., 1980). These studies are of particular significance because of the centrality of language deficits to children with autism. Only half of all children with autism fail to develop functional speech (Lord & Rutter, 1994). Even amongst those with good expressive vocabulary there are persisting impairments in the communicative use of language and in understanding complex or abstract concepts (Howlin, 1998).

Harris et al. (1983) investigated the impact of training parents in speech therapy techniques to enhance their autistic children's speech on parent–child communication and children's language usage. The programme included modules on the principles of speech therapy with non-verbal children, eye contact and sitting, non-verbal imitation, shaping sounds, teaching nouns, teaching adjectives and verbs, and generalization of language behaviour. The programme is based on Harris's (1976) text *Teaching Speech to the Non-verbal Child*. In this multiple baseline across-groups study, nine autistic preschool children referred by outside agencies were divided into two groups. Each group completed a no-treatment baseline period followed by a behavioural parent training programme, and finally a parental speech therapy training programme. The rate at which these three elements were completed was staggered, so that in the section of the design of particular interest here, the parents of the first group participated in a seven-session speech therapy training programme while the parents of the second group completed a six-session behavioural parent training programme. Both programmes were conducted across a two-month period by experienced clinicians and in each programme a series of fortnightly home-visits were conducted by co-therapists to aid generalization of skills parents were taught in the clinic-based sessions. Ratings of videotapes of parent–child interaction showed that parental speech-oriented language increased after parents received speech therapy training but not after behavioural parent training. Both before and after speech therapy training, the parents of more verbal children emitted more speech-oriented language than the parents of mute children. There was no significant change in child speech after behavioural parent training but there was an increase after their parents had completed the speech therapy training programme. The changes in the two groups were accounted for by the verbal children, with the mute children showing little evidence of change.

In a subsequent study, Harris et al. (1990) evaluated the impact of an intensive speech and language therapy programme provided within the context of integrated and segregated classroom settings over a period of five to eleven months. The curriculum for both classes was developmentally organized and language-focused. Children in both classes were set individual speech and language goals and were exposed to formal, structured group language instruction in the classroom including a weekly group led by the speech and language specialist. The five children in the segregated class were provided with more individualized instruction, worked in smaller groups and had a higher adult to child ratio. The five children in the integrated class were taught with four normally developing peers. The autistic children participating in the study were relatively high functioning and the groups were matched for chronological age, IQ and language development but those in the segregated class had more behavioural problems. Participants in both groups made significant progress, but intergroup differences in improvements in language development were not statistically significant. On the Preschool Language Scale (Zimmerman et al., 1979) scores of the segregated class improved from 38 to 47 and those for the integrated class improved from 40 to 53 over the course of the programme.

Bloch et al. (1980) carried out a retrospective study comparing the effects of language remediation on 12 preschool autistic with the impact of a routine school curriculum on 14 matched controls. Children in the language remediation programme received twice-weekly half-hour sessions with a speech and language pathologist to supplement their routine school placement. Data on communicative speech recorded two years after the start of the programme yielded an effect size of 0.7, which indicated that the average youngster who received language remediation was functioning better than 76% of controls. At the end of the second year of the programme 58% of children treated with language remediation showed clinically significant improvement in eye contact and relatedness, auditory comprehension, non-verbal imitation, vocal play, vocal imitation, expressive speech, and communicative speech. Only 14% of children in the control group showed such gains.

Conclusions concerning speech and language programmes

The three studies reviewed in this section indicate that autistic children can benefit from speech and language training and show clinically significant improvement in language, speech and communication. Relatively brief interventions can be effective. In the three studies reviewed here, the duration of the programmes ranged from two months to two years. Direct and indirect training were both effective. That is, programmes in which speech therapy is offered directly and involves one-to-one contact between professional speech and language therapists and children are effective and so are programmes in which parents are trained to implement speech therapy programmes at home with their children. These parent speech therapy training programmes have the additional benefit of improving the quality of parent–child speech-based communication. Training parents to teach their children speech and language skills is more effective than training them in the general principles of behaviour modification for improving their children's communicative skills. Both integrated and segregated preschool-based speech and language programmes are equally effective. Greatest gains in speech and language programmes are made by children with some verbal skills at the start of the programme.

Conclusions

From this review it may concluded that Lovaas's behavioural intervention programme, Schopler's TEACCH programme, and speech- and language-focused programmes all hold promise as secondary preventative interventions for children with autism. The review also suggests seven further conclusions about effective programmes in this domain which deserve highlighting, particularly because they are consistent with the views of previous reviewers of this literature (Dawson & Osterling, 1997; Green, 1996; Howlin, 1997, 1998; Rogers, 1998). First, psychological interventions can have marked impact on the cognitive, behavioural and social adjustment of children with autism in the short and long term. Second, effective interventions are intensive (20–40 hours per week) and protracted (six months to two years in duration). Third, effective intervention programmes occur across multiple contexts including the home and the school or preschool setting, with highly collaborative working relationships between parents, teachers and clinical staff. Fourth, effective interventions have a high adult to child ratio varying from 1:1 to 1:3. Fifth, effective interventions are highly structured and based on theoretically derived procedural treatment manuals. Sixth, effective intervention programmes are sufficiently flexible to address the unique profile of needs of each child. Seventh, effective programmes are designed to enhance skills in five key areas: (1) attending to aspects of the environment essential for learning; (2) imitation; (3) language usage; (4) imaginative play; and (5) social interaction.

Implications for policy and practice

The implications of this review for policy and practice are clear. In order to prevent adjustment problems in children with autism, screening and assessment systems which allow for the early detection of autism are vital. A list of assessment instruments is included at the end of the chapter. Once identified, youngsters with autism require intensive intervention on a 1:1–3 basis for 20–40 hours per week over an extended period. Assessment programmes should be highly structured and modelled on Lovaas's behavioural approach, Schopler's TEACCH approach, and speech and language programmes that have been shown to be effective for children with autism. In addition, psycho-educational and relief-care support services for parents may be required, although research on this issue is lacking.

A central issue in the treatment of youngsters with autism is whether they should be placed in special schools exclusively for children with autism or whether they should be placed in mainstream schools attended by children without disabilities and provided with additional support (Harris & Handleman, 1997). Only very limited data are available on this issue in the area of language development and this shows that both approaches are effective. Because of the limited available data, policy and practice decisions on this issue are influenced by ethical and pragmatic considerations. Ethically, there is widespread agreement that children with disabilities such as autism should be provided with every opportunity to live as normal a life as possible, and for this reason autistic children should be educated in mainstream schools with additional support provided. However, pragmatically, it is often difficult to arrange for sufficient support within mainstream schools to be provided to allow a child with autism to received an adequate education within that context. It is often easier to centralize the special educational resources required for children with autism. Of course, national policy, the views of autism advocacy groups, and the way in which funding from statutory and voluntary sources is allocated all determine the availability of mainstream or centralized special educational placements.

Implications for future research

Well-designed programme evaluation studies which meet the method-ological criteria set out in Table 6.3 are required in this area. These multisite studies should include large numbers of cases ($N = 100$) in intervention and control groups and extensive follow-up periods of 5–10 years. The behavioural, structured learning and speech and language programmes described in this chapter need to be rigorously evaluated within the context of such studies.

Assessment resources

Gilliam, J. (1991). *Gilliam Autism Rating Scale*. Odessa, FL: Psychological Assessment Resources. (PAR, PO Box 998, Odessa Florida, 33556.)

Krug, D., Arick, J., Almond, P. (1980). Behaviour checklist for identifying severely handicapped children with high levels of autistic behaviour. *Journal of Child Psychology and Psychiatry*, 21, 221–229.

Krug, D., Arick, J. & Almond, P. (1996). *Autism Screening Instrument For Educational Planning*. Second Edition. Odessa, FL: Psychological Assessment Resources. (PAR, PO Box 998, Odessa Florida, 33556.)

Lord, C., Rutter, M. & Le Couteur, A. (1994). Autism Diagnostic Interview – Revised. *Journal of Autism and Developmental Disorders*, 24, 659–685.

Lord, C., Rutter, M., Goode, S., Heemsbergen, J., Jordan, H. & Mawhood, L. (1989). Autism diagnostic observation schedule: A standardized observation of communicative and social behaviour. *Journal of Autism and Developmental Disorders*, 19, 185–212. (Training is required for ADOS & ADI-R. Contact Catherine Lord, Child and Adolescent Psychiatry, University of Chicago, 5841 S. Marylan Avenue, Chicago, Illinois 60637.)

Mesibov, G., Schopler, E. & Caison, W. (1989). *Adolescent and Adult Psycho-Educational Profile (AAPEP)*. Austin, TX: Pro-ed.

Schopler, E. Richler, R. & Renner, B. (1986). *The Childhood Autism Rating Scale (CARS) for Diagnostic Screening and Classification of Autism*. New York: Irvington. (Order CARS from Western Psychological Services 12031 Wilshire Boulevard, Los Angeles, California 90025–1251. Tel 1–800–648–8857. Order a CARS training video from Health Sciences Consortium 201 Silver Cedar Court, Chapel Hill, NC, 27514–1517. Tel 919–942–8731.)

Schopler, E., Reichler, R., Bashford, A., Lansing, M. & Marcus, L. (1990). *Psychoeducational Profile Revised (PEP-R)*. Austin, TX: Pro-ed. (Order from PRO-ED, 8700 Shoal Creek Blvd, Austin TX 78758. Tel 512–451–3246.)

Wing, L. (2000). *DISCO: The Diagnostic Interview Schedule for Social and Communication Disorders*. UK: National Autistic Society. (Available from The Centre for Social and Communication Disorders, Elliott House. 113 Masons Hill, Bromley, Kent BR2 9HT. Tel +44–20–8466–0098. Email: elliot.house@nas.org.uk.)

Programme resources

Cohen, D. & Volkmar, F. (1997). *Handbook of Autism and Pervasive Developmental Disorders* (Second Edition). New York: Wiley.

Harris, S. (1976). *Teaching Speech to a Non-verbal Child*. Lawrence, KS: H & H Enterprises.

Howlin, P. & Rutter, M. (1987). *Treatment of Autistic Children*. New York: Wiley.

Lovaas, O.I., Ackerman, A.B., Alexander, D., Firestone, P., Perkins, J., & Young, D. (1980). *Teaching Developmentally Disabled Children: The Me Book*. Austin, TX: Pro-Ed.

Lovaas, O.I. & Leaf, R.I. (1981). Five video tapes for teaching developmentally disabled children. Baltimore: University Park Press.

Maurice, C. (Ed.) *Behavioral Intervention for Young Children with Autism. A Manual for Parents and Professionals*. Austin, TX: Pro-Ed.

Rumsey, J. & Vitiello, B. (2000). Treatments for people with autism and other pervasive developmental disorders. Special issue of *Journal of Autism and Developmental Disorders*, Volume 30, Whole of Number 5, 369–508.

Schopler, E. (1980). Demonstration tape on using the Childhood Autism Rating Scale (CARS). TEACCH (*T*reatment and *E*ducation of *A*utistic and related *C*ommunication handicapped *CH*ildren) Videotapes. Health Sciences Consortium Distribution Department, 201 Silver Cedar Court, Chapel Hill, NC, 27514–1517.

Schopler, E. (1980) Video of TEACCH Programme for Parents. Chapel Hill, NC: Health Sciences Consortium Distribution Department.

Schopler, E. (1980). Demonstration videotape on scoring the Psychoeducational Profile (PEP). Chapel Hill, NC: Health Sciences Consortium Distribution Department.

Schopler, E. (1980). Video of TEACCH Programme for Teachers. Chapel Hill, NC: Health Sciences Consortium Distribution Department.

Schopler, E. (1980). Videotape of an individualised education programme. Conversion of a psychoeducational profile (PEP) into an individualised teaching programmes. Chapel Hill, NC: Health Sciences Consortium Distribution Department.

Schopler, E., Lansing, M. & Reichler, R. (1979). *Individualised Assessment And Treatment For Autistic And Developmentally Disabled Children. Teaching Strategies for Parents and Professionals Volume 11*. Austin, TX: Pro-ed.

Schopler, E., Lansing, M. & Waters, L. (1980). *Individualised Assessment And Treatment For Autistic And Developmentally Disabled Children. Teaching Strategies for Parents and Professionals Volume 111*. Austin, TX: Pro-ed.

Resources for parents with autistic children

Grandin, T. & Scariano, M. (1986). *Emergence, Labelled Autistic*. London: Costello. (Biographical account of autism.)

Harris, S. (1994). *Siblings of Children with Autism. A Guide for Families*. Bethesda, MD: Woodbine House.

Jordon, R. & Powell, S. (1995). *Understanding and Teaching Children with Autism*. New York: Wiley.

Maurice, C. (1993). *Let me Hear Your Voice*. New York: Knopf. (A mother's story of children's recovery following behavioural treatment.)

National Autistic Society (1993). *Approaches to Autism* (Second Edition). London: National Autistic Society.

Williams, D. (1992). *Nobody Nowhere*. London: Doubleday. (Biographical account of autism.)

Wing, L. (1996). *The Autistic Spectrum: A Guide for Parents and Professionals*. Constable: London.

7 Prevention of challenging behaviour in children with intellectual disabilities

Bronagh Kennedy and Alan Carr

Challenging behaviour refers to activities which could be harmful to the individual or challenging for carers or care staff to deal with. Self-injury, aggression, temper tantrums and property destruction are among the more common types of challenging behaviour (Emerson, 1995; Psychological Society of Ireland, 1998; Schneider et al., 1996). Self-injury, a particularly significant subcategory of challenging behaviour, refers to repeated, self-inflicted, non-accidental injury, producing temporary or permanent tissue damage and can include head-banging, biting, and cutting or severely scratching skin so as to inflict wounds. Aggression towards others refers to all forms of hitting, kicking and biting or attacking others barehanded or with objects. Temper tantrums refer to uncontrolled displays of aggression which may include shouting, self-injury or aggression. Property destruction refers to all forms of destructive behaviour directed towards objects rather than the self or other people, for example, breaking furniture or crockery by kicking or throwing them.

From this account of common forms of challenging behaviour, it is clear that such behaviour may be directed towards the self, others or objects. It may vary in frequency from occasional incidents to high-rate behaviour. It may vary in intensity from minimally harmful to extremely dangerous. There may also be variation in chronicity from recent onset to long-standing problems. There may also be considerable variation in associated contextual factors. Thus, some challenging behaviour occurs in a limited number of situations while others may occur across multiple contexts.

Epidemiology

There are few accurate data on the epidemiology of challenging behaviour. However, a number of broad trends may be noted (Emerson, 1995; Psychological Society of Ireland, 1998; Schneider et al., 1996). Challenging behaviour is most common among children with intellectual disabilities and pervasive developmental disorders such as autism. Boys are more likely to be identified as showing challenging behaviour than girls and challenging behaviour is most frequently seen in individuals between the ages of 15 and

30. The prevalence of challenging behaviour increases with the level of intellectual impairment and is positively related to the level of restrictiveness in a person's residential placement. Thus, challenging behaviour is more commonly found in institutions and residential services than community settings and day services.

Aetiology

Empirically supported psychological intervention programmes to prevent challenging behaviour are grounded in behavioural theory and applied behavioural analysis (Carr et al., 1990). Within this framework, challenging behaviour is viewed as being maintained by the occurrence of specific antecedent conditions and/or by specific consequences which follow challenging behaviour.

Antecedents of challenging behaviour may be proximal or distal. Proximal antecedents (referred to as discriminative stimuli) include such events as instructions to complete difficult tasks, changes in routine, or lack of stimulation. Establishing operations are one particular class of distal antecedent events which have been shown to be of particular significance for the maintenance of challenging behaviour (Wilder & Carr, 1998). Establishing operations may momentarily increase the reinforcing value of a stimulus. So, for example, food deprivation, sleep deprivation, disruption of routines, and pain are all establishing operations whereby specific consequences (food, attention, provision of comfort, or escape) can be established as effective reinforcers for specific challenging behaviours (such as aggression or self-injury).

Challenging behaviour may be maintained by two specific classes of consequences: positive reinforcement and negative reinforcement. Positive reinforcement refers to situations where challenging behaviour is followed by a desired stimulus and this increases the probability that the challenging behaviour will recur. For example, self-injury may invariably lead to attention. Negative reinforcement refers to situations where the challenging behaviour leads to escape from, or removal of, an aversive stimulus. For example, aggression may invariably lead to no further demands being placed on a person.

Challenging behaviour has been viewed as occupying a range of functional categories in terms of the reinforcers it gives the individual access to, with some theorists emphasizing the communicative function of challenging behaviour (Carr & Durand, 1985) and others emphasizing the positive self-stimulatory function (Harris, 1992). Carr and Durand (1985) argue that self-injurious behaviour serves a communication function such as looking for attention, looking for a break, or requesting access to a desired object or situation. Luiselli (1986) attributes the maintenance of self-injurious behaviour to the sensory reinforcement derived from head-hitting or face-scratching. Similarly, Harris (1992) argues that self-injurious behaviour is reinforced by the euphoria which results from stress-induced endogenous opiate release during episodes of self-injury.

Developmental accounts of self-injurious challenging behaviour hold much in common with Harris' position in highlighting the self-stimulatory role of these types of behaviour in normal development. For example, Schneider et al. (1996) suggest that self-injurious behaviour occurs in all children as a transitory self-stimulatory behaviour during early develop-ment and later these are replaced by safer behaviours which fulfil the same function. However, due to the developmental lag which typifies children with intellectual disabilities and pervasive developmental disorders, less harmful behaviours such as hand-mouthing do not develop as safer replacement self-stimulatory behaviours and self-injurious behaviours persist.

Behavioural interventions to prevent the persistence of challenging behaviours focus on altering the proximal and distal antecedents of such behaviours and their consequences. A range of behavioural interventions have been developed and reviews of studies which have evaluated the effectiveness of these will be addressed below.

Previous reviews

Didden et al. (1997) reviewed 482 studies in which single case design methodologies were used to evaluate the impact of 64 different behavioural interventions on 34 different challenging behaviours. With respect to specific categories of challenging behaviours, they found that behaviours involving property destruction were more responsive to treatment than self-injurious behaviours or socially disruptive behaviours such as public disrobing or inappropriate shouting and swearing. With respect to treatment, they found that response-contingent treatment procedures were more effective than non-contingent procedures, antecedent control procedures and pharmacological interventions. Finally they found that performing a detailed experimental functional analysis was the main significant predictor of treatment effective-ness. Functional analysis aims to identify the functional properties of a prob-lem behaviour, i.e. the antecedents and consequences that maintain it and the function it serves for the individual (O'Neill et al., 1997). In addition to careful interviewing about typical episodes of challenging behaviour and observing these in their natural setting, a thorough functional analysis involves observing clients with challenging behaviour in a series of analogue experimental situations. Iwata et al. (1994a, b) have developed an analogue functional analysis procedure which permits clinicians to determine if a prob-lem behaviour is maintained by social positive reinforcement (attention, access to food or materials), social negative reinforcement (escape from demanding tasks or other sources of aversive stimulation), automatic (sensory) reinforcement or a combination of these variables by observing individuals in series of carefully designed experimental situations.

A variety of different procedures for preventing challenging behaviour have been developed, notably: functional communication training, neutralizing routines, over-correction and restraint. All of these procedures have been the focus of major review papers which deserve mention.

Functional communication training

This involves assessing the function of youngsters' challenging behaviours and teaching them more appropriate behaviours which serve the same functions as the challenging behaviour (Mirenda, 1997). For example, screaming to gain attention might be replaced by a simple signing procedure or displaying a card to signify that attention is needed. Functions of challenging behaviour vary from case to case, but commonly include escaping from an aversive situation; soliciting attention from a caregiver; obtaining access to a preferred tangible object such as food, drink or toys; and providing sensory stimulation (Iwata et al., 1994a, b). In a review of 21 single case design studies, Mirenda (1997) found that functional communication training resulted in immediate and substantial reduction in the frequency of problem behaviour for 44 of the 52 (85%) participants. In the 15% of cases where interventions were ineffective, this could be attributed to staff resistance to implementing the intervention procedures in a consistent manner. There was some evidence for generalization of treatment gains to other contexts and the maintenance of treatment gains over time, but data on generalization were only available in 25% of cases and follow-up data were only available for 46% of cases.

Neutralizing routines

Wilder and Carr (1998), in a review of interventions that focus on neutralizing antecedent establishing operations, concluded that such neutralizing routines can be effective in preventing challenging behaviour. Establishing operations momentarily increase the reinforcing value of a stimulus. So, for example, food deprivation may be an establishing operation whereby specific consequences (food) can be established as an effective reinforcer for specific challenging behaviours (such as aggression) following a specific discriminative stimulus (such as an instruction to complete a task). Neutralizing routines are applied before the discriminative stimulus and the predicted display of challenging behaviour and aim to reduce the value of any subsequent reinforcement of the challenging behaviour. For example, a youngster who engages in challenging aggressive behaviour when asked to follow an instruction (the discriminative stimulus), but only when hungry (following the establishing operation of food deprivation), might show a reduction in challenging behaviour if the neutralizing routine of feeding occurred before the discriminative stimulus of asking him to follow an instruction.

Overcorrection

Overcorrection involves restitution and positive practice (Carter & Ward, 1987). With restitution youngsters are required to restore the area around them to the state it was in before they disrupted it through engaging in challenging behaviour. With positive practice, youngsters are required to rehearse appropriate alternative responses to replace their challenging behaviour. Carter and Ward (1987) reviewed 32 studies consisting of 47 discrete single case design experiments with 80 participants ranging in age from 3 to 46. Successful outcomes in terms of short-term suppression of self-injurious behaviour were reported for 76 of the 80 participants, indicating that overcorrection is a promising intervention for preventing further challenging behaviour.

Physical restraint

Physical restraint refers to actions or procedures which are designed to limit or suppress movement or mobility (Harris, 1996). Both non-contingent (continuous application of restraint procedure) and contingent (restraint procedure only applied when problem behaviour occurs) restraint fall into this category. Harris (1996) reviewed data from 25 reports consisting of 32 separate studies of restraint with 73 participants ranging in age from 6 to 37. He concluded that both non-contingent (continuous application of restraint procedure) and contingent (restraint procedure only applied when problem behaviour occurs) restraint can result in long-term reductions in challenging behaviour. The non-contingent application of physical restraint was found by Harris to be most effective when fading was involved (relaxing of procedures) and contingent application was found to be most effective when care-staff were involved in the treatment plans.

Other interventions

Other interventions such as negative reinforcement (withdrawing an aversive stimulus or providing a means of escape from an aversive situation), instructional manipulation, and punishment have been used to prevent challenging behaviour (Carr et al., 1990). However, major recent review papers on the impact of these procedures have not been published. A wide variety of pharmacological interventions have been used to prevent challenging behaviour. Reviews of this literature conclude that pharmacological interventions are less effective than behavioural interventions in modifying challenging behaviour (Didden et al., 1997; Ellis et al., 1997).

The major review papers cited in this section included studies involving both adults and children. In addition many included studies where intervention programmes were implemented without a thorough functional analysis first being conducted. The present review focused on studies where participants were children or adolescents and (in most instances) where intervention programmes were based on a functional analysis of challenging behaviour.

Method

The aim of the present review was to identify effective psychological intervention programmes for preventing challenging behaviour from persisting in youngsters with intellectual disabilities. A PsychLit search of English language journals for the years 1977 to 2000 was conducted in which the terms *challenging behaviour* and *self-injurious behaviour* were combined with terms such as *treatment*, *intervention*, *behaviour modification*, *applied behavioural analysis* and so forth. These searches were limited to the terms *child* and *adolescent*. In addition Database Problem Behavior 4.0, which includes studies of a wide variety of behaviour problems in children and adults with a variety of disability profiles, was searched for intervention studies conducted specifically with children or adolescents (Duker et al., 1996). The bibliographies of recent review articles on the topic were also consulted to complement the database literature searches. Studies were selected for inclusion in this review if participants were children or adolescents with moderate, severe or profound intellectual disabilities and if the studies met at least two of the following criteria:

- The dependent variable (challenging behaviour) and the independent variable (treatment procedure) were clearly operationally defined and assessed in a reliable manner.
- The intervention programmes were based on a functional analysis of challenging behaviour.
- Clear readable graphs of changes in the dependent variable as a function of the independent variable were presented in the report.

In all, fifteen studies containing a total of twenty-two cases were selected for inclusion in the review.

Overview of studies

Table 7.1 gives an overview of the fifteen studies selected for review. The majority of the studies were conducted in the USA. Two were conducted in Australia and one each in New Zealand and Ireland. All of the studies were published between 1981 and 1998. The fifteen studies include twenty-two cases ranging in age from three to seventeen years old. Only six of the twenty-two cases were female. In all cases youngsters had intellectual disabilities in the moderate, severe or profound ranges. Seven of the cases had been diagnosed with autism and no specific diagnoses were given for the other fifteen cases. Self-injurious behaviour was present in seventeen cases; aggression in

Table 7.1 Characteristics of challenging behaviour prevention studies

Case no.	Author	Year	Country	N	Partici- pant's name	Age	Gender	Level of intellectual disability or diagnosis	Target behaviour	Programme settings
1	Campbell & Lutzker	1993	USA	1	Don	8	M	Autism	TT PD	Home and community outings
2	Durand	1993	USA	3	Michelle	5	F	Moderate	SIB Agg	Special school for students with DD
3					Peter	15	M	Severe	SIB Agg TT	Day school for students with DD
4					Joshua	3	M	Severe	SIB Agg TT	Community preschool
5	Fisher et al.	1998	USA	2	Ike	13	M	Mild- moderate	Agg PD	Inpatient unit for assessment and treatment of severe behaviour disorders
6					Tina	14	F	Severe	Agg	
7	Horner et al.	1990	USA	1	David	14	M	Moderate	Agg	Self-contained special class in mainstream school
8	Sigafoos & Meikle	1996	Australia	2	Dale	8	M	Autism Severe– moderate	SIB Agg PD	Therapy centre and special class for children with autism
9					Pete	8	M	Autism Severe– moderate	SIB Agg PD	
10	Steege et al.	1990	USA	2	Ann	5	F	Profound	SIB	Classroom of hospital inpatient unit
11					Dennis	6	M	Profound	SIB	
12	Horner et al.	1997	USA	3	Clay	12	M	Severe	SIB Agg	Family home with full-time staff support
13					Patrick	17	M	Severe	Agg	
14					Karl	14	M	Autism Severe	SIB Agg	

Table 7.1 continued

Case no.	Author	Year	Country	N	Partici- pant's name	Age	Gender	Level of intellectual disability or diagnosis	Target behaviour	Programme settings
15	Taylor et al.	1996	Ireland	1	Mike	5	M	Autism	SIB Agg	Special school for moderate intellectual disability
16	Agosta et al.	1980	USA	1	Tom	3	M	Severe	SIB	Preschool classroom for multiply handicapped Foster home
17	Luiselli et al.	1981	USA	1	John	10	M	Autism	SIB	Special class in mainstream school
18	Luiselli	1986	USA	1	Ken	16	M	Severe	SIB	Private residential facilities for DD
19	Neufeld & Fantuzzo	1984	USA	1	–	9	F	Moderate Autism	SIB	Community-based short-term residential treatment facility
20	Radler et al.	1985	Australia	1	Joanne	14	F	Severe	SIB	Large residential institution
21	Singh et al.	1981	New Zealand	1	–	16	F	Profound	SIB	Patients' residential unit
22	Linscheid et al.	1994	USA	1	Stan	8	M	Severe–profound	SIB	Acute care hospital

Notes
Agg = aggression. DD = developmental disabilities. PD = property destruction. SIB = self-injurious behaviour. TT = temper tantrums.

twelve; property destruction in four; and temper tantrums in three. In ten cases there were multiple challenging behaviours. Only three of the studies applied the intervention techniques in the family home setting. The remaining studies were conducted in special schools, residential institutions or inpatient treatment centres.

The teams who conducted the fifteen studies reviewed here were largely university-based and were invited by schools or health care agencies to provide alternative treatment programmes for severe forms of challenging behaviour which had not responded to routine management procedures. In one study only (Campbell & Lutzker, 1993) an independent service – Project Ecosystems – which specialized in providing home-based services conducted the intervention which was then recorded by the university team. Behavioural assessments involved trained students attached to senior members of the research team or staff from the referring agency recording rates of specified target challenging behaviours (and alternative behaviours in the case of functional communication training) before and during intervention trials at specified time points. In all studies, parents, teachers or residential staff were trained to implement the intervention procedures by the research team concerned.

Methodological features

An overview of the methodological features is presented in Table 7.2. All but three of the studies gave detailed operational definitions of the target behaviour under consideration. This fine detail is a necessary prerequisite to accurate behaviour observation and recording. Only one study failed to provide any evidence of conducting some form of functional analysis prior to intervention. Three of the studies combined three or four methods of functional analysis to yield a more comprehensive explanation as to why a particular behaviour might occur and thus give direction as to how the behaviour could be prevented. In fourteen of the fifteen studies experienced observers or trainers were employed to conduct the behaviour observations or to train staff to conduct the observations. Inter-observer reliability was calculated in every study except one. In all cases inter-observer reliability was found to meet or exceed the standard criteria of 80%. Implementation reliability checks were conducted in only six of the fifteen studies. Carter and Ward (1987) have highlighted the need to provide independent evaluation of the implementation of behaviour modification programmes as a means to improving research in the field. All fifteen studies gave precise details of the treatment procedures used so that the study could be replicated. If special equipment or materials were necessary these were well documented in the studies concerned. A generalization probe was included in ten of the fifteen studies. Follow-up data with collection points ranging from four months to one year were reported in eight studies. All three reviews cited earlier (Mirenda, 1997; Harris, 1996; Carter and Ward, 1987) mentioned the lack of generalization sessions and follow-up data as general shortcomings of studies

Table 7.2 Methodological features of challenging behaviour prevention studies

Feature	Case number																					
	S1	S2	S3	S4	S5	S6	S7	S8	S9	S10	S11	S12	S13	S14	S15	S16	S17	S18	S19	S20	S21	S22
Operational definitions of target behaviour	1	1	1	1	1	1	1	1	1	0	1	1	1	1	1	1	1	1	1	0	1	1
Operational procedural descriptions	1	1	1	1	1	1	1	1	1	1	1	1	1	1	1	1	1	1	1	1	1	1
Structured behavourial interview	0	0	0	0	1	1	0	0	0	0	0	0	0	0	1	0	0	0	0	0	0	0
Motivation assessment scale	0	1	1	0	0	1	0	0	0	0	0	0	0	0	0	0	0	0	0	0	0	0
Analogue functional analysis	0	0	0	0	1	1	0	0	1	0	1	1	0	1	0	0	0	0	0	1	0	0
ABC analysis	1	0	0	0	1	0	0	0	0	1	1	1	1	1	1	1	0	0	0	1	0	0
Scatterplot observational assessment	0	0	0	0	0	1	0	0	0	0	0	0	0	0	1	0	0	0	0	0	0	0
Pre-experimental informal observation or interview	1	0	1	0	1	0	1	1	1	1	0	0	0	0	1	1	1	1	1	1	1	1
Experienced observers or trainers used	1	1	1	1	1	1	1	1	1	1	1	1	1	1	1	0	0	1	1	1	1	1
Inter-observer reliability for assessment > 80%	1	1	1	1	0	1	0	0	1	1	1	1	1	1	1	1	1	1	0	1	1	1
Implementation reliability checks	1	0	0	0	0	1	0	0	0	1	1	0	0	1	0	0	0	1	0	0	0	0
Generalization probe	1	1	1	1	1	0	1	1	0	0	0	0	0	0	1	1	0	1	1	1	1	1
Follow-up	0	0	0	0	0	0	0	1	1	1	0	0	0	0	0	0	0	1	1	1	1	1
Supplementary objective	0	1	0	1	0	0	0	0	0	0	0	0	0	1	1	0	0	0	1	0	0	0
Total	8	7	7	7	9	9	6	6	7	7	8	8	8	8	10	5	4	9	7	7	7	7

Notes

S = case study. 1 = design feature was present. 0 = design feature was absent. ABC = antecedent, behaviour, consequence.

in this field. Although generalization was quite well covered in ten of the studies, follow-up data were less commonly reported. Three of the studies provided supplementary ratings in their reports, two of which were acceptability questionnaires and one rated increases in positive facial expression. The other studies gave anecdotal accounts of caregivers' satisfaction with the programmes or general verbal reports about improvements in behaviour of the participant who underwent treatment. Overall, the fifteen studies met the methodological criteria for robust single case design treatment outcome research and employed one of the following single case research designs: AB, ABAB reversal, alternating treatments, or multiple baseline across subjects (Kazdin, 1982).

Effectiveness ratings

In order to quantitatively compare and synthesize the results of the fifteen studies reviewed here, three types of effectiveness ratings were calculated for each case:

- percentage non-overlapping data
- the percentage zero data
- mean percentage reduction in challenging behaviour

Each of these metrics, which are defined in Chapter 1, have been used in other quantitative reviews of single case design studies. Because no one of these has been established as the 'gold standard' in the field, in Table 7.3 all three are reported.

Substantive findings

Effectiveness ratings for the treatments used with the twenty-two cases involved in the fifteen studies reviewed here are presented in Table 7.3 and a narrative summary is given in Table 7.4. For convenience, in these tables, treatments have been grouped into proactive and suppressive interventions. Proactive interventions include functional communication training, negative reinforcement, neutralizing routines and instructional manipulation. Suppressive interventions include overcorrection, restraint and punishment.

Proactive interventions

Proactive interventions were used to treat different forms of challenging behaviour, including property destruction, aggression, temper tantrums and self-injurious behaviour, in fifteen cases involved in eight studies. In nine cases from five studies the effectiveness of functional communication training was evaluated (Campbell & Lutzker, 1993; Durand, 1993; Fisher et al., 1998; Horner et al., 1990; Sigafoos & Meikle, 1996). In one study involving two

Table 7.3 Summary of effectiveness rates from challenging behaviour prevention studies

	Main intervention and case number															Suppressive interventions						
	Proactive interventions																					
	FCT									*NR*		*NRO*			*IM*	*OC*		*R*				*P*
Variable	S1	S2	S3	S4	S5	S6	S7	S8	S9	S10	S11	S12	S13	S14	S15	S16	S17	S18	S19	S20	S21	S22
% Non-overlapping data	82.3	93.8	100	94.1	93.8	100	100	100	88.2	92.9	100	100	100	75.0	88.2	100	55.6	70.4	100	97.0	96.0	48.0
% Zero data	88.9	63.6	100	25.0	26.7	61.5	75.0	90.9	80.0	66.7	78.8	40	100	75.0	75.0	33.3	00.0	00.0	100	17.2	31.5	37.0
Mean % reduction in CB	95.8	95.8	100	88.4	87.5	94.8	92.9	100	88.9	94.8	94.0	81.2	100	89.2	100	93.7	90.5	83.5	100	90.0	82.6	91.0

Note
FCT = functional communication training. NR = negative reinforcement. NRO = neutralizing routine. IM = instructional manipulation. OC = overcorrection. R = restraint. P = punishment. All values are percentages.

Table 7.4 Summary of key findings of challenging behaviour prevention studies

Author	Year	Programme settings	N	Case no.	Age	Gender	Level of intellectual disability or diagnosis	Target behaviour	Intervention class	Intervention type	Key findings
Campbell & Lutzker	1993	Home and community outings	1	1	8	M	Autism	TT PD	P	FCT	• The child was successful in learning functional communication using a simple signing gesture • Level of challenging behaviour reduced as an indirect consequence of functional communication training • Functional communication skills transferred from therapist to parent and generalized successfully to community settings
Durand	1993	Special school for students with DD	3	2	5	F	Moderate	SIB Agg	P	FCT	• The unprompted rate of use of a functional communication voice-output device improved for all 3 children • The level of challenging behaviour reduced for all 3 children
		Day-school for students with DD		3	15	M	Severe	SIB Agg TT	P	FCT	• The 3 children appeared happier and showed increases in rates of positive facial expression
		Community preschool		4	3	M	Severe	SIB Agg TT	P	FCT	
Fisher et al.	1998	Inpatient unit for assessment and treatment of severe behaviour disorders	2	5	13	M	Mild–moderate	Agg PD	P	FCT	• For both children, functional communication training combined with extinction led to a marked improvement in appropriate communication using communication cards and a reduction in destructive and aggressive behaviour
				6	14	F	Severe	Agg	P	FCT	
Horner et al.	1990	Self-contained special class in MS school	1	7	14	M	Moderate	Agg	P	FCT	• The child showed a high efficiency response, once trained in functional communication using a canon communicator machine and this was associated with substantial decreases in aggression
Sigafoos & Meikle	1996	Therapy centre and special class for children with autism	2	8	8	M	Autism Severe–moderate	SIB Agg PD	P	FCT	• Both cases made significant improvements in functional communication by pointing to line drawings of preferred objects, tapping their teacher's hand as a signal, or using single-word verbal requests
				9	8	M	Autism Severe–moderate	SIB Agg PD	P	FCT	• Challenging behaviour decreased as communicative alternatives increased for both cases • These gains were maintained at follow-up although children still required prompting to elicit alternative communicative responses
Steege et al.	1990	Classroom of hospital in-patient unit	2	10	5	F	Profound	SIB	P	NR	• Negative reinforcement combined with functional communication training using a microswitch operated output device and guided compliance led to a marked decrease in self-injurious behaviour for both children
				11	6	M	Profound	SIB	P	NR	• At follow-up low rates of self-injurious behaviour were reported for one child but high rates were reported for the other
Horner et al.	1997	Family home with full-time staff support	3	12	12	M	Severe	SIB Agg	P	NRO	• Level of problem behaviour decreased for all three children following the introduction of neutralizing routines which involved engaging in preferred activities (case 12); reviewing a personal yearbook (case 13); and having a nap (case 14)
				13	17	M	Severe	Agg	P	NRO	• All three children were less agitated during instructional sessions
				14	14	M	Autism Severe	SIB Agg	P	NRO	• Neutralizing routines increased the reinforcing value of praise and decreased the reinforcing value of escape for 2 of the 3 children

Table 7.4 continued

Author	Year	N	Case no.	Age	Gender	Level of intellectual disability or diagnosis	Target behaviour	Intervention class	Intervention type	Key findings
Taylor et al.	1996	1	15	5	M	Autism	SIB Agg	P	IM	• Instructional manipulation with positive reinforcement, pre-task requesting, pacing and task choice led to a gradual decline in challenging behaviour to negligible levels • The positive effects were apparent in the child's classroom and activity hall and to a lesser extent in the swimming pool (generalization probe) • Teachers' questionnaire responses confirmed the reduction in challenging behaviour, improvement in response in class, and increased mixing with other children
Agosta et al.	1980	1	16	3	M	Severe	SIB	S	OC	• Overcorrection with restitution and positive practice led to significant reductions in self-injurious behaviour but not to zero levels and improvements did not generalize to the home setting
Luiselli et al.	1981	1	17	10	M	Autism	SIB	S	OC	• Overcorrection reduced self-injurious behaviour to near zero levels and the effect was maintained at six-month follow-up • Continuous application of overcorrection was more effective than intermittent application • Improved engagement in classroom instruction occurred as consequence of reduced self-injurious behaviour
Luiselli	1986	1	18	16	M	Severe	SIB	S	R	• Restraint with two protective devices led to rapid substantial reductions in self-injurious behaviour and these gains were maintained at follow-up • Staff rated restraint as effective, acceptable and easy to implement
Neufeld & Fantuzzo	1984	1	19	9	F	Moderate	SIB	S	R	• Restraint with a protective device combined with positive reinforcement and time-out greatly reduced levels of self-injurious behaviour • Gains were maintained at follow-up and generalized to a new residential setting • Time-out was less effective than the restraint intervention in reducing the level of self-injurious behaviour
Radler et al.	1985	1	20	14	F	Severe	SIB	S	R	• Physical restraint by holding arms or legs down combined with positive reinforcement for avoiding self-injury and structured training led to a clinically significant reduction in self-injurious behaviour during intervention and at follow-up • Full-time 1:1 care was discontinued due to improvement in self-injurious behaviour
Singh et al.	1981	1	21	16	F	Profound	SIB	S	R	• Physical restraint led to a clinically significant reduction in self-injurious behaviour • One minute of physical restraint with a soft jacket was more successful than three minutes of restraint in reducing self-injurious behaviour • The impact of the restraint procedure generalized across different staff and settings
Linscheid et al.	1994	1	22	8	M	Severe–profound	SIB	S	P	• Punishment with a SIBIS electric-shock device led to rapid suppression of fatal self-injurious behaviour • Gains generalized to home and school settings and were maintained at one-year follow-up • Parents reported that they were satisfied with the outcome and that their son was more content and making more progress in school

Author	Year		Case no.	Age	Gender					Programme settings
Taylor et al.	1996		15	5	M					Special school for moderate intellectual disability
Agosta et al.	1980		16	3	M					Preschool classroom for multiply handicapped Foster home
Luiselli et al.	1981		17	10	M					Special class in MS school
Luiselli	1986		18	16	M					Private residential facilities for DD
Neufeld & Fantuzzo	1984		19	9	F					Community-based short-term residential treatment facility
Radler et al.	1985		20	14	F					Large residential institution
Singh et al.	1981		21	16	F					Patients' residential unit
Linscheid et al.	1994		22	8	M					Acute care hospital

Note

m = male. f = female. Agg = aggression. DD = developmental disability. PD = property destruction. SIB = self-injurious behaviour. CB = challenging behaviour. P = Proactive intervention. S = Suppressive intervention. FCT = Functional communication training. NR = negative reinforcement. NRO = neutralising routine. IM = instructional manipulation. OC = overcorrection. R = restraint. P = punishment.

cases, the effectiveness of negative reinforcement (coupled with functional communication training) was assessed (Steege et al., 1990). In one study involving three cases, the effectiveness of neutralizing routines was evaluated (Horner et al., 1997), and in one study the impact of instructional manipulation was assessed (Taylor et al., 1996).

Functional communication training

In each of the nine cases where the effectiveness of functional communication training was the central concern, an in-depth functional analysis was conducted initially to establish the function that the challenging behaviour fulfilled for the child (Campbell & Lutzker, 1993; Durand, 1993; Fisher et al., 1998; Horner et al., 1990; Sigafoos & Meikle, 1996). Establishing the function of challenging behaviour (such as escaping from a noxious situation, obtaining attention, getting a preferred object, or producing sensory stimulation) was essential so that a suitable replacement communication skill that would be functionally equivalent to the target challenging behaviour could be selected and taught.

Campbell and Lutzker (1993) trained an eight-year-old boy who presented with severe tantrums and property destruction to use simple hand-signs to communicate with his parent in a more appropriate way. The communication system was at first successfully applied in the home setting and then transferred to community outings. The challenging behaviour was not directly treated in this case but decreases in challenging behaviour were associated with increased use of simple signs as a form of communication. The authors suggested that the appropriate communication skill was found by the boy to be favourable because it achieved the desired response more efficiently than the challenging behaviour.

Durand (1993) used functional communication training to prevent three youngsters with severely limited communication skills from persisting with self-injurious behaviour, aggression and temper tantrums. He trained them to use computerized voice-output devices which required minimal input to produce a fully recognizable output. All three participants were successfully trained to use their devices with minimal prompting. During the programme, challenging behaviour was blocked and an emergency procedure applied if the challenging behaviour was deemed to be dangerous. Increased rates of positive facial expression occurred after the programme, which was interpreted as evidence that the three youngsters were more content following the intervention. Durand argues that these devices, which emit clear output, can facilitate the inclusion of severely impaired individuals in their communities. Steege et al. (1990) agree that microswitches which activate pre-taped messages which are easily interpreted by caregivers may be more efficient than hand-signs which can go unnoticed in busy classrooms or noisy homes.

Fisher et al. (1998) coupled functional communication training with extinction in the treatment of two teenagers who presented with aggression and property destruction. The youngsters were trained to use signalling cards (a stop-sign card and a green card) to communicate their needs in a more appropriate manner and their carers were trained to respond to these signals by meeting specific needs communicated by the cards. In addition, carers were trained not to respond with attention to challenging behaviour. This was the extinction procedure. The training took place in an inpatient unit specializing in the assessment and treatment of severe challenging behaviour and was later applied to the participant's daily routines in their natural environment. Levels of challenging behaviour decreased when functional communication using the cards was practised and challenging behaviour was put on extinction.

Horner et al. (1990) tested the hypothesis that to be adopted as an alternative, a functional communication response designed to replace the challenging behaviour must be more efficient than the challenging behaviour in achieving the required outcome for the client, and that where alternatives are available the most efficient alternative will be preferred and lead to the greatest reduction in challenging behaviour. They trained a fourteen-year-old boy who presented with aggression to input two different responses on a Canon Communication Device. One was a 'high effort – low efficiency' response which involved typing 'please help' on the device and the other was a 'low effort – high efficiency' response, where a single key press produced the same message. They found that the 'low effort – high efficiency' response was associated with larger decreases in challenging behaviour than the 'high effort – low efficiency' response. Horner et al. also found that the boy used other non-aggressive forms of communication, such as pointing at a desired object, as an indirect consequence of functional communication training. This suggests that he had learned about the principles of communication from being taught how to use a communication device to elicit desired responses from caregivers.

Sigafoos and Meikle (1996) taught two autistic boys who presented with self-injurious behaviour, aggression and property destruction that were maintained by both attention and giving access to preferred objects, to use two separate functional communication strategies as alternatives to challenging behaviour to fulfil these two functions, i.e. soliciting attention and gaining access to preferred objects. They taught the youngsters to tap the teacher's hand three times to gain attention. They also taught them to point to line drawings of food, drink or toys or to say 'want food/drink/toy' to obtain access to preferred objects. During the training trials the boys were prompted to use the functional communication skills so that learning was errorless and no episodes of challenging behaviour occurred during the training trials.

From Table 7.3 it is clear that in each of the nine cases where functional communication training was the main intervention, a substantial reduction in challenging behaviour was achieved. Percentages of non-overlapping data ranged from 82.3 to 100% across the nine cases with a mean of 95%. Percentage of zero data ranged from 25 to 100% with a mean of 68%. Mean percentage reduction in problem behaviour ranged from 87.5 to 100%

with a mean of 94%. Collectively these results indicate that functional communication training is a highly effective method for preventing challenging behaviour from persisting.

Negative reinforcement

To prevent self-injury that was maintained by escaping from grooming activities in two multiply handicapped children, Steege et al. (1990) used an intervention that involved brief escape from grooming activities (negative reinforcement) contingent upon a response that was incompatible with self-injury. This was a functional communication-like response, of pressing a microswitch which activated a prerecorded message of 'stop'. This response allowed the youngsters to obtain a brief break from the grooming procedures. Guided compliance was introduced if either participant displayed any self-injurious behaviour during intervention.

From Table 7.3 it is clear that in each case where negative reinforcement (combined with functional communication training) was the main intervention a substantial reduction in self-injury was initially achieved. Percentages of non-overlapping data ranged from 92.9 to 100% across the two cases with a mean of 96%. Percentage of zero data ranged from 66.7 to 78.8% with a mean of 73%. Mean percentage reduction in problem behaviour ranged from 94 to 94.8% with a mean of 94%. Collectively these results indicate that negative reinforcement (combined with functional communication training) in the short term is a highly effective method for preventing challenging behaviour from persisting.

The programme was conducted in an inpatient treatment centre and before discharge parents, teachers and carers attended a training workshop and also received a demonstration video of the techniques involved. In one case the programme was reliably implemented in the home setting; follow-up home visits were made to ensure that the intervention was reliably implemented; and gains made during the initial treatment programme were maintained at six-month follow-up. In the second case, initial gains were not maintained at follow-up. The teacher and parents did not persist with the programme and did not received home visits and follow-up contacts from the treatment team, which probably accounted for the relapse. This finding highlights the importance of maintaining close follow-up contact and investigating if the suggested interventions are both acceptable and appropriate to the participants and carers concerned.

Neutralizing routines

Horner et al. (1997) prevented the persistence of aggression and self-injurious behaviours in three adolescents with severe intellectual disabilities with programmes involving neutralizing routines as their central procedure. In each of the three cases a detailed functional analysis interview pinpointed the type of consequence that typically followed the challenging behaviour, the proximal antecedents (discriminative stimuli) that triggered the challenging behaviour and the distal antecedents (establishing operations) which momentarily increased the reinforcing value of the typical consequences of the challenging behaviour (O'Neill et al., 1990, 1997). In each case, specific neutralizing routines were developed and applied before the discriminative stimulus and the predicted display of challenging behaviour with the aim of reducing the reinforcement value of the normal consequences of challenging behaviour. In the first case, when a preferred planned event was delayed more than fifteen minutes, the youngster showed more intense challenging behaviour (kicking, screaming, hair-pulling) in response to instructions to correct handwriting mistakes at school, a response which was maintained by negative reinforcement, in that he escaped from completing the task. The neutralizing routine applied thirty to forty minutes prior to the instructional session was to allow the youngster to engage in a highly preferred calming activity consisting of drawing pictures and writing repetitive phrases with a staff member for ten minutes. In the second case, when a preferred planned event was postponed for a day, the youngster showed more intense challenging behaviour (kicking, hitting himself, head butting) in response to corrective feedback when errors in his school work were pointed out by a teacher, a response which was maintained by negative reinforcement, in that he escaped from completing the task. The neutralizing routine applied thirty to forty minutes prior to the instructional session was to allow the youngster to engage in a calming activity consisting of reviewing a year-book with a staff member for ten minutes. In the third case, when the youngster had less than five hours' sleep on the preceding night, he showed more intense challenging behaviour in response to being physically interrupted when reaching for a food item on the reinforcement tray at school, a response which was maintained by positive reinforcement, in that he usually got the preferred object from the reinforcement tray. The neutralizing routine applied 30–40 minutes prior to the instructional session was to allow the youngster to have a one hour nap.

From Table 7.3 it is clear that in the three cases where neutralizing routines were the main intervention a substantial reduction in challenging behaviour occurred. Percentages of non-overlapping data ranged from 75 to 100% across the three cases with a mean of 92%. Percentage of zero data ranged from 40 to 100% with a mean of 72%. Mean percentage reduction in problem behaviour ranged from 81.2 to 100% with a mean of 90%. Collectively these results indicate that neutralizing routines in the short term are a highly effective method for preventing challenging behaviour from persisting.

Instructional manipulation

Taylor et al. (1996) found that a programme based on instructional manipulation techniques was effective in reducing levels of self-injurious behaviour and aggression in a young boy in a classroom setting. This study combined techniques of pre-task requesting (favourable request presented before unfavourable request), pacing (continual explanation of desired behaviour and associated reinforcement) and task choice (participant is offered a choice from possible acceptable behaviours). Specific verbal praise for appropriate behaviour was also given throughout the intervention. The teacher concerned successfully applied these techniques in the classroom and activity hall and rated the intervention as acceptable and effective.

From Table 7.3 it is clear that a substantial reduction in challenging behaviour occurred in this case where a programme based on instructional manipulation was the main intervention. Percentage of non-overlapping data was 88%. Percentage of zero data was 75%. Mean percentage reduction in problem behaviour was 100%.

Suppressive interventions

Suppressive interventions were used to treat self-injurious behaviour in seven studies involving seven cases. Two studies evaluated overcorrection (Agosta et al., 1980; Luiselli et al., 1981); four evaluated restraint (Luiselli, 1986; Neufeld & Fantuzzo, 1984; Radler et al., 1985; Singh et al., 1981); and in one study the effectiveness of punishment was assessed (Linsheid et al., 1994).

Overcorrection

Agosta et al. (1980) applied an overcorrection procedure to prevent persisting hand-biting in a three-year-old child in a preschool setting for children with severe intellectual disabilities. Each time the child bit himself, he received a verbal reprimand; instructions to brush his teeth and wash his hands with prompting where necessary as restitution for his hand-biting; and positive practice which entailed instructions in how to work with a peg-board as an alternative response to hand-biting but which also involved 'doing things with his hands'. Rates of self-injurious behaviour decreased rapidly in the school setting but did not generalize to the home setting because the boy's parents had not been trained in the overcorrection procedures. School staff found the intervention acceptable.

Luiselli et al. (1981) also applied an overcorrection procedure to help reduce the hand-biting behaviour of a ten-year-old boy with autism in a school setting. The procedure consisted of a verbal reprimand and positive practice which entailed the boy following three instructions to put his hands over his head, in front of him, and at his sides. Only after the positive practice had been completed could the boy return to his original activity. Furthermore, Luiselli found that continuous application of this overcorrection procedure was more effective than intermittent application, although it was more time-consuming for school staff. Under the continuous application condition, hand-biting was reduced to near zero levels and these lower levels were maintained at the six-month follow-up.

From Table 7.3 it is clear that in the two cases where overcorrection was the main intervention a substantial reduction in self-injurious behaviour occurred. Percentages of non-overlapping data ranged from 55.6 to 100% across the two cases with a mean of 78%. Percentage of zero data ranged from 0 to 33.3% with a mean of 17%. Mean percentage reduction in problem behaviour ranged from 90.5 to 93.7% with a mean of 92%. Collectively these results indicate that overcorrection is a moderately effective method for preventing self-injurious behaviour from persisting.

Physical restraint

To prevent self-injury through head-banging and self-hitting in a sixteen-year-old deaf-blind boy with severe intellectual disability, Luiselli (1986) applied a protective helmet with a face guard and cotton padded mittens each time self-injurious behaviour occurred. The boy remained seated and stationary while the protective equipment was worn until self-injurious behaviour and resistance subsided for at least thirty seconds. Thereafter, the boy was allowed to return to ongoing activity. Throughout this programme of contingently applied restraint, the boy was also reinforced for appropriate behaviour. Short-term reductions in self-injurious behaviour were maintained at six-month follow-up. Furthermore staff at the residential unit where the boy was placed rated the intervention as acceptable and effective and found it easier to apply than the direct physical immobilization procedures that they had used in the past. The application of the helmet and mittens protected the boy from harm but did not impede movement. The procedure may have been effective because it served as a form of time-out or impeded sensory stimulation associated with self-injury.

To prevent self-injury through arm-biting in a nine-year-old autistic girl with moderate intellectual disability, Neufeld and Fantuzzo (1984) applied a protective plastic bubble-like helmet every time self-injurious behaviour occurred. The self-biting typically occurred in response to directives given during educational or recreational activities. In these situations, if the girl followed the directions she was reinforced for compliance with praise and a gentle touch. If she engaged in self-injury, staff briefly restrained her, put the protective helmet in place and then the girl was permitted to continue with activities as usual. The helmet was removed after two minutes of no further attempts at self-injury or resistance. Short-term gains were maintained at six-week follow-up. The protective helmet used in this programme has a number of advantages. It was not necessary to remove the girl from her usual setting when applying the helmet. The device did not physically prevent appropriate behaviour nor did it restrict sensory stimulation. It was highly acceptable to staff as it was easy to apply and the girl offered little resistance to its application.

To prevent self-injury through arm-biting, head-banging and self-hitting in a fourteen-year-old visually impaired girl with severe intellectual disability and moderate hearing loss, Radler et al. (1985) implemented a programme involving a hierarchical schedule of contingent restraint. The programme was conducted in a residential facility and a school setting, and the hierarchy of restraints was applied by staff at the two facilities. Each time the girl engaged in self-injury (e.g. hitting her head with her knee or biting her arm) initially her hands or legs were held down without staff speaking or making any eye contact. The girl was released after fifteen seconds or until a period of five seconds elapsed without resistance. This was the first level of restraint in the hierarchy. The second level of restraint was applied if the girl successfully engaged in self-injury while at the first level of restraint or if she showed two or more self-injurious behaviours at the same time (e.g. self-biting and self-hitting). There were two variants of the second level of restraint in the hierarchy, one of which was used in the residential facility and one of which was used in the school. At the residential facility, the second level of restraint involved the girl's wrists being held while she was led at a quick walking pace until resistance stopped for at least five seconds. At the school, the second level of restraint involved the girl lying face down on a bean bag with her hands held by staff behind her back until resistance stopped for at least five seconds. As with the first level of restraint, staff did not speak or make any eye contact while applying both variations of the second level of restraint. Two variants of the second level of restraint were necessary because staff at the residential and school facilities expressed preferences for the variants described. Throughout the first two weeks of the restraint programme, the girl was reinforced with a piece of chocolate every fifteen minutes if she had not engaged in self-injurious behaviour in the preceding fifteen seconds. Staff at the school and residential unit were trained to do this and to verbally reinforce her for engaging in appropriate educational activities and daily living skills throughout the restraint programme. Finally, throughout the restraint programme, the girl received three periods of structured training each day at school. These focused on developing skills for completing preferred tasks (riding an adult size tricycle, changing towels in the bathrooms, and collecting a jug of milk for morning tea). For a four-month period one-to-one staffing was required to implement the programme. Short-term gains were maintained at eight-month follow-up.

To prevent self-injury through face-punching in a sixteen-year-old deaf-blind girl with profound intellectual disability Singh et al. (1981) applied a restraining soft jacket for either one or three minutes each time a self-injurious behaviour occurred. The jacket was loose fitting, made from calico, with buttons down the back, closed sleeves and ties attached to the end of each sleeve. The jacket was put on sleeves first, buttoned and the arms crossed at the front and tied at the back. The one-minute application of the restraint procedure was found to be more effective than the three-minute application. The application was found to generalize across different staff members and different settings. At follow-up, however, short-term gains were not fully maintained because the girl was placed in a class with eight other pupils and staff had insufficient time to ensure a consistent approach to behaviour management.

From Table 7.3 it is clear that in the four cases where restraint was the main intervention a substantial reduction in self-injurious behaviour occurred. Percentages of non-overlapping data ranged from 70.4 to 100% across the four cases with a mean of 91%. Percentage of zero data ranged from 0 to 100% with a mean of 37%. Mean percentage reduction in problem behaviour ranged from 82.6 to 100% with a mean of 89%. Collectively these results indicate that restraint is an effective method for preventing self-injurious behaviour from persisting.

Punishment

To prevent fatal head-banging in an eight-year-old non-ambulatory micro-cephalic boy with severe or profound intellectual disability and cerebral palsy, Linscheid et al. (1994) administered a programme involving the Self-Injurious Behaviour Inhibiting System (SIBIS). Through repeated head-banging, the boy risked damaging a ventricular peritoneal shunt which had been fitted to prevent brain damage secondary to hydrocephalus. Damage to the shunt could lead to brain damage and possible death. The SIBIS is a device designed to administer brief electrical stimulation to the leg each time head-banging occurs. It includes a helmet which contains a sensor that detects head-banging and emits a signal to a stimulus module worn on the leg. The stimulus module administers a 200 ms, 3.5 mA electrical charge at 85 volts to the leg each time head-banging occurs. The pro-gramme was conducted over a five-day period for two to six hours per day. The programme was effective. From Table 7.3 it may be seen that there were 48% non-overlapping data points; 37% zero data; and 91% mean reduction in problem behaviour. Short-term gains were maintained at one-year follow-up

Conclusions

Challenging behaviour, particularly self-injury, aggression, temper tantrums and property destruction, are of central concern to parents and carers of people with intellectual and other developmental disabilities because they are particularly unresponsive to routine care practices and because they place clients, parents and carers at risk of injury. Substantial reductions in challenging behaviour may be achieved using proactive and suppres-sive interventions, following detailed functional analysis of challenging behaviour.

Proactive interventions include functional communication training, nega-tive reinforcement, neutralizing routines and instructional manipulation. Functional communication training involves assessing the function of young-sters' challenging behaviour and teaching them more appropriate behaviour which serves the same function as the challenging behaviour. Negative reinforcement refers to withdrawing an aversive stimulus or providing a means of escape from an aversive situation that triggers challenging behaviour. Neutralizing routines are brief calming interventions, that are applied after events that render individuals vulnerable to challenging behaviour (such as sleep or food deprivation or disruption of routines) and before events that trigger the onset of challenging behaviour such as demanding instructions. Instructional manipulation involves attempting to control challenging behaviour by modifying both the way in which teaching and instruction occur and the content of the curriculum. Here favourable requests may be presented before unfavourable requests, continual explanation of desired behaviour and associated reinforcement may be given, and youngsters may be offered a choice of possible acceptable behaviours.

Suppressive interventions include overcorrection, restraint and punishment. Overcorrection refers to the intense practice of a series of acceptable behaviours each time the target challenging behaviour occurs. During this procedure clients might also be required to restore the area around them to an improved state if they have caused any disruption. Physical restraint and punishment have been used to prevent challenging behaviour. Physical restraint refers to actions or procedures which are designed to limit or suppress movement or mobility. Both non-contingent (continuous application of restraint procedure) and contingent (restraint procedure only applied when problem behaviour occurs) restraint fall into this category. Punishment refers to the use of aversive stimuli, such as administering electric shock when challenging behaviour occurs.

Implications for practice

This review has clear implications for clinical practice in preventing challenging behaviour. One central practice issue is how to decide which category of intervention to consider in any particular case. Interventions that focus on antecedents of challenging behaviour, such as functional communication training, neutralizing routines and instructional manipulation, have been used to good effect with challenging behaviour that is directed at others (such as aggression) and the self (self-injurious behaviour) and in a wide range of community and institutional settings. These interventions, because of their non-coercive and non-aversive nature and their suitability to multiple settings, may be the interventions of first choice when youngsters present with challenging behaviour. In contrast, interventions which focus predominantly on altering the consequences of challenging behaviour such as overcorrection, restraint and punishment have been used exclusively with self-injurious behaviours in predominantly institutional settings in the studies reviewed in this chapter. These may therefore be viewed as second-line interventions to consider when functional communication training, neutralizing routines and instructional manipulation have not been effective, particularly within institutional settings, and particularly with self-injurious behaviour. Strong ethical justification is required in using these more coercive interventions. For example, where youngsters are engaging in potentially fatal self-injurious behaviour, their use may be ethically justified.

Implications for research

The studies reviewed in this chapter, while the best currently available, are not without their limitations. Generalization and follow-up data were not widely reported. Future studies should incorporate generalization probes into the design and report long-term follow-up data, aggregated across series of case studies.

Assessment resources

Interview and informant report methods

Durand, V.M. & Crimmins, D. (1992). *Motivation Assessment Scale*. Topeka, KS: Monaco & Associates (Available from Monaco & Associates 531 NE 35th, Topeka, KS 66617–1445, USA. Contains 16 questions rated on a 7-point Likert scale assessing the likelihood of a particular behaviour occurring in different situations, for example situations involving social attention, presentation of tangible objects, sensory feedback, demands.).

Iwata, B.A., Wong, S.E., Riordan, M.M., Dorsey, M.F. & Lou, M.M. (1982). Assessment and training of clinical interviewer skills: analogue analysis and field replication. *Journal of Applied Behavior Analysis*, 15, 191–203.

O'Neill, R.E., Horner, R.H., Albin, R.W., Storey, K. & Sprague, J. (1990). *Functional Analysis: A Practical Assessment Guide*. Pacific Grove, CA: Brookes Cole.

O'Neill, R.E., Horner, R. H., Albin, R.W., Sprague, J., Storey, K. & Newton, J. (1997). *Functional Assessment and Programme Development for Problem Behaviour: A Practical Handbook* (Second Edition). Pacific Grove, CA: Brookes Cole.

Observational methods

Analogue functional analysis tests behaviour reactions in experimentally controlled conditions including: demand, social attention, play and tangibles to find out what types of situations tend to maintain the problem behaviour and are described in Iwata et al. (1994a, b).

Iwata, B.A., Dorsey, J.R, Slifer, K.J., et al. (1994a). Towards a functional analysis of self-injury. *Journal of Applied Behavior Analysis*, 27(2), 197–209.

Iwata, B.A., Pace, G.M., Dorsey, J.R., et al. (1994b). The functions of self-injurious behaviour: an experimental-epidemiological analysis. *Journal of Applied Behavior Analysis*, 27(2), 215–240.

Programme resources

Carr, E., Levin, L., McConnachie, G., Carlson, J., Kemp, D. & Smith, C. (1994). *Communication Based Intervention for Problem Behaviour. A Users Guide for Producing Positive Change.* Baltimore, MD: Paul H. Brookes.

Duker, P.C., Didden, R., Korzilius et al. (1996). Database problem behavior: a literature retrieval system for professionals dealing with problem behaviours of individuals with intellectual disabilities. *International Journal of Disability, Development and Education*, 43(3), 197–202. (Database Problem Behavior 4.0 contains information from 885 empirical studies encompassing information about behaviour topography, intervention procedures used, functional analyses as well as descriptive details about each study. Available from Behavioural Software, PO Box 31310, 6530 CH Nijmegen, The Netherlands.)

Durand, V.M. (1990). *Severe Behaviour Problems: A Functional Communication Training Approach.* New York: Guilford.

Luiselli, J.K., Maston, J. & Singh, N. (1992). *Self-Injurious Behaviour: Analysis, Assessment and Treatment.* New York: Springer Verlag.

McBrien, J., & Felce, D. (1992). *Working with People who have Severe Learning Difficulty and Challenging Behaviour.* England: The Cookley Printers, A BIMH Publication.

Reichle, J., York, J. & Sigafoos, J. (1991). *Implementing Augmentative and Alternative Communication.* Baltimore, MD: Paul H. Brookes.

Singh, N. (1997). *Prevention and Treatment of Severe Behavior Problems: Models and Methods in Developmental Disabilities.* Pacific Grove, CA: Brooks/Cole.

Policy document

Psychological Society of Ireland: Learning Disability Group (April 1998). *Responding to Behaviour that Challenges.* (Contains the results of surveys which examine the nature and prevalence of challenging behaviour among people with intellectual disabilities in Ireland. This document also proposes a framework for effective individual intervention.)

8   Prevention of physical abuse

Beth O'Riordan and Alan Carr

Since the publication of Henry Kempe's seminal paper on the battered child syndrome (Kempe et al., 1962), there has been a growing awareness that the physical abuse of children is a problem of significant proportions requiring preventative action. While many preventative programmes have been developed, the effectiveness of most of these remains untested. The aim of this chapter is to review methodologically robust research studies on the effectiveness of physical abuse prevention programmes which target high-risk groups, draw reliable conclusions about the effectiveness of these, and outline the implications of these conclusions for policy and practice.

Physical abuse refers to the physical injury of a child or the failure to prevent physical injury (or suffering) to a child, including deliberate poisoning, suffocation and Munchausen's syndrome by proxy (Browne & Herbert, 1997). Physical abuse leads to short-term psychological effects in almost all cases and significant long-term effects on psychological development in a proportion of cases exposed to severe abuse in the absence of personal or contextual protective factors, such as good coping strategies or the availability of social support (Briere et al., 1996; Browne & Herbert, 1997; Browne & Peterson, 1997; Guterman, 1997). The psychological consequences of physical abuse include increased rates of internalizing and externalizing behaviour problems, lowered self-esteem, relationship problems, and academic or cognitive difficulties.

Epidemiology

Estimates of the incidence of physical abuse range from less than 1% to more than 60%, depending on the definitions used (Gelles, 1987). With narrow definitions, estimates for the prevalence of serious physical abuse range from 1% to 10% (Browne & Herbert, 1997).

Aetiology

Within complex systemic conceptualizations of physical abuse it is argued that physical abuse occurs in families characterized by high levels of stress and low levels of support when children place demands on their parents which outstrip their parents' coping resources, and parents in frustration injure their children (Carr, 1999). There is considerable agreement now concerning the risk factors for physical child abuse (Briere et al., 1996; Browne & Herbert, 1997; Browne & Peterson, 1997; Guterman, 1997). Child-related risk factors include prematurity, low birth weight, difficult temperament, child misbehaviour and insecure attachment. All of these child-related risk factors increase the demands that children place upon their parents. Parental risk factors include parental immaturity, criminality, chronic physical and mental health problems and a personal history of abuse. All of these parental risk factors compromise parents' capacity to tolerate frustration and meet their children's needs in an appropriately sensitive manner. Contextual risk factors include conflictual marital relationships, inadequate social support networks, high levels of life stress and poverty. These contextual risk factors compromise a family's capacity to sustain co-operative parent–child relationships.

Previous reviews

Previous reviews of the literature on the prevention of physical child abuse have reached a number of important conclusions (Browne & Peterson, 1997; Guterman, 1997; MacMillan et al., 1994a; Olsen & Widom, 1993). First, a range of risk factors are typically considered in screening families for inclusion in physical child abuse prevention programmes. Some of these factors are listed in Table 8.1. Second, only some of a wide range of preventative programmes currently in operation have been subjected to evaluation. Those whose effectiveness has been assessed have focused predominantly on parents and in doing so have aimed to enhance the parenting received by children. Some of the common goals of physical abuse prevention programmes are listed in Table 8.1 along with outlines of common components of programmes which have been systematically evaluated. Third, home visiting has been a central feature of many programmes, where programme staff visit parents and children in their homes and deliver an intervention programme within the home context. In contrast, a minority of evaluated programmes have involved parents attending outpatient clinics or community centres on the one hand or inpatient-residential facilities on the other. Fourth, there has been considerable variability in the timing and duration of programmes. Some are offered to parents at risk before the birth of their first child while others are not offered until shortly after the birth of the child. Some programmes are short term while others are long term and are offered over a number of years. Fifth, some programmes aim to provide parents at risk with supportive relationships with professionals while others aim to train parents in specific skills such as parenting skills, life skills or stress management skills. Sixth, some preventative programmes have had a relatively narrow focus and exclusively targeted one specific aspect of the family while others are more

Table 8.1 Components of physical child abuse prevention programmes

Screening	• *Child characteristics*: prematurity, low birth weight and difficult temperament • *Maternal characteristics*: teenage pregnancy, physical or mental health problems, substance abuse, chaotic lifestyle, personal adjustment difficulties, personal history of abuse or neglect, previously suspected of child abuse • *Family factors*: insecure mother–child attachment, being a single parent, lack of father involvement, lack of family support • *Social factors*: high levels of life stress, poverty, homelessness, and under-use of appropriate health and social services
Goals	• To increase parental knowledge of child development so as to modify unrealistic expectations • To help parents recognize and understand infants' signals when they require basic needs to be met • To help parents develop feeding, sleeping, cleaning, and playing/stimulating routines with their infants • To help parents maintain socially supportive relationships with their partners and members of the extended family • To help parents maintain supportive relationships with health and social services professionals • To provide crisis intervention to help parents cope with psychosocial and economic crises that interfere with providing quality infant care • To help parents develop stress management skills so that stress related anger will not lead parents to injure their children • To monitor children's health and development
Home visiting	• Professionals, para-professionals or trained volunteers visit mothers and infants frequently at the family home • Visiting, ideally, being before the birth of the child • The home visitor provides information about child development and child care; helps with the development of parenting skills; and offers social support • The non-judgmental, supportive and empathic quality of the relationship that typifies the relationship between the home visitor and the mother is central to its effectiveness as a source of support for vulnerable or at-risk parents

Behavioural parent training	• The parent and child regularly visit an outpatient centre and the parent develops specific parenting skills by engaging in behavioural parent training with a professional • Behavioural parent training may be provided on a group or individual basis • The clear, precise procedures for developing feeding, sleeping, cleaning, and playing/stimulating routines which are based on well-established behavioural principles are central to the effectiveness of behavioural parent training
Life skills training	• In life skills training parents, through modelling, instruction and guided practice, acquire the skills necessary to manage certain psychosocial and economic life stresses that compromise their capacity to provide quality infant care • These skills include money and household management; budgeting; dealing with health, social services, educational and financial agencies; enhancing problem-solving and communication skills
Stress management training	• In stress management training parents, through modelling, instruction and guided practice, acquire the skills necessary to manage negative mood states such as anger, anxiety and depression that may compromise their capacity to provide quality infant care • These skills include recognizing the signs of stress early; challenging thoughts that maintain negative mood states; learning relaxation skills; changing potentially stressful situations so that they are less demanding; and using social support to reduce stress
Multimodal programmes	• These contain combinations of home visiting, supportive counselling, behavioural parent training, life skills training, stress management training and routine monitoring of children's health and development • They may be offered on an inpatient or outpatient basis

wide ranging and aim to address many features of families at risk. For example, behavioural parent training programmes specifically target parenting skills while multimodal programmes may aim to provide parents with support and parenting skills training and to provide children with day care and intellectual stimulation. Seventh, some programmes involve regular contact with professionals (such as nurses, social workers or care workers) while others involve contact with paraprofessionals such as trained volunteers or lay counsellors. Eighth, the weight of available evidence suggests that prevention programmes which include long-term home visiting by paraprofessionals are the most effective. Finally, at a methodological level, many studies which evaluate the effectiveness of physical abuse prevention programmes have had serious methodological shortcomings which compromise the confidence that may be placed in their results. Common shortcomings include the absence of control groups, failure to randomly assign cases to groups, failure to match groups on demographic or other variables to ensure group homogeneity, and the use of post-test-only designs. In this chapter our focus was exclusively on well-designed evaluation studies.

Method

The aim of the present review was to identify effective physical abuse prevention programmes. A PsychLit database search of English language journals for the years 1977 to 2000 was conducted to identify studies of the effectiveness of physical child abuse prevention programmes. The search combined the problem area of *child physical abuse* as the main term with a range of other terms including *primary* and *secondary prevention*, *treatment* and *intervention*. A manual search through bibliographies of recent review papers of the area was also conducted. Single case designs and studies reported in dissertations or convention papers were not included in the review. Twenty well-designed studies were selected. Each of these included a control or comparison group and reliable pre- and post-intervention assessment batteries which assessed abuse or abuse potential.

Characteristics of the studies

Characteristics of the twenty studies reviewed in this chapter are set out in Table 8.2. All the chosen studies were conducted between 1979 and 1994. Fifteen studies were conducted in the USA, four in Canada and one in Great Britain. All of the studies evaluated secondary prevention programmes for families containing children at risk of physical child abuse. Mothers were the primary focus of intervention in all studies. Mothers ranged in age from 14 to 45 years, with younger mothers being targeted in most studies. Black mothers, single mothers, and women of lower socioeconomic status were over-represented in some studies, since these were identified as being from families at risk of child abuse. Over 2,500 families participated in these

Table 8.2 Characteristics of physical child abuse prevention studies

Study no.	Study type	Authors	Year	N per group	Mean age and range	Family characteristics	Programme setting	Programme duration
1	HV	Gray et al.	1979	1. HV-N(pre + post) = 50 2. C = 50			Community OP Home	324 sess over 2.25 y 108 OP sess HV sess
2	HV	Olds et al.	1986	1. HV-N(pre + post) = 216 2. C = 184	Mothers 47% <19 y	62% unmarr 89% white lower SES	Home	42 sess over 2 y
3	HV	Affleck et al.	1989	1. HV-N (post) = 47 2. C = 47	Mothers 28 y	83% marr	Home	30 sess over 4 m
4	HV	Infante-Rivard et al.	1989	1. HV-N (pre + post) + SUP = 21 2. C = 26	Mothers 24 y	56% lower SES	Home	8 sess over 7 m
5	HV	Barth et al.	1988	1. HV (pre + post) = 24 2. C = 26	Mothers 22 y	lower SES	Home	12 sess over 6 m
6	HV	Barth	1991	HV-P(peri + post) 97 C = 94	Mothers 23 y	45% white 31% latino 17% black 7% other	Home	12 sess over 6 m
7	HV	Hardy & Street	1989	1. HV-P(post) = 131 2. C = 132	Mothers 23 y	78% SPF 100% black lower SES	Home	46 sess over 2 y
8	HV	Larson	1980	1. HV-P(pre + post) = 35 2. HV(post) = 36 3. C = 37	Mothers 18–35 y	lower SES 56–63% white	Home	72 sess over 1.5 y
9	BPT	Field et al.	1982	1. BPT-HV (post) = 40 2. BPT = 40 3. C = 40	Mothers 16 y	lower SES	Home	48 sess over 6 m or 120 sess over 6 m
10	BPT	Burch & Mohr	1980	1. BPT-G = 21 2. C = 10	Mothers 19 y		Community OP	32 sess over 4 m
11	BPT	Wolfe et al.	1988	1. BPT-G = 16 2. C = 14	Mothers 16–25 y Children 9–60 m	lower SES SPF	Community OP	29 sess over 20 w

Table 8.2 continued

Study no.	Study type	Authors	Year	N per group	Mean age and range	Family characteristics	Programme setting	Programme duration
12	BPT	Resnick	1985	1. BPT + LST = 18 2. C = 18	Mothers 27 y 18–45 y	lower SES	Community OP	28 sess over 14 w
13	BPT	Barth et al.	1983	1. BPT-G + SMT = 10 2. C = 10		lower SES	Community OP	8 sess over 4 m
14	SMT	Schinke et al.	1986	1. SMT = 33 2. C = 37	Mothers 16 y		Community OP	12 sess over 3 m
15	MCI	Lutzker & Rice	1984	1. MCI (pre + post) = 50 2. C = 47			Home	>40 sessions over 1 y
16	MCI	Marchenko & Spence	1994	1. M CI + HV (pre + post) = 110 2. C = 77	Mothers 23 y	89% unmarr, 94% black 4% hispanic , 2% white 80% unplanned pregnancy	Home	>30 sess over 10 m
17	MCI	Lealman et al.	1983	1. MCI (post) = 103 2. C = 209	Children 18 m		Community OP	1 dpw over 18 m
18	MIT	Siegel et al.	1980	1. MIT + HV (post) = 88 2. C = 149	Mothers 21 y	24–31% white	Hospital inpatient Home	15 sess over 3 m
19	MIT	Taylor & Beauchamp	1988	1. MIT + HV (post) = 16 2. C = 16	Mothers 24 y	57% marr 47% lower SES 47% black	Home Hospital inpatient	4 sess over 3 w
20	MIT	O'Connor et al.	1980	1. MIT = 143 2. C = 158	Mothers 18 y 14–31 y	56–63% white	Hospital inpatient	17 m

Notes

HV = home visitation. HV-N = home visiting by nurses. HV-P = home visiting by paraprofessionals. BPT = behavioural parent training. BPT-G = group behavioural parent training. SMT = stress management training. LST = life skills training. MIT = multimodal inpatient intervention. MCI = multimodal community intervention. pre = prenatal. post = postnatal. peri = perinatal. C = control group. OP = outpatient. SW = social work. SES = socioeconomic status. SPF = single parent family. marr = married. unmarr = unmarried. w = weeks. m = months. y = years. sess = sessions. dpw = days per week.

studies, with 1,377 allocated to prevention programmes and 1,381 allocated to control groups. In eight studies home visitation was the main intervention. In five studies behavioural parent training was evaluated. Stress management training was evaluated as a focal intervention in one study. Community-based multimodal programmes were evaluated in three studies and in three studies the effectiveness of inpatient multimodal programmes was assessed. The duration of interventions ranged from four sessions over three weeks to more than 300 sessions over 2.25 years.

Methodological features

Methodological features of the twenty studies are summarized in Table 8.3. All twenty studies contained a control or comparison group. Cases were randomly assigned to intervention and control groups in fifteen studies and cases in different groups were demographically similar in seventeen studies. In twelve studies cases were evaluated before the prevention programme and in all studies post-programme data were collected. Follow-up data collected at least three months following the intervention programme were reported in thirteen studies. All studies included multiple outcome measures completed by a combination of parents, therapists and researchers to assess pre- and post-intervention status. In ten studies parents and therapists were the principal informants while researcher ratings were used in eighteen studies. Intervention was guided by a manual in only two studies, but ten studies checked the integrity of the programme. Experienced professionals were involved in delivering the prevention programme in all twenty studies. Ongoing supervision was provided to therapists or key-workers in nine studies. While dropout rates were assessed in fourteen studies, only two studies reported deterioration data and four studies gave information on engagement in concurrent or further intervention programmes. The statistical significance of the gains following intervention was reported in all twenty studies. Nine studies offered data on the clinical significance of the effects of the intervention in terms of the number of cases judged to be clinically improved following participation in the prevention programme. From a methodological viewpoint, it may be concluded that the studies reviewed here are sufficiently well designed to allow relatively reliable conclusions to be drawn about the types of preventive interventions evaluated.

Screening procedures

In almost all of these studies screening procedures were used to identify families at risk of physical child abuse. The screening procedures included interviews with mothers, questionnaires completed by mothers, and observations of mother–child interaction. Criteria for selecting parents for inclusion in prevention programmes varied across studies, but in most instances criteria included some combination of specific child characteristics, specific maternal

Table 8.3 Methodological features of physical child abuse prevention studies

Feature	Study number																			
	S1	S2	S3	S4	S5	S6	S7	S8	S9	S10	S11	S12	S13	S14	S15	S16	S17	S18	S19	S20
Control or comparison group	1	1	1	1	1	1	1	0	1	1	1	1	1	1	1	1	1	1	1	1
Random assignment	1	1	1	1	1	1	1	1	1	1	0	1	1	0	1	1	1	1	1	1
Demographic similarity	0	1	1	1	1	1	1	0	0	1	0	0	1	0	1	1	1	0	1	1
Pre-treatment assessment	1	1	0	0	1	0	1	1	1	1	1	1	1	1	1	0	0	0	0	0
Post-treatment assessment	1	1	1	1	1	1	1	1	1	1	1	1	1	1	1	1	1	1	1	1
3-month follow-up assessment	0	1	1	0	1	1	1	0	0	1	1	1	0	0	1	0	1	1	0	1
Parents' ratings	0	1	0	0	0	0	0	0	0	1	1	0	1	0	1	0	0	0	0	0
Therapists' or trainers' ratings	1	1	0	0	1	0	0	1	1	1	1	1	0	1	0	0	0	1	0	0
Researcher ratings	1	1	1	1	0	1	1	1	1	0	1	1	1	0	0	1	1	1	1	1
Deterioration assessed	0	0	0	0	0	1	0	0	0	0	0	0	0	0	0	0	0	0	0	0
Drop-out assessed	0	1	0	1	1	1	1	1	1	1	0	0	0	1	1	1	1	1	1	1
Clinical significance of change assessed	1	0	0	0	0	0	0	0	1	1	1	1	1	1	1	1	0	1	0	1
Experienced professionals used	1	1	1	1	1	1	1	1	1	1	1	1	0	1	1	1	1	1	1	1
Programmes were equally valued	0	1	0	0	0	0	0	0	0	0	0	0	0	0	1	0	0	0	0	0
Programmes were manualized	0	1	0	0	0	0	0	0	0	0	0	0	0	0	0	0	1	0	0	0
Supervision was provided	0	1	0	1	0	0	0	0	1	1	0	0	1	1	0	0	0	1	0	1
Programme integrity checked	0	0	1	1	1	1	0	0	0	1	1	1	1	0	0	0	1	1	0	0
Data on concurrent treatment given	0	0	0	0	0	0	0	0	0	0	0	0	0	0	1	1	1	0	0	0
Data on subsequent treatment given	0	0	0	0	1	1	0	0	0	1	0	0	0	0	0	1	0	0	0	0
Total	7	14	10	9	10	14	11	9	9	16	13	7	10	8	12	9	13	11	11	8

Notes
S = study. 1 = design feature was present. 0 = design feature was absent.

characteristics, and particular family and social characteristics indicative of vulnerability to physical child abuse. Child characteristics included prematurity, low birth weight and difficult temperament. Maternal characteristics included teenage pregnancy, physical or mental health problems, substance abuse, chaotic lifestyle, personal adjustment difficulties, personal history of abuse or neglect and previously suspected of child abuse. Family and social factors included insecure mother–child attachment, being a single parent, lack of father involvement, lack of family support, high levels of life stress, poverty, homelessness, and underuse of appropriate health and social services. For example, Gray et al. (1979) used a predictive questionnaire (Schneider et al., 1972) along with a postpartum interview and perinatal nursing observations. Barth et al. (1988) used a nine-item screening instrument based on the work of Murphy et al. (1985) and Schneider et al. (1972). Wolfe et al. used the Child Abuse Inventory (Milner, 1980) along with mothers' and children's ages.

Outcome measures

In these studies the number of child abuse reports or hospitalizations were the most important distal outcome measures and one or other of these were only reported in eight of the twenty studies reviewed here. Proximal outcome measures included parental reports of personal well-being as evaluated by measures of anxiety, depression, coping, social support; parental reports of child welfare; researcher ratings of parenting child care skills and behaviour; researcher ratings of parenting of knowledge and attitudes. The Home Observation for Measurement of the Environment (HOME; Caldwell & Bradley, 1979) was the most commonly used instrument for making researcher ratings in this group of studies.

Substantive findings

Treatment effect sizes and outcome rates for the twenty studies are presented in Table 8.4. A narrative summary of key findings from each study is given in Table 8.5.

Studies of home visitation

Physical abuse prevention programmes in which home visitation was the central intervention were evaluated in eight studies (Affleck et al., 1989; Barth et al., 1988; Barth, 1991; Gray et al., 1979; Hardy & Street, 1989; Infante-Rivard et al., 1989; Larson, 1980; Olds et al., 1986). In half of these, home visiting was conducted by a professional nurse and in the remainder a paraprofessional visited participants in their homes. Paraprofessionals were typically women with personal parenting experience, in many instances from culturally similar backgrounds to programme participants, specifically

Table 8.4 Summary of results of treatment effects and outcome rates from physical child abuse prevention studies

	Study number and condition								
	Study 1	Study 2	Study 3	Study 4	Study 5	Study 6	Study 7	Study 8	
Variable	HV-N (pre + post) v C	HV-N (pre + post) v C	HV-N (post) v C	HV-N (pre + post) v C	HV-P (pre + post) v C	HV-P (peri + post) v C	HV-P (post) v C	HV-P (pre + post) v C	HV-P (post) v C
Improvement after programme									
Parents' ratings									
Parent well-being	—	0.2	0.5	—	0.2	0.1	—	—	—
Child welfare	0.0	0.2	—	—	1.2	0.1	—	0.5	0.0
Researchers' ratings									
Parenting skills and behaviour	0.0	0.2	0.5	0.4†	—	—	—	0.4	0.0
Parents' knowledge and attitudes	—	—	—	—	—	—	—	—	—
Improvement at follow-up									
Parents' ratings									
Parents' well-being									
Child welfare									
Researchers' ratings									
Parenting skills and behaviour									
Parents' knowledge and attitudes									
Negative clinical outcomes									
Child abuse reports	0% v 10%	4% v 19%*	—	14% v 19%	8% v 12%	15% v 15%	2% v 10%	—	—
Hospitalizations	—	—	—	—	—	—	6% v 15%	—	—
% Drop-out	—	15–21%	—	33%	16%	20%	8% v 10%	22%	22%

Notes

HV-N = home visiting by nurses. HV-P = home visiting by paraprofessionals. pre = prenatal. post = postnatal. peri = perinatal. C = control group.

*For poor unmarried teenagers. † For cases with low social support.

Table 8.4 (Continued) Summary of results of treatment effects and outcome rates from physical child abuse prevention studies

Study type, number and condition

	BPT						SMT	MCI			MIT		
Variable	*Study 9* BPT-HV (post) v C	BPT v C	*Stud 10* BPT-G v C	*Study 11* BPT-G v C	*Study 12* BPT + LST v C	*Study 13* BPT-G + SMT v C	*Study 14* SMT v C	*Study 15* MCI (pre + post) v C	*Study 16* MCI + HV (pre + post) v C	*Study 17* MCI (post) v C	*Study 18* MIT + HV (post) v C	*Study 19* MIT + HV (post) v C	*Study 20* MIT v C
Improvement after programme													
Parents' ratings													
Parent well-being	—	0.6	—	0.7	—	1.4	0.6	—	0.4	—	—	—	—
Child welfare	0.6	0.6	—	0.3	—	—	—	—	—	—	—	—	—
Researchers' ratings													
Parenting skills and behaviour	0.6	0.6	—	0.0	0.7	1.3	0.0	—	—	—	0.9	2.6	0.9
Parents' knowledge and attitudes	—	—	0.9	—	—	—	—	—	—	—	—	0.9	—
Improvement at follow-up													
Parents' ratings													
Parents' well-being	0.5	0.7	—	1.0	—	—	0.6	—	—	—	—	—	—
Child welfare	0.5	0.7	—	3.2	—	—	—	—	—	—	—	—	—
Researchers' ratings													
Parenting skills and behaviour	0.0	0.0	—	0.0	0.0	—	—	—	—	—	—	1.1	—
Parents' knowledge and attitudes	—	—	—	—	—	—	0.5	—	—	—	—	—	—
Negative clinical outcomes													
Child abuse reports	—	—	—	—	—	—	—	10% v 32%	—	1% v 1%	9% v 6%	—	1% v 4%
Hospitalizations	—	—	—	—	—	—	—	—	—	4% v 19%	9% v 6%	—	14% v 17%
% Drop-out	—	—	69%	43%	39%	—	—	6%	17%	27%	—	6%	15%

Notes
HV = home visitation. HV-N = home visiting by nurses. HV-P = home visiting by paraprofessionals. BPT = behavioural parent training. BPT-G = group behavioural parent training. SMT = stress management training. LST = life skills training. MIT = multimodal inpatient intervention. MCI = multimodal community intervention. pre = prenatal. post = postnatal. peri = perinatal. C = control group.

Table 8.5 Summary of key findings of prevention studies for physical child abuse

Study no.	Study type	Authors	Year	N per group	No. of sessions	Group differences	Key findings
1	HV	Gray et al.	1979	1. HV-N (pre + post) = 50 2. C = 50	324 sess over 2.25 y 108 OP sess 216 HV sess	1 > 2	• Five (10%) of controls sustained serious injuries requiring hospitalization, potentially attributable to child abuse, while none of the children in the child abuse prevention programme that received weekly home visiting by a nurse and bi-monthly paediatric consultations had sustained any such serious injuries at 2 years of age • After 2 years the high-risk intervention group did not differ significantly from the high risk control group in rates of abnormal parenting or scores on the Denver Developmental screening test
2	HV	Olds et al.	1986	1. HV-N (pre + post) = 216 2. C = 184	42 sess over 2 y	1 > 2	• The group that received intensive home visiting had fewer confirmed child abuse reports than controls • The accident rate leading to emergency hospital attendance was lower for children in the group who received home visiting • Compared with controls, the group that received intensive home visiting punished and restricted their children less frequently; reported more childrearing options; and provided their children with more verbal stimulation and these gains were maintained at follow-up • Differences in child abuse and accident rates across treatment and control groups were greater for those women who had a lower sense of control over their lives
3	HV	Affleck et al.	1989	1. HV-N = 47 2. C = 47	30 sess over 4 m	1 > 2	• For mothers of high-risk infants discharged from newborn intensive care units in greatest need of postnatal support, the home-visiting programme led to increases in parents' responsiveness to their children; their sense of competence as parents; and their perceived control compared to controls
4	HV	Infante-Rivard et al.	1989	1. HV-N (pre + post) + SUP = 21 2. C = 26	8 sess over 7 m	1 > 2	• Home visiting and control groups showed similar improvements in parenting but the treatment group showed lower child hospitalisation rates
5	HV	Barth et al.	1988	1. HV-P (pre + post) = 24 2. C = 26	12 sess over 6 m	1 > 2	• After 6 months compared with controls, the home-visiting group showed significantly fewer child welfare problems, enhanced parental well-being and marginally lower rates of substantiated reports of physical child abuse
6	HV	Barth	1991	HV-P(peri + post) = 97 C = 94	12 sess over 6 m	1 = 2	• After 6 months the intervention and control groups did not differ significantly in levels of parental wellbeing or child welfare • Rates of substantiated reports of physical child abuse were 15% for both groups
7	HV	Hardy & Street	1989	1. HV-P (post) = 131 2. C = 132	46 sess over 2 y	1 > 2	• The group that received intensive home visiting plus support showed a significant reduction in hospitalizations for serious injury and abuse and neglect compared with controls • Compared with controls, parents in the home-visiting group brought their children for fewer medical consultations for routine childhood illnesses and they also showed improvements in parenting practices • For parents to benefit from home-visiting parenting education, the home visitor had to help parents manage life psychosocial and economic stresses and crises which distracted parents from focusing on providing quality infant care
8	HV	Larson	1980	1. HV-P (pre + post) = 35 2. HV-P(post) = 36 3. C = 37	72 sess over 1.5 y	1 > 2 = 3	• Home visiting was only effective for the group that received the intervention both prenatally and postnatally. Those who received postnatal home visiting only did not differ from controls in their adjustment • The accident rate leading to emergency hospital attendance was lower for children in the group who received both pre- and postnatal home visiting • Ratings of the quality of the home environment and the quality of maternal behaviour was best for the group who received home visits before and after the birth of the child

9	BPT	Field et al.	1982	1. BPT-HV (post) = 40 2. BPT = 40 3. C = 40	48 sess over 6 m or 120 sess over 6 m	1 = 2 > 3	• Infants whose parents received behavioural parent training in a home visiting or nursery setting showed greater growth and development than those in the control group during the first 2 years of life • Families in both programmes also showed greater improvement in parent–child interaction than controls but this was not maintained at follow-up • Repeat pregnancy rates were lower and return to school or work rates were higher for mothers who participated in the programmes • On indices of child welfare and development; mother–child interaction; and maternal adjustment families in the programme conducted in the day care facility fared better than families in the home-visiting programme
10	BPT	Burch & Mohr	1980	1. BPT-G = 21 2. C = 10	32 sess over 4 m	1 > 2	• Behavioural parent training led to significant positive changes in parenting attitudes and knowledge compared with controls
11	BPT	Wolfe et al.	1988	1. BPT-G = 16 2. C = 14	29 sess over 20 w	1 > 2	• Behavioural parent training led to a reduction in behavioural problems and fewer problems associated with parenting-risk during follow-up
12	BPT	Resnick, G	1985	1. BPT + LST = 18 2. C = 18	28 sess over 14 w	1 = 2 > 3	• Behavioural parent training led to improvements in parenting attitudes and skills, but only skills gains were maintained at follow-up
13	BPT	Barth et al.	1983	1. BPT-G + SMT = 10 2. C = 10	8 sess over 4 m	1 > 2	• Parents who received group-based behavioural parent training and stress management training showed a decline in anger levels; a decline in negative self-statements; an improvement in parenting attitudes and knowledge; and an improvement in parenting skills
14	SMT	Schinke et al.	1986	1. SMT = 33 2. C = 37	12sess over 3 m	1 > 2	• Stress management training led to improvements in parent well-being and parenting skills, but only improvements in well-being were maintained at follow-up
15	MCI	Lutzker & Rice	1984	1. MCI (pre + post) = 50 2. C = 47	> 40 sess over 1 y	1 > 2	• Significantly fewer incidents of child abuse were reported among the families who participated in the multimodal community intervention programme compared with controls who received routine services
16	MCI	Marchenko & Spence	1994	1. M CI + HV (pre + post) = 110 2. C = 77	> 30 sess over 10 m	1 > 2	• Mothers who participated in the multimodal community-based programme reported a significant decrease in their overall psychological distress and increased access to services and social support from baseline to follow-up, but control group cases did not make similar gains
17	MCI	Lealman et al.	1983	1. MCI (post) = 103 2. C = 209	1 dpw over 18 m	1 = 2	• Families who participated in a multimodal community programme had fewer hospital admissions and fewer admissions for major trauma, but not lower rates of child abuse or neglect
18	MIT	Siegel et al.	1980	1. MIT + HV (post) = 88 2. C = 149	15 sess over 3 m	1 > 2	• Compared with controls, the group who participated in the multimodal inpatient programme showed improvements in mother–infant attachment
19	MIT	Taylor & Beauchamp	1988	1. MIT + HV (post) = 16 2. C = 16	4 sess over 3 w	1 > 2	• The group that received multimodal inpatient treatment followed by home visiting showed improvements in parental attitudes; parental problem-solving; and the quality of parent–child interaction on measures of verbal interaction, discipline and nurturance • These improvements were maintained at 3-month follow-up
20	MIT	O'Connor et al.	1980	1. MIT = 143 2. C = 158	17 m	1 > 2	• Compared with cases in the control group, there were fewer families from the multimodal programme with child hospitalizations, parenting problems, children hospitalized due to parenting problems, cases of suspected child abuse, and children placed in care away from their parents

Notes
HV = home visitation. HV-N = home visiting by nurses. HV-P = home visiting by paraprofessionals. BPT = behavioural parent training. BPT-G = group behavioural parent training. SMT = stress management training. LST = life skills training. MIT = multimodal inpatient intervention. pre = prenatal. post = postnatal. peri = perinatal. C = control group. OP = outpatient. w = weeks. m = months. y = years. sess = sessions.

trained in home visiting procedures, but without formal professional qualifications.

In these studies the mothers participating in the home visitation programmes were visited by a nurse or paraprofessional on a regular basis, usually weekly, for a period of four months to two and a quarter years. In some instances the home visiting began shortly before the birth of the child and in all cases it extended over the infant's first months of life. During these home visits the mothers were provided with social support, advice and education about child care and child development. Furthermore, home visitors modelled and encouraged effective parenting. In some instances home visitors provided respite care and allowed the mothers to have a break from the demanding routine of caring for their infants. The non-judgmental, supportive and empathic quality of the relationship between the home visitor and the mother was central to its effectiveness as a source of support for vulnerable parents at risk of involvement in child abuse.

Gray et al. (1979) provided fifty high-risk mothers with weekly home visits from nurses and bi-monthly consultations with a paediatrician over a period of two and a quarter years and compared the outcome of this group with that of fifty high-risk mothers who received routine services. After two years, participants in the prevention programme fared no better than controls in rates of abnormal parenting as assessed by researcher ratings or child welfare as assessed by the Denver Developmental Screening test (Frankenburg et al., 1970). However, the groups differed in rates of hospitalization for serious accidents potentially attributable to physical child abuse. Five (10%) controls sustained serious injuries (fractured femur, fractured scull, subdural haematoma, third degree burns and barbiturate poisoning) while none of the children in the child abuse prevention programme had sustained any serious injuries at two years of age.

Olds et al. (1986) evaluated a home visitation programme conducted by nurses. All mothers in this programme received home visits prior to their child's birth and half of the mothers received regular visits until their child was two years of age. After two years, for that subgroup of mothers particularly at risk (due to teenage pregnancy, poverty and being a single parent) only 4% of those who participated in the home-visiting programme had substantiated reports of child abuse compared with 19% of their counterparts in the control group. The accident rate leading to emergency hospital attendance was lower for children in the group who received home visiting. Compared with controls, the mothers in the group that received intensive home visiting punished and restricted their children less frequently; reported more child-rearing options; and provided their children with more verbal stimulation. Differences in child abuse and accident rates across treatment and control groups were greater for those women who had a lower sense of control over their lives.

Affleck et al. (1989) evaluated the effects of a home-visiting programme conducted by nurses for mothers of high-risk infants discharged from newborn intensive care units. The programme began with an initial consultation session a few days before discharge. Subsequently, home visits were provided for 15 weeks. For mothers in greatest need of postnatal social and informational support, the home-visiting programme led to increases in parents' responsiveness to their children as assessed by a subscale of the HOME Inventory (Caldwell & Bradley, 1979); increases in their sense of competence as parents as assessed by the Competence Scale of the Parenting Stress Index (Abidin, 1983); and increases in their perceived control over their children's health.

Infante-Rivard et al. (1989) evaluated the effects of a home-visiting programme conducted by nurses for low-SES mothers. Mothers participating in the programme received three prenatal and five postnatal visits while those in the control group only received a routine postnatal visit. Compared with controls, mothers who participated in the home-visiting programme fared better at the end of the programme on those subscales of the HOME inventory (Caldwell & Bradley, 1979) which evaluated avoidance of children and restriction of their activity and the provision of play materials for stimulation of children. The beneficial effects of the programme were greater for parents with more than one child.

In a series of two studies, Barth et al. (1988; Barth, 1991) evaluated the Child Parent Enrichment Project, a home-visiting intervention provided by paraprofessionals to high-risk mothers for a six-month period beginning prenatally. Child welfare was assessed in terms of both the child's history of illness and accidents and also the use of social and health services. In the 1988 study, but not the 1991 study, the programme led to significant improvement in child welfare and reduced rates of child abuse. Substantiated rates of physical child abuse were 8% and 12% in the intervention and control group respectively in the 1988 study and 15% in both groups in the 1991 study. In both studies the programme had no positive impact on maternal well-being as assessed by self-report measures of anxiety (State-Trait Anxiety Inventory; Spielberger, 1973), depression (Center for Epidemiological Studies of Depression Scale; Radloff, 1977), coping (Pearlin & Schooler, 1978) and child abuse potential (Milner, 1980).

Hardy and Street (1989) evaluated a programme in which low-SES families received home visits on a biweekly basis from a paraprofessional, and regular paediatric consultations and support at two- to three-month intervals over two years following the birth of a child. After two years, the group that participated in the home-visiting programme had lower rates of substantiated child abuse reports (2% v 10%) and lower rates of hospitalization (6% v 15%).

Larson (1980) compared the effectiveness of two paraprofessional home visitation programmes one of which began prenatally and the other of which did not commence until six weeks after the birth of the child. Both programmes concluded when children reached fifteen months. When children were eighteen months, the cumulative accident rate for the group that participated in the pre- and postnatal home-visiting programme was significantly lower than that of participants in the postnatal home-visiting programme and the control group. In addition, the emotional and verbal responsiveness of mothers as assessed by the HOME Inventory (Caldwell & Bradley, 1985) from the pre- and postnatal home-visiting programme was significantly higher than that of the other two groups and there was a trend for their maternal behaviour to be more positive.

From the results of the eight studies summarized above and in Tables 8.4 and 8.5, the following conclusions may be drawn. First, programmes for preventing child abuse in which home visiting is a central component have a positive effect on the adjustment of young families. Second, participating in home-visiting programmes can reduce the risk of physical child abuse by half. Averaging across the four studies for which there are data, in only 7% of families that received home visiting were substantiated reports of physical child abuse made after the programmes had concluded compared with 14% of families that did not participate in home-visiting child abuse prevention programmes. Mothers at greater risk (poor, unmarried teenagers) may have derived greatest benefit from home-visiting programmes. Third, participating in home-visiting programmes can reduce the risk of hospitalization by half. Averaging across the three studies for which there are data, in 7% of families that received home visiting children were hospitalized for illnesses or injuries after the programmes had concluded compared with 15% of families that did not participate in home-visiting child abuse prevention programmes. Fourth, home-visiting child abuse prevention programmes had a limited positive effect on self-reported parental well-being. Effect sizes ranged from 0.1 to 0.5 with a mean of 0.3, indicating that the average mother who participated in a home-visiting programme reported a better sense of well-being afterwards than 62% of controls. Fifth, home-visiting child abuse prevention programmes had a limited effect on parents' reports of their children's health, well-being and welfare. Effect sizes ranged from 0 to 1.2 with a mean of 0.3, indicating that the average mother who participated in a home-visiting programme reported that their children fared no better afterwards than 62% of controls. Sixth, programmes in which home visiting began prenatally were probably more effective than those that commenced after the birth of the child. Seventh, there were no consistent differences between programmes in which home visiting was carried out by nurses and those where paraprofessionals conducted home visits. Eighth, most families completed child abuse prevention programmes in which visiting was the central component without dropping out. Drop-out rates from home-visiting programmes ranged from 15% to 33% with a mean of only 20%. Thus, on average, only one in five families dropped out. Drop-out rates were unrelated to programme duration and it is worth noting that some programmes lasted for more than two years. Unfortunately long-term follow-up data were not reported in any of these studies so the durability of the positive effects remains a matter of conjecture and a potential focus for future research.

Behavioural parent training programmes

Five studies in this review examined the effectiveness of child abuse prevention programmes in which behavioural parent training was the central intervention (Barth et al., 1983; Burch & Mohr, 1980; Field et al., 1982; Resnick, 1985; Wolfe et al., 1988). Parent training programmes aim to improve practical parenting skills and parents' knowledge of child development. In most programmes normative information on the physical and psychological development of children is given with particular emphasis on children's needs and abilities at different developmental stages. This is particularly important in child abuse prevention programmes, because inaccurate expectations of infants and lack of awareness of age-appropriate capabilities of young children have repeatedly been found to typify perpetrators of physical child abuse (Carr, 1999). Alongside the acquisition of this intellectual understanding of child development, parents are helped to develop the practical skills required to interpret their infants' preverbal and early verbal communications and respond appropriately to these. Skills for meeting needs for feeding, toileting, sleeping, comforting, communication, stimulation, behavioural limits, relationships with others, and daily routines are taught. Teaching methods based in social learning theory are typically used to train parents. These include modelling, rehearsal, shaping and social reinforcement. Furthermore, the parenting skills taught in these programmes are based on the principles of behavioural psychology and social learning theory also. In the studies reviewed here, programmes ran from four to six months and varied in intensity from daily to weekly sessions.

Field et al., (1982) compared the effectiveness of a child abuse prevention programme which included behavioural parent training offered on a home-visiting basis, and a similar programme that was offered to young mothers while they were being trained as nursery assistants in a day-care facility. These programmes for low-SES, teenage mothers and their infants were conducted postnatally over a six-month period. Infants whose parents participated in both programmes showed greater growth and development than those in the control group during the first two years of life in terms of their body weight and their status on the Denver Developmental Screening Test (Frankenburg et al., 1970) and the Bayley (1969) Scales of Infant Development. Families who participated in the two programmes also showed greater improvement in mother–child interaction, as assessed by researcher ratings, than controls four months into the programme but this improvement was not maintained on the HOME (Caldwell & Bradley, 1979) at follow-up. Repeat pregnancy rates were lower and return to school or work rates were higher for mothers who participated in the programmes. On indices of child welfare and development, mother–child interaction and maternal adjustment, families in the programme conducted in the day care facility fared better than families in the home-visiting programme.

Burch and Mohr (1980) evaluated a behavioural parent training programme for mothers at risk of child abuse. The programme was conducted over four months on an outpatient basis. Compared with a control group, after the programme participants showed increased child development knowledge and more positive parental attitudes.

Wolfe et al. (1988) compared the effectiveness of a behavioural parent training programme with that of routine parent education classes offered at a child protection agency for young at-risk families. The training programme was based on Forehand and McMahon's (1981) manual. As part of the parent training process parents were given video-feedback of their interactions with their children and offered opportunities to discuss constructive criticism with the programme trainers. Parents also received home visits throughout the programme and routine parent education. After the intervention and at three-month follow-up families who participated in the behavioural training programme showed greater improvement on indices of maternal well-being (as assessed by the Child Abuse Inventory (Milner, 1980) and Beck Depression Inventory (Beck et al., 1961)) and child behaviour problems (as assessed by the Behaviour Rating Scales (Coen et al., 1970).

Resnick (1985) evaluated the effectiveness of a behavioural parent training programme combined with life-skills training for an at-risk group of mothers with pre-school children. After the programme, compared with controls participants showed improvements in parent–child relationships as assessed by the Parental Attitudes Research Instrument (Schaefer & Bell, 1958) and behavioural observation. Only the behaviourally observed gains were maintained at one-year follow-up. A third group of mothers in this study completed a self-esteem-building programme. Because this programme was ineffective, data from this aspect of the study have been omitted from Table 8.4.

Barth et al. (1983) evaluated the effectiveness of a behavioural parent training programme combined with a stress management training which included training in self-relaxation and anger management strategies. Following treatment, parents showed a decline in anger levels as assessed by Novaco's (1975) Anger Inventory, more positive self-statements, and improvements in parent–child communication skills.

From the results of the five studies summarized above and in Tables 8.4 and 8.5, the following conclusions may be drawn. First, programmes for preventing child abuse in which behavioural parent training is a central component have a positive effect on the adjustment of young families. Second, behavioural parent training child abuse prevention programmes lead to marked improvements in parental well-being and this is sustained at follow-up. Effect sizes ranged from 0.7 to 1.4 with a mean of 1.0 after training and from 0.5 to 1.0 with a mean of 0.7 at follow-up. This indicates that the average mother who participated in a behavioural parent training programme reported a better sense of well-being afterwards than 84% of controls after training and 76% of controls at follow-up. Third, behavioural parent training child abuse prevention programmes lead to marked improvements in parent reported child welfare and this is sustained at follow-up. Effect sizes ranged from 0.3 to 0.6 with a mean of 0.5 after training and from 0.5 to 3.2 with a mean of 1.5 at follow-up. This indicates that the average mother who participated in a behavioural parent training programme reported better child welfare than 69% of controls after training and 93% of controls at follow-up. Fourth, behavioural parent training child abuse prevention programmes lead to marked short-term improvements in parenting skills. Effect sizes ranged from 0 to 1.3 with a mean of 0.6 after training, indicating that the average mother who participated in a behavioural parent training programme was judged by researchers to have better parenting skills than 69% of controls after training. Fifth, short-term gains in parenting skills arising from participation in behavioural parenting training programmes are not maintained at follow-up and there is significant attrition from these programmes. The average effect size at follow-up is 0 and the average drop-out rate is 50%. Future research should focus on finding ways to help parents remain engaged in behavioural parent training programmes and to continue to use the skills they learn in these programmes after completion. It is also imperative that research in this area routinely includes rates of child abuse and hospitalization as outcome variables. No data on the impact of behavioural parent training programmes on these outcome variables were reported in the studies reviewed here.

Stress management training

Schinke et al. (1986) evaluated the effectiveness of a stress management programme designed to lower the risk of family violence for a group of teenage parents. The programme included training in problem-solving skills, communication skills, self-instructional coping strategies, relaxation skills, and the skills necessary for developing a social support network. After treatment and at follow-up significant improvements in parental well-being occurred on a range of indices of personal adjustment and stress management skills. At three-month follow-up, improvements in parenting competence also occurred. From this study it may be concluded that stress management training may have an important role to play in child abuse prevention programmes for young parents. Effect sizes of 0.5 for parental well-being after training and at follow-up indicate that the average mother who participated in this stress management training programme fared better than 69% of controls after training and three months later. The effect size of 0.6 for parenting competence which occurred at follow-up indicates that the average mother who participated in this stress management training programme fared better than 69% of controls three months after completing the programme.

Multimodal community-based intervention

In three studies multimodal community-based prevention programmes for physical child abuse were evaluated (Lealman et al., 1983; Lutzker & Rice, 1984; Marchenko & Spence, 1994). These all involved the provision of a range of health care, social and educative services on an outpatient basis to families at risk for physical child abuse.

Lutzker & Rice (1984) evaluated the Project 12 Ways ecobehavioural phys-ical child abuse prevention programme. At-risk families referred from a child protection agency in southern Illinois were referred to this multimodal pro-gramme which incorporated home visiting. Families who participated in this programme received tailormade home-based behavioural intervention pro-grammes to help them solve a wide range of child care problems, family difficulties and personal problems. Programmes included parent education, behavioural parent training, parental stress management training, life skills training, and supportive counselling. Data from the State Central Registry for child abuse showed that the programme significantly reduced the rate of child abuse and neglect. Compared with control group families who received routine services, those in the multimodal programme showed lower rates of child abuse and neglect during the programme (2% v 11%); lower rates of child abuse and neglect in the year following the programme (8% v 11%); lower rates of children who were abused two or more times (0% v 6%); and lower overall rates of abuse and neglect incidents during and after the programme (10% v 32%).

Marchenko & Spence (1994) evaluated the effectiveness of a multimodal community-based child abuse prevention programme for women and their newborns in which families received a range of services from the time of the mother's first prenatal visit until the child was a year old. The programme was delivered by a social worker, a nurse and a paraprofessional home visitor. The social worker helped mothers access services and conducted individual and family counselling. The nurse addressed the infant's and family's physical health care needs. The home visitor conducted parent training and provided young mothers with a socially supportive relationship. After ten months compared with families in the control group, those in the programme reported receiving more help in accessing a range of services including baby clothing, baby furniture and toys, transportation and personal clothing. They also reported experiencing an increased level of social support during the programme especially from members of the extended family and friends. Compared with controls, mothers who participated in the programme also experienced fewer psychological problems.

Lealman et al. (1983) evaluated a multimodal programme for at-risk fam-ilies with young children in Bradford, UK. The programme involved postna-tal contact with social worker and access to a drop-in centre where help could be sought from a health visitor on demand. Data from medical and social service records and the child abuse register collected when children were eighteen months showed that compared with an untreated control group infants whose families participated in the multimodal programme had fewer hospital admissions (4% v 19%), fewer admissions for major trauma (1% v 2%) but not lower rates of child abuse (1% v 1%) or neglect (12% v 2%).

From the results of the three studies summarized above and in Tables 8.4 and 8.5, the following conclusions may be drawn. First, multimodal community-based programmes for preventing physical child abuse have a positive effect on the adjustment of young families. Second, participating in multimodal programmes can reduce the risk of physical child abuse by more than half. Averaging across the two studies for which there are data, in only 6% of families that participated in multimodal programmes were substantiated reports of physical child abuse made after the programmes had concluded compared with 17% of families that did not participate in multimodal child abuse prevention programmes. Third, participating in multimodal community-based programmes can reduce the risk of hospitalization by a factor of four. However, this is a tentative finding based upon a single study in which hospitalization rates were 4% for families that participated in the multimodal programme and 19% for controls. Fourth, multimodal child abuse prevention programmes increase self-reported parental well-being. However, this is a tentative finding based upon a single study in which the effect size for parental distress was 0.4, indicating that the average mother who participated in a multimodal programme reported a better sense of well-being afterwards than only 66% of controls. Fifth, most families completed multimodal prevention programmes without dropping out. Drop-out rates from multimodal community-based programmes ranged from 6% to 27% with a mean of only 17%. Thus, on average, fewer than one in five families dropped out. The highest drop-out rate occurred in the study where home visiting was not a central part of the multimodal programme. Unfortunately long-term follow-up data were not reported in any of these studies so the durability of the positive effects remains a matter of conjecture and a potential focus for future research.

Multimodal inpatient intervention

In three studies multimodal inpatient prevention programmes for physical child abuse were evaluated (O'Connor et al., 1980; Siegel et al., 1980; Taylor & Beauchamp, 1988). These all involved the provision of a range of health care, social and educative services on an inpatient basis to young mothers and their infants at risk for physical child abuse.

Siegel et al. (1980) evaluated an intensive multimodal inpatient programme for low SES mothers who had perinatal complications and their newborn infants. The programme involved early and extended physical mother–infant contact to promote bonding and following discharge an intensive home-visiting programme. Mothers had a minimum of 45 minutes of contact with their infants during the first three hours postpartum and subsequently five hours contact per day until discharge. Thereafter they received regular weekly home visits from a paraprofessional for three months with a focus on parent education, fostering positive mother–child interaction, providing support, and stress management training. At four months, the quality of attachment shown by mothers and infants was better for the group that participated in the multimodal programme and this was accounted for by the early and extended mother–infant contact, not the home-visiting programme. At twelve months, the amount of positive behaviour shown by infants was greater in the group that participated in the multimodal programme and this too was accounted for by the early and extended mother–infant contact, not the home-visiting programme. The groups did not differ in their rates of child abuse or hospitalization a year after the programme.

Taylor and Beauchamp (1988) evaluated a brief one-month multimodal inpatient child-abuse prevention programme. Mothers participating in this programme received intensive support, parent education, stress management, help accessing services in a series of sessions that began while in hospital and continued on a home-visiting basis after discharge. At the conclusion of the programme, compared with controls participants showed significant gains in self-reported knowledge of child development, parenting attitudes, and parenting skills as assessed by an observational rating scale. These gains were maintained at three-month follow-up.

O'Connor et al. (1980) evaluated the effectiveness of a multimodal inpatient programme which involved increased mother–infant contact during the postpartum period. Mothers and infants spent up to eight hours together per day until discharge in a special rooming-in suite in a maternity hospital. Seventeen months later hospital and social service records showed that mothers and infants who participated in the multimodal inpatient programme fared better than controls who received routine care. Compared with mothers in the control group, there were fewer families from the multimodal programme with child hospitalizations (14% v 17%), parenting problems (2% v 7%), children hospitalized due to parenting problems (1% v 6%), cases of suspected child abuse (1% v 4%), and children placed in care away from their parents (0% v 4%).

From the results of the three studies summarized above and in Tables 8.4 and 8.5, the following conclusions may be drawn. First, multimodal inpatient programmes for preventing physical child abuse have a positive effect on the adjustment of young families. Second, multimodal inpatient programmes lead to marked short-term improvements in parenting skills, knowledge and attitudes. Effect sizes ranged from 0.9 to 2.6 with a mean of 1.3 after programme completion, indicating that the average mother who participated in a multimodal inpatient programme was judged by researchers to have better parenting skills than 90% of controls. There is some evidence to suggest that gains in parenting knowledge are maintained at follow-up. Third, the evidence from two studies provides no support for the view that multimodal inpatient programmes of the type described in this review prevent child abuse or child hospitalization. Averaging across the two studies, child abuse rates for cases that participated in multimodal inpatient programmes and controls were 5% and child hospitalization rates for intervention and control groups were 12%. Fourth, most mothers completed multimodal inpatient prevention programmes without dropping out. Drop-out rates from multimodal inpatient programmes ranged from 6% to 15% with a mean of only 11%. Thus, on average, about one in ten families dropped out. Unfortunately long-term follow-up data were not reported in any of these studies so the durability of the positive effects remains a matter of conjecture and a potential focus for future research.

Conclusions

Because physical child abuse is a violation of children's rights, because it leads to deleterious short- and long-term psychological consequences, and because the prevalence of serious physical abuse is about 10%, the prevention of physical child abuse is imperative. Physical abuse occurs in families characterized by high levels of stress and low levels of support when children place demands on their parents which outstrip parental coping resources, and parents in frustration injure their children. Criteria for selecting parents for inclusion in prevention programmes include some combination of specific child characteristics, specific maternal characteristics and particular family and social characteristics indicative of vulnerability to physical child abuse. Programmes designed to prevent physical child abuse aim to reduce stress, increase support, enhance parenting knowledge and skills, and promote child health so as to reduce demands children place on vulnerable parents. The child abuse prevention programmes reviewed here involved home-visiting, behavioural parent training, life skills training, stress management training and the provision of paediatric medical care for children. In some instances these interventions were offered in isolation, while in others they were combined into complex multimodal inpatient or community-based programmes.

From the results of the twenty studies reviewed here it may be concluded that home-visiting programmes, behavioural parent training programmes, and both inpatient and community-based multimodal programmes all either modify risk factors for physical child abuse or reduce the risk for physical child abuse or both. Participating in home-visiting programmes, particularly those that begin prenatally, can reduce the risk of physical child abuse and child hospitalization by half. Poor, unmarried teenage mothers may derive greatest benefit from home-visiting programmes. Both nurses and paraprofessional home visitors can deliver effective home-visiting interventions. But home-visiting programmes have minimal impact on parents' self-reports of well-being or child welfare. In contrast both stress management training programmes and behavioural parent training child abuse prevention programmes lead to marked short-term improvements in parental well-being and in parent-reported child welfare and this is sustained at follow-up.

Unfortunately the marked short-term improvements in parenting skills which arise from participation in behavioural parent training child abuse prevention programmes are not maintained at follow-up. The studies reviewed here suggest that, to some degree, multimodal community-based programmes confer the benefits of both home-visiting programmes and behavioural parent training in that they can reduce the risk of physical child abuse by more than half and can reduce the risk of hospitalization by a factor of four, but in addition increase self-reported parental well-being. Attrition is a problem in all physical child abuse prevention programmes. The evidence reviewed in this chapter shows that the lowest drop-out rates occur in home-visiting and multimodal programmes and the highest drop-out rates occur in behavioural parent training programmes conducted on a group basis in community centres rather than in parents' homes or inpatient settings.

Implications for policy and practice

The implications of these conclusions for policy and practice are clear. Families at risk for physical child abuse should be identified by screening mothers prenatally using the criteria listed in Table 8.1. Subsequently they should be engaged in multimodal community-based programmes which begin prenatally and which include home visiting conducted by nurses or paraprofessionals, behavioural parent training, stress management and life skills training until a comprehensive multidisciplinary assessment of risk factors indicates that the risk of physical abuse has been substantially reduced. It is acknowledged that this approach may be coupled in a comprehensive prevention policy with primary prevention approaches that focus on the whole population by, for example, reducing poverty.

Implications for research

The studies reviewed in this chapter have implications for future research. There is a need to evaluate not only immediate indicators of post-programme improvements on indices of abuse potential such as parental well-being, child welfare, parenting skills and parents' knowledge of child development, but also the long-term impact of such programmes on child abuse rates, child hospitalization rates and child development.

There is considerable evidence that fathers may play an important role in the aetiology of physical child abuse and also that father involvement in family therapy can have a significant impact on outcome (Carr, 2001c). Despite this, physical child abuse prevention programmes, such as those evaluated in the studies reviewed in this chapter, have rarely involved fathers. Future research should evaluate the impact of programmes that target both fathers and mothers as programme participants.

Future research should evaluate manualized intervention programmes in which checks for programme integrity are made. In such studies, training sessions are recorded and blind raters use programme integrity checklists to evaluate the degree to which sessions approximate manualized training curricula. Such integrity checks allow researchers to say with confidence the degree to which a pure and potent version of their programme has been evaluated.

Studies that examine the impact of design features that may make programmes more effective are required. Specifically research is needed on the effects of including different components in multimodal programmes (home visiting, behavioural parent training, stress management and life skills training, personal counselling, family therapy and so forth) and the effects of programmes of differing durations.

Studies are required which investigate the mechanisms and processes that underpin programme effectiveness. Improvements probably occur through a variety of complex mechanisms including increasing support to parents; enhancing parental child care knowledge and skills; empowering parents to manage external stresses and internal negative mood states which precipitate abusive actions; and supporting the development of secure parent–child attachments.

Not all families respond equally to physical child abuse prevention programmes. There is a need to design and evaluate programmes for families that have particular difficulties in responding to routine multimodal prevention programmes. There is also a need to research ways to help parents remain engaged in certain types of interventions, particularly behavioural parent training programmes, and to continue to use the skills they learn in these programmes after programme completion.

Assessment resources

Abidin, R. (1983). *Parenting Stress Index*. Charlottesville, VA: Pediatric Psychology Press.

Barth, R., Hacking, S. & Ash, J.R. (1988). Preventing child abuse: An experimental evaluation of the Child Parent Enrichment Project. *Journal of Primary Prevention*, 8(4), 201–217.

Bromwich, R. (1983). *Parent Behaviour Progression*. Unpublished manual, California State University, Northridge, CA.

Caldwell, B. & Bradley, R. (1985). *Home Observation for Measurement of the Environment*. New York: Dorsey Press.

Carey, W.B. (1970). A simplified method for measuring infant temperament. *Journal of Pediatrics*, 77, 188–194.

Clark-Stewart, K. (1973). Interactions between mothers and their young children: Characteristics and consequences. *Monograph of Social Research on Child Development*, 153, 1–100.

Helfer, R., Hoffmeister, J. & Schneider, C. (1978). *The Michigan Screening Profile of Parenting*. Boulder, CO: Manual Test Analyis and Development Corporation.

Milner, J.S. (1980). *The Child Abuse Inventory: Manual*. Webster, NC: Psytec.

Murphy, S., Orkow, B. & Nicola, R. (1985). Prenatal prediction of child abuse and neglect: A prospective study. *Child Abuse and Neglect*, 9, 225–235.

Schaefer, E. & Bell, R. (1958). Development of a Parental Attitudes Research Instrument (PARI). *Child Development*, 29, 337–361.

Schneider, C., Helfer, R. & Pollock, E. (1972). The predictive questionnaire: A preliminary report. In C. Hempe & R. Helfer (Ed.), *Helping the Battered Child and His Family*. Philadelphia: JB Lippincott.

Programme resources

Kelly, J. (1983). *Treating Abusive Families: Interventions Based on Skills Training Principles*. New York: Plenum.

Schaefer, C. & Friemeister, J. (1989). *Handbook of Parent Training*. New York: Wiley.

Willis, D., Holden, E. & Rosenberg, M. (1992). *Prevention of Child Maltreatment: Developmental and Ecological Perspectives*. New York: Wiley.

Wolfe, D. (1991). *Preventing Physical and Emotional Abuse of Children*. New York: Guilford.

Wolfe, D. & McMahon, R. (1997). *Child Abuse: New Directions in Prevention and Treatment Across the Lifespan*. Thousand Oaks, CA: Sage.

9 Prevention of child sexual abuse

Yvonne Duane and Alan Carr

Child sexual abuse (CSA) is now recognized as a problem of significant proportions in most industrialized cultures, a problem requiring urgent preventative action (Briere et al., 1996). From the results of a national survey, Finkelhor and Dziuba-Leatherman (1995) concluded that two-thirds of children in the USA participate in school-based CSA prevention programmes. In Ireland *The Stay Safe Programme*, a CSA prevention programme specifically designed for the Irish educational context, is conducted in almost all schools in the Republic of Ireland (MacIntyre & Lawlor, 1991; MacIntyre & Carr, 2000). While the ubiquity of CSA prevention programmes is a laudable response to the growing recognition of CSA as an important problem, the effectiveness of much CSA prevention remains untested (MacIntyre & Carr, 2000). The aim of this chapter is to review methodologically robust research studies on the effectiveness of CSA prevention programmes, draw reliable conclusions about the effectiveness of these, and outline the implications of these conclusions for policy and practice.

Child sexual abuse refers to any sexual activity involving a child and adult, or significantly older child, where activities are intended for sexual stimulation of the perpetrator and which constitute an abusive condition, such as when the child is coerced or tricked into the activity, or when there is a discrepancy in age between the participants, indicating a lack of consensuality (Wurtele, 1997). Sexual abuse may vary in intrusiveness (from viewing or exposure to penetration) and frequency (from a single episode to frequent and chronic abuse). A distinction is made between intrafamilial sexual abuse, the most common form of which is father–daughter incest, and extrafamilial sexual abuse where the abuser resides outside the family home.

Epidemiology

Reliably establishing the number of children who experience sexual abuse is difficult. In Ireland, McKeown and Gilligan's study (1991) found the number of confirmed cases of CSA to be 1.2 per 1,000 children. However, this is likely to be a considerable underestimate of the problem, as most cases of CSA are never officially reported (Finkelhor, 1984). Estimates of prevalence rates vary from 2 to 30% in males and 4 to 30% in females depending on definitions used and population studied (Carr, 1999).

Sexual abuse has profound short- and long-term effects on psychological functioning (Berliner & Elliott, 1996; Kendall-Tackett et al., 1993; Wolfe & Birt, 1995). About two-thirds of sexually abused children develop psychological symptoms. Behaviour problems shown by children who have experienced sexual abuse typically include sexualized behaviour, excessive internalizing or externalizing behaviour problems, school-based attainment problems and relationship difficulties. In the eighteen-month period following the cessation of abuse in about two-thirds of cases behaviour problems abate. Up to a quarter of cases develop more severe problems. About a fifth of cases show clinically significant long-term problems which persist into adulthood.

Aetiology

Finkelhor (1984) has argued that four preconditions must be met for CSA to occur. The abuser must be motivated to abuse, overcome internal inhibitions, overcome external inhibitions and finally the child must be unable to resist the abuser's actions. Tutty (1991) has shown that prevention programmes for child sexual abuse may be classified in terms of the particular preconditions, identified in Finkelhor's (1984) model, they target. Some programmes, focusing largely on treatment of offenders, target the perpetrator's motivation to abuse children and on offenders' lax internal inhibitions. Others aim to increase external inhibitions by promoting awareness concerning sexual abuse in key groups such as parents and teachers. A third approach to prevention is to increase children's capacity to resist abuse by training them in appropriate skills. In this chapter our main concern is with prevention programmes which target children, parents and teachers, that is programmes which are largely concerned with tackling the third and fourth preconditions from Finkelhor's (1984) model.

Previous reviews

Evaluation studies addressing programme efficacy have been summarized in a few narrative reviews (Carrol et al., 1992; Finkelhor & Strapko, 1992; MacMillan et al., 1994a, 1994b; MacIntyre & Carr, 2000). The broad conclusions of these are that most children benefit from participation in CSA prevention programmes. They acquire self-protective knowledge and skills which may help them prevent perpetrators from sexually abusing them.

Rispens et al. (1997) in their meta-analysis of studies which evaluated the effectiveness of CSA prevention programmes reported a large post-intervention mean effect size of 0.7. This suggests that, immediately after programme participation, the average child has better prevention skill and knowledge than 76% of untreated control cases. The follow-up mean effect size in this meta-analysis was 0.6. Rispens concluded that programmes were effective in teaching sexual abuse concepts and self-protection skills and that children who participate in CSA prevention programmes retain their self-protective knowledge even after a number of months have elapsed. It was also found that this held true even for relatively young children. Programmes with explicit training were more effective in increasing self-protection skill than were less explicit skills oriented programmes.

The curricula of prevention programmes considered in previous reviews covered the topics listed in Table 9.1, although not all topics were covered in all programmes. Child-focused training methods varied from programme to programme with some programmes using traditional 'talk and chalk' didactic methods and others using multimedia active behavioural skills training procedures such as video modelling, role-playing, rehearsal and discussion. Some programmes were multisystemic, insofar as they included modules for significant members of children's social systems such as teachers and parents in addition to child-focused training. Most reviewers found that

Table 9.1 Core concepts in curricula of CSA school-based prevention programmes

Body ownership	• The child's body belongs to her or him and the child has a right to control access to her or his body
Touch	• A distinction may be made between 'good', 'bad' and 'confusing' touches • A child may permit a good touch and reject a bad or confusing touch from an adult or another child
Saying 'NO'	• A child has right to say 'No' when approached or touched inappropriately and the skill of saying 'No' should be practised
Escape	• It is important to escape from potential perpetrators and skills for escaping must be practised so the child will be prepared if the need to escape arises
Secrecy	• A distinction may be made between appropriate surprises (which are fun) and inappropriate secrets (which are scary) • A child should talk about any touch he or she is asked to keep a secret
Intuition	• A child should trust his or her own feelings when he or she feels something is not quite right
Support systems	• Children should identify adults that they can turn to for help when they wish to make a disclosure of abuse or attempted abuse • A child should seek help from another adult if the first adult does not listen or believe his or her disclosure
Blame	• A child is not to blame if he or she is abused or victimized
Bullying	• Bullying is unfair and wrong • Be assertive with bullies and tell trusted adults about them • Support your friends if they are bullied

multisystemic programmes which targeted children, parents and teachers and which incorporated multimedia active behavioural skills training methods were particularly effective. However, there was considerable variability in the methodological quality of the studies included in these previous reviews. One goal of the present review was to focus exclusively on well-designed studies, so that conclusions about the most effective approach to prevention of CSA could be drawn with considerable confidence.

Method

The aim of the present review was to identify effective classroom-based CSA prevention programmes. A PsychLit database search of English language journals for the years 1977 to 2000 was conducted to identify studies in which CSA prevention programmes were evaluated. The term *sexual abuse prevention*, limited to the term *child*, was combined with terms such as *programme*, *study*, *evaluation*, *school-based* and *effect*. A manual search through the bibliographies of all recent reviews, and relevant journals on child sexual abuse prevention was also conducted. Studies were selected for review if they had a group design, which included a classroom-based treatment and control or comparison group; if at least ten cases were included in each group; and if reliable pre- and post-treatment measures were included. Using these criteria sixteen studies were initially selected. One study, which used post-treatment measures only, was added to this group of studies because of the large number of participants and its significance in the CSA prevention literature, i.e. Oldfield et al., 1996. Thus a total of seventeen studies were selected for inclusion in this review.

Characteristics of studies

An overview of the characteristics of the seventeen selected studies is set out in Table 9.2. The studies were classified in terms of the main intervention they evaluated or their design features. The first two studies examined the effects of observing a play in which self-protective skills were modelled by actors. The next four studies evaluated the impact of child-focused self-protective behavioural skills training programmes. The next three studies were comparative in design, with one comparing different types of prevention programmes and two comparing the effects of different types of instructors on the outcome of the prevention programmes. Eight of the studies evaluated complex prevention programmes. These programmes used multimodal training methods or targeted multiple systems or both. All studies were published between 1985 and 1997. Of the studies, fourteen were conducted in the USA, two in Canada and one in Ireland.

Aggregating across all seventeen studies there were 3,623 programme participants and 2,186 controls in total. In programmes using a single, dedicated type of intervention there were 2,217 participants with 1,296 controls. In

Table 9.2 Characteristics of CSA prevention studies

Study no.	Authors	Year	N per group	Mean age and range	Gender	Family characteristics	Programme setting	Programme duration
1	Oldfield et al.	1996	Play	1. PL-C = 658 2. C = 611	6–12 y	M = 47% F = 53%	Low SES = 22% Cauc = 86%	Schools	1 × 45 min
2	Tutty	1992	Play	1. PL-C = 100 2. PL-C = 100 3. C = 100 4. C = 100	4–12 y	—	Low SES	8 Schools	1 × 45 min
3	Nemerofsky et al.	1994	Behavioural skills training	1. BT-C = 1,044 2. C = 295	4.5 y 3–6 y	M = 48% F = 52%	—	Day-care centres	5 d
4	Sarno and Wurtele	1997	Behavioural skills training	1. BT-C = 41 2. P = 34	4.6 y 3–5 y	M = 52% F = 48%	2-parent families = 44% SPF = 45% Other = 12% Low SES	Preschool	5 d
5	Wurtele & Sarno-Owens	1997	Behavioural skills training	1. BT-C = 262 2. C = 144	4.5 y 3–5 y	F = 52% M = 48%	2-parent families = 55% SPF = 40% Other = 5%	Preschools	5 d
6	Wurtele	1990	Behavioural skills training	1. BT-C = 12 2. C = 12	4.2 y	M = 71% F = 29%	Majority 2-parent families Mid SES	YMCA pre-school	3 d × 25 min
7	Wurtele et al.	1989	Comparative	1. BT-C = 32 2. GT-C = 37 3. P = 31	5 y 4–6 y	M = 49% F = 51%	Low SES	2 Preschools	3 d × 5 h
8	Wurtele et al.	1992a	Comparative	1. BT-C(T) = 21 2. BT-C(P) = 18 3. C = 22	4.8 y	M = 54% F = 46%	2-parent families = 56% SPF = 33% Other = 11% Low SES	Preschool Home Combination	1. 3 × 5 h 2. 1.5 h over 1 w
9	Wurtele et al.	1992b	Comparative	1. BT-C(T) = 41 2. BT-C(P) = 44 3. BT-C(T + P) = 43 4. P = 44	4.6 y	M = 43% F = 57%	2-parent families = 48% SPF = 51% Other = 1% Low SES	Preschool Home Combination	1. 4 × 15 min 2. 2.5 h over 4 d 3. Combination
10	Conte	1985	Multimodal	1. GT-C + BT-C = 20 2. C = 20	4–5 y 6–10 y	M = 60% F = 40%	—	Day-care centre	3 × 1 h
11	Fryer et al.	1987 a,b	Multimodal	1. GT-C + BT-C = 23 2. C = 21	4–7 y	—	—	School	8 × 20 min

Table 9.2 continued

Study no.	Authors	Year		N per group	Mean age and range	Gender	Family characteristics	Programme setting	Programme duration
12	Harvey	1988	Multimodal	1. VT-C + GT-C + BT-C = 35 2. C = 36	5.8 y 5–6 y	M = 46.5% F = 53.5%	Low–mid SES	4 Schools	3 × .5 h
13	Saslawsky and Wurtele	1986	Multimodal	1. VT-C + GT-C = 33 2. C = 34	J = 6.2 y S = 11.1 y	M = 52% F = 48%	Low–mid SES	Schools	1 × 50 min
14	Tutty	1997	Multimodal	1. VT-C + GT-C + BT-C = 117 2. C = 114	4–12 y	—	Majority 2-parent families	2 Schools	2 × 45–60 min
15	Hazzard et al.	1991	Multisystemic Multimodal	1. VT-C + GT-C + BT-C + GT-T = 286 2. C = 113	8–9 y	M = 50% F = 50%	Mid SES.	6 Schools	1. 3 × 1 h + 6 h workshop 2. 3 × 1 h 3. 6 h workshop
16	Kolko et al.	1987	Multisystemic Multimodal	1. VT-C + GT-C + GT-T + GT-P = 125 2. VT-C + GT-C + GT-T + GT-P = 173 3. C = 41	9 y 7–10 y	M = 53% F = 47%	Low–mid SES	3 Schools	2 × 1.5h
17	MacIntyrre and Carr	2000	Multisystemic Multimodal	1. VT-C + GT-C + BT-C + GT-T + VT-T + GT-P + VT-P = 358 2. C = 414	J = 8 y S = 10 y	M = 55% F = 45%	Married parents = 96%	Schools	12 × 30–40 min

Notes
C = control group. P = attention placebo control group. PL-C = children, observing a play. GT-C = instructional group training for children based on discussion. GT-P = instructional group training for parents based on discussion. GT-T = instructional group training for teachers based on discussion. BT-C = behavioural skills training for children involving role-play and rehearsal. BT-P = behavioural skills training for parents. BT-C(P) = behavioural skills training for children involving role-play and rehearsal, taught by parents. BT-C(T) = behavioural skills training for children involving role-play and rehearsal, taught by teachers. VT-C = video-based training for children. VT-P = video-based training for parents. VT-T = video-based training for teachers. y = year. SES = socioeconomic status. SPF = single parent family. h = hour. min = minutes. d = day. w = week. m = month. S = senior. J = junior.

studies comparing interventions there were 355 participants and 135 controls. In programmes that compared instructors there were 167 participants and 66 controls. In the multi-component/multisystemic interventions group there were 1,170 participants and 793 controls.

The duration of interventions ranged from one to twelve sessions with length of sessions ranging from fifteen minutes to six hours. Across studies participants' ages ranged from three to twelve years. The mean age of children was six and a half years. For the fourteen studies in which gender data was given 52% were male and 48% were female.

From the twelve studies in which data on socioeconomic status (SES) were given, it may be concluded that the majority of children came from either low or low to middle income families. Six studies gave data on family characteristics. From these is may be concluded that the majority of children came from two-parent families and a sizeable minority (around 40%) came from single-parent families. CSA prevention programmes evaluated in the seventeen studies reviewed here were conducted in primary schools, preschools or day care centre settings.

Methodological features

The methodological features for the seventeen studies are given in Table 9.3. All studies included demographically similar participants and controls. Fourteen of seventeen studies randomly assigned participants to treatment and control or comparison groups. With one exception (Oldfield et al., 1996), all studies conducted assessments immediately before intervention. Post-intervention assessments were used in all studies and in twelve of the seventeen studies follow-up assessments were conducted at time periods ranging from six weeks to twelve months after the end of the prevention programme. The studies evaluated the effectiveness of prevention programmes using measures of child, parent and teacher knowledge, and child behaviour and skill. Only one of the studies evaluated programme effectiveness using actual behavioural responses to simulated situations (Fryer et al., 1987a, 1987b). Child self-report measures were employed in all studies. Some studies used combinations of parent, teacher and child reports. Three studies included therapist or trainer ratings and only one included researcher ratings. Eight studies reported data on the number of drop-outs. Nine of the studies examined negative outcomes of participation in programmes, including increased fear and anxiety, behaviour problems, negative sense of sexuality and over-generalization of concepts to benign touches. Six studies collected data on child sexual abuse disclosures. Programme integrity was checked in six of the studies and in only three studies were programmes delivered by experienced trainers. However, this possible shortcoming may be offset by the fact that in all but three of the studies interventions were explicitly manualized so that they could be reliably delivered by teachers, preschool and day care staff. Therefore consistency of content and format was more likely in these

Table 9.3 Methodological features of CSA prevention studies

Feature	Study number																
	S1	S2	S3	S4	S5	S6	S7	S8	S9	S10	S11	S12	S13	S14	S15	S16	S17
Control or comparison group	1	1	1	1	1	1	1	1	1	1	1	1	1	1	1	0	1
Random assignment	1	0	1	1	1	1	1	1	1	1	1	1	1	1	1	0	0
Demographic similarity	1	1	1	1	1	1	1	1	1	1	1	1	1	1	1	1	1
Pre-treatment assessment	0	1	1	1	1	1	1	1	1	1	1	1	1	1	1	1	1
Post-treatment assessment	1	1	1	1	1	1	1	1	1	1	1	1	1	1	1	1	1
1 month + follow-up assessment	1	1	0	0	0	1	1	1	1	0	1	1	1	0	1	1	1
Children's self-report	1	1	1	0	1	1	1	1	1	1	1	1	1	1	1	1	1
Parents' ratings	0	0	0	0	0	1	1	1	1	0	0	0	0	1	1	0	1
Teachers' ratings	0	0	0	0	0	0	0	1	1	0	0	0	0	0	0	0	1
Therapist or trainer ratings	0	0	0	0	0	0	0	1	1	0	0	0	0	1	0	0	0
Researcher ratings	0	0	0	0	0	1	0	0	0	1	1	0	1	1	0	0	0
Negative effects assessed	1	0	0	0	0	1	1	1	1	1	0	1	1	1	1	1	1
Drop-out assessed	0	1	1	0	0	0	0	1	1	0	0	0	0	0	0	0	1
Clinical significance of change assessed	0	1	0	1	1	1	1	0	1	0	0	0	0	1	1	1	0
Experienced therapists or trainers used	0	0	0	0	0	0	1	0	0	0	0	0	0	1	1	0	0
Programmes were equally valued	0	0	0	1	1	0	0	1	0	0	0	0	1	0	0	0	0
Programmes were manualized	1	1	1	1	1	1	0	1	1	1	0	1	1	0	1	1	1
Supervision was provided	0	0	0	0	0	0	0	0	0	0	0	0	0	0	0	0	0
Programme integrity checked	0	0	1	0	0	0	1	0	1	1	0	0	0	0	0	1	1
Subsequent disclosure data given	1	0	0	1	0	0	0	1	0	0	0	0	0	0	1	1	1
Total	9	9	8	9	8	13	14	16	17	8	11	9	8	10	12	12	13

Notes

S = study. 1 = design feature was present. 0 = design feature was absent.

programmes. In three of the programmes supervision of trainers was provided. The statistical significance of changes in self-protective knowledge and skill was reported in all studies. In eight studies data on the clinical significance of intervention effects were reported. Overall this was a methodologically robust group of studies.

Substantive findings

A summary of the effect sizes and outcome rates for the seventeen studies is presented in Table 9.4 and Table 9.5 summarizes, in narrative form, the key findings of each of the studies.

Self-protection modelled through drama

Different plays with similar themes were used in the two studies which examined the effect of observing a play which modelled self-protective skills. Oldfield et al. (1996) used the Project TRUST play *Touch* (Riestenberg, 1993) and Tutty (1992) used the play *Touching* by Michael Adkin. In both plays the central characters were placed in situations where they could model the self-protective knowledge and skills curriculum outlined in Table 9.1. In each study, plays were followed by participative question and answer discussions in which points raised in the plays were elaborated. Effect sizes based on scores from Tutty's (1995) Children's Knowledge of Abuse Questionnaire completed after watching the play were 0.2 and 0.5 with a mean of 0.4, indicating that following these programmes the average participant had more self-protective knowledge and skills than 66% of children in the control group. Three- to five-month follow-up data from these studies yielded effect sizes of 0.1 (Tutty, 1992) and 0.9 (Oldfield et al., 1996). The effects of Oldfield et al.'s (1996) programme were particularly durable, with the average child's self-protective knowledge score being higher than 82% of those of children in the control group three months after the programme. Disclosure data were also collected and a higher number of disclosures of sexual abuse were found in the intervention group (0.6%) compared with the control group (0.2%) during the follow-up period. Oldfield et al. (1996) found that knowledge acquisition was greater for older children and also that the programme did not lead to increased anxiety.

The results of these two studies confirm that CSA prevention programmes which involve observing a play that models self-protective skills and discussing its implications can effectively improve knowledge about sexual abuse and this improved knowledge persists over time, with greatest gains being made by older children.

Table 9.4 Summary of results of treatment effects and outcome rates from CSA prevention studies

Variable	Play studies — Study 1 BT-C v P	Play studies — Study 2 PL-C v C	BST — Study 3 GT-C v C	BST — Study 4 BT-C v P	BST — Study 5 BT-C v C	BST — Study 6 PL-C v C	Comparative — Study 7 BT-C v P	Comparative — Study 7 GT-C v P	Comparative — Study 8 BT-C(T) v C	Comparative — Study 8 BT-C(P) v C	Comparative — Study 9 BT-C(T) v P	Comparative — Study 9 BT-C(P) v P	Comparative — Study 9 BT-C(T+P) v P
Improvement after programme													
Children's self-report skill	1.2	—	2.7	1.1	1.2	—	0.7	0.5	1.0	1.4	0.8	1.3	1.4
Children's self-reported knowledge	0.8	0.2	—	0.0	0.5	0.5	—	—	1.0	1.2	0.6	1.0	1.0
Researcher rating	—	—	—	—	—	—	—	—	—	—	—	—	—
Parents' self-rating of knowledge	—	—	—	—	—	—	—	—	—	—	—	—	—
Teachers' self-rating of knowledge	—	—	—	—	—	—	—	—	—	—	—	—	—
Improvement at follow-up													
Children's self-reported skill	1.0	—	—	—	—	—	0.6	0.2	0.7	1.0	0.7	1.1	1.0
Children's self-report knowledge	0.9	—	—	—	—	—	—	—	0.8	0.7	0.5	0.7	0.9
Parents' self-rating of knowledge	—	—	—	—	—	—	—	—	—	—	—	—	—
Teachers' self-rating of knowledge	—	—	—	—	—	—	—	—	—	—	—	—	—
Positive clinical outcomes													
% improved after treatment	74%	—	—	—	—	—	—	—	—	—	—	—	—
% improved at follow-up	—	—	74%	—	—	—	—	—	—	—	—	—	—
% of parents who rated positive effects	—	—	—	—	—	—	—	—	67%	67%	89%	89%	89%
% of subsequent disclosures	—	—	—	3%	—	0.6%	—	—	7%	7%	0%	0%	0%
Negative clinical outcomes													
Teacher ratings of negative effects	0.0	—	—	—	—	—	—	—	0.0	0.0	0.0	0.0	0.0
Parent ratings of negative effects	0.0	—	—	—	—	—	0.0	0.0	0.0	0.0	—	—	—
% Deteriorated	—	—	—	—	—	0%	0%	—	0%	0%	0%	0%	0%
% Drop-out	0%	20%	—	—	—	—	0%	—	0%	0%	0%	0%	0%

Notes

C = control group. P = attention placebo control group. PL-C = children, observing a play. GT-C = instructional group training for children based on discussion. GT-P = instructional group training for parents based on discussion. GT-T = instructional group training for teachers based on discussion. BT-C = behavioural skills training for children involving role-play and rehearsal. BT-P = behavioural skills training for parents. BT-T = behavioural skills training for teachers. BT-C(P) = behavioural skills training for children, taught by parents. BT-C(T) = behavioural skills training for children involving role, play and rehearsal, taught by teachers. VT-C = video-based training for children. VT-P = video-based training for parents. VT-T = video-based training for teachers.

Table 9.4 *(continued)* Summary of results of treatment effects and outcome rates from CSA prevention studies

Study type, number and condition

Variable	Studies of multimodal interventions						Studies of multimodal-multisystemic interventions		
	Study 10 GT-C+ BT-C- older v C	GT-C+ BT-C- younger v C	Study 11 GT-C+ BT-C v C	Study 12 VT-C+ GT-C+ BT-C v P	Study 13 VT-C+ GT-C v P	Study 14 VT-C+ GT-C+ BT-C v C	Study 15 VT-C+ GT-C+ BT-C+ GT-T v C	Study 16 VT-C+ GT-C+ GT-T+ GT-P v C	Study 17 VT-C+ GT-C+ BT-C+ GT-T+ GT-P+ VT-P+ VT-P v C
Improvement after programme									
Children's self-report skill	—	—	—	0.3	0.6	—	0.1	2.0	1.4
Children's self-reported abstract knowledge	—	0.4	—	1.3	0.6	0.4	1.0	0.7	—
Children's self-reported explicit knowledge	1.1	1.1	0.6	—	—	—	—	—	—
Researcher rating	1.3	—	—	—	—	—	—	—	—
Parents' self-rating of knowledge	—	—	—	—	—	—	—	0.6	—
Teachers' self-rating of knowledge	—	—	—	—	—	—	—	0.0	—
Improvement at follow-up									
Children's self-reported skill	—	—	—	0.7	0.1	—	0.1	0.5	—
Children's self-report knowledge	—	—	—	1.3	0.4	—	0.7	0.5	—
Parents' self-rating of knowledge	—	—	—	—	—	—	—	0.6	—
Teachers' self-rating of knowledge	—	—	—	—	—	—	—	0.0	—
Positive clinical outcomes									
% improved after treatment	—	—	—	—	—	71%	—	—	—
% improved at follow-up	—	—	—	—	—	—	—	—	—
% of parents who rated positive effects	—	—	—	—	—	—	69%	—	45%
% of subsequent disclosures	—	—	—	—	—	—	5%	7%	—

Table 9.4 (continued) Summary of results of treatment effects and outcome rates from CSA prevention studies

	Study type, number and condition							
	Studies of multimodal interventions					Studies of multimodal-multisystemic interventions		
Variable	Study 10	Study 11	Study 12	Study 13	Study 14	Study 15	Study 16	Study 17
	GT-C+ BT-C- older / GT-C+ BT-C- younger v C	GT-C+ BT-C v C	VT-+ GT-C+ BT-C v P	VT-C+ GT-C v P	VT-C+ GT-C+ BT-C v C	VT-C+ GT-C+ BT-C+ GT-T v C	VT-C+ GT-C+ GT-T+ GT-P v C	VT-C+ GT-C+ BT-C+ GT-T+ GT-P+ VT-T+ VT-P v C
Negative clinical outcomes								
Teacher ratings of negative effects	—	—	—	—	—	—	—	16%
Parent ratings of negative effects	—	—	—	—	—	—	—	23%
% deteriorated	5%	—	—	—	9%	—	—	—
% drop-out	5%	8%	18%	0%	—	18%	15%	—

Note
C = control group. P = attention placebo control group. PL-C = children, observing a play. GT-C = instructional group training for children based on discussion. GT-P = instructional group training for parents based on discussion. GT-T = instructional group training for teachers based on discussion. BT-C = behavioural skills training for children involving role-play and rehearsal. BT-T = behavioural skills training for parents. BT-P = behavioural skills training for parents. BT-C(T) = behavioural skills training for children involving role-play and rehearsal, taught by parents. BT-C(P) = behavioural skills training for children involving role-play and rehearsal, taught by teachers. VT-C = video-based training for children. VT-P = video-based training for parents. VT-T = video-based training for teachers.

Table 9.5 Summary of key findings from CSA prevention studies

Study no.	Authors	Year	N per group	No. of sessions	Group differences	Key findings
1	Oldfield et al.	1996	1. PL-C = 658 2. C = 611	1 × 45 min	1 > 2	• Children who observed the play 'Touch' demonstrated significantly greater knowledge gain than controls. Three months later this gain was maintained. Anxiety scores were equal between those who did and did not see the play
2	Tutty	1992	1. PL-C = 100 2. PL-C = 100 3. C = 100 4. C = 100	1 × 45 min	1 = 2>3 = 4	• Following programme children who viewed a play demonstrated greater prevention knowledge than controls. This knowledge was maintained 5 months later • Older children made the greatest gains
3	Nemerofsky et al.	1994	1. BT-C = 1,044 2. C = 295	5 d	1 > 2	• Following programme the children who received group training with discussion demonstrated greater knowledge of prevention skills and concepts compared to matched controls • Benefit from training varied with age. 4-, 5- and 6-year-old children demonstrated significantly greater knowledge and skills than 3-year-olds. Similarly 6-year-olds demonstrated significantly greater knowledge and skills than 4-year-olds
4	Sarno and Wurtele	1997	1. BT-C = 41 2. P = 34	5 d	1 > 2	• Children, who received behavioural skills training showed significant gains in prevention knowledge and skills.
5	Wurtele & Sarno-Owens (findings of 5 combined studies)	1997	1. BT-C = 262 2. C = 144	5 d	1 > 2	• Children who received behavioural skills training demonstrated greater knowledge about sexual abuse and improved skill in recognizing, resisting and reporting inappropriate touch requests than controls • Training did not have differential effects on children within this specific age range, i.e., 3.4 to 5.6 years. Similarly, it did not have differential effects on boys and girls
6	Wurtele	1990	1. BT-C = 12 2. C = 12	3 d × 25 min	1 > 2	• Following programme and one month later children who received behavioural skills training demonstrated greater knowledge about sexual abuse and higher levels of personal safety skills compared to controls
7	Wurtele et al.	1989	1. BT-C = 32 2. GT-C = 37 3. P = 31	3 d ×.5	1 = 2 > 3 1 > 2	• Following programme and one month later both training groups showed enhanced knowledge and prevention skills • Children in the feelings-based programme (2) had difficulty recognizing the appropriateness of certain touch requests, whereas those in the behavioural skills training programme (1) did not
8	Wurtele et al.	1992a	1. BT-C(T) = 21 2. BT-C(P) = 18 3. C = 22	1. 3 × .5 h 2. 1.5 h over 1 w	1 = 2 > 3	• Following programme and two months later, children who received behavioural skills training demonstrated greater knowledge about sexual abuse and higher levels of personal safety skill than controls • No significant differences were found between children taught by teachers or parents
9	Wurtele et al.	1992b	1. BT-C(T) = 41 2. BT-C(P) = 44 3. BT-C(T + P) = 43 4. P = 44	1. 4 × 15 min 2. 2.5 h over 4 d 3. combination	1, 2 and 3 > 4 2 > 1 3 > 1	• Following programme and 5 months later, children with behavioural skills training demonstrated greater knowledge about sexual abuse and higher levels of personal safety skills than controls • Children taught by parents only showed enhanced recognition of inappropriate-touch requests and improved personal safety skills compared with those taught by teachers only • Children taught both by parent and teacher, were better able to recognize appropriate-touch requests and demonstrated higher personal safety skills compared with those taught by teacher only

Table 9.5 continued

Study no.	Authors	Year	N per group	No. of sessions	Group differences	Key findings
10	Conte	1985	1. GT-C + BT-C = 20 2. C = 20	3 × 1 h	1 > 2	• 1 week following programme children who received group training with discussion and role play showed a significantly greater knowledge of prevention concepts than the control group • Older children learned more concepts than younger children • Both younger and older children had greater difficulty with abstract than explicit concepts
11	Fryer et al.	1987, a,b	1. GT-C + BT-C = 23 2. C = 21	8 × 20 min	1 > 2	• Children who received instruction and behavioural skills training demonstrated improved behavioural responses under simulated conditions, compared with controls. These skills were maintained 6 months after programme completion
12	Harvey	1988	1. VT-C + GT-C + BT-C = 35 2. C = 36	3 × .5 h	1 > 2	• Three and seven weeks following programme, the group trained with behaviour skills, role-play and video, demonstrated more knowledge about preventing abuse and performed better on simulated scenes involving sexual abuse than controls
13	Saslawsky & Wurtele	1986	1. VT-C + GT-C = 33 2. C = 34	1 × 50 min	1 > 2	• Children who viewed the film and took part in subsequent discussion demonstrated greater knowledge gain and enhanced personal safety skills compared with controls. These gains were maintained 3 months later • Older children learned more than younger ones
14	Tutty	1997	1. VT-C + GT-C + BT-C = 117 2. C = 114	2 × 45-60 min	1 > 2	• The group trained with discussion, video and role-play showed increased knowledge of both Appropriate and Inappropriate Touch, to a significantly greater degree than controls • Age significantly differentiated knowledge levels, regarding inappropriate touch, with younger children knowing fewer concepts than older
15	Hazzard et al.	1991	1. VT-C + GT-C + BT-C + GT-T = 286 2. C = 113	1. 3 × 1 h + 6 h workshop 2. 3 × 1 h 3. 6 h workshop	1 > 2	• Following programme and 6 weeks later the children who received multimedia training exhibited significantly greater knowledge and were better able to discriminate safe from unsafe situations on a video measure than controls. These gains were maintained one year later
16	Kolko et al.	1987	1. VT-C + GT-C + GT-T + GT-P = 125 2. VT-C + GT-C + GT-T + GT-P = 173 3. C = 41	2 × 1.5 h	1 = 2 > 3	• Following programme, children who received multimodal training reported learning more about the differences between good and bad touching, and being more likely to both report episodes of sexual victimization and utilise programme-specific preventive skills, relative to controls • Six months later knowledge gains were not maintained
17	MacIntyre and Carr	2000	1. VT-C + GT-C + BT-C + GT-T + VT-T + GT-P + VT-P = 358 2. C = 414	12 × 30-40 min	1 > 2	• The group trained with discussion, video, role-play and behavioural skills training made large and significant gains in safety knowledge and skills as well as self-esteem, compared with controls. These gains were largely maintained 3 months later • Greatest gains were made by younger children • Parents and teachers showed significant gains in knowledge and attitudes about protection

Notes

C = control group. P = attention placebo control group. PL-C = children, observing a play. GT-C = instructional group training for children based on discussion. GT-P = instructional group training for parents based on discussion. GT-T = instructional group training for teachers based on discussion. BT-C = behavioural skills training for children based on discussion. BT-P = behavioural skills training for parents. BT-T = behavioural skills training for teachers. BT-C(P) = behavioural skills training for children involving role-play and rehearsal, taught by parents. BT-C(T) = behavioural skills training for children involving role-play and rehearsal, taught by teachers. VT-C = video-based training for children. VT-P = video-based training for parents. VT-T = video-based training for teachers. h = hour. min = minutes. d = day. w = week

Behavioural skills training

Four studies assessed the impact of self-protective behavioural skills training (Nemerofsky et al., 1994; Sarno & Wurtele, 1997; Wurtele, 1990; Wurtele & Sarno-Owens, 1997). Nemerofsky et al. (1994) evaluated the impact of the Children's Primary Prevention Training Programme (Nemerofsky et al., 1986) on preschool children. The programme comprises five story books: *1. Let's talk about touch, 2. Private parts, 3. Surprises, 4. Tell someone* and *5. Remember*. These books cover most of the curriculum set out in Table 9.1. Teachers who delivered the programme underwent extensive training in how to use the books as a basis for discussion, role-play and rehearsal of self-protective skills. In a series of studies, Wurtele and colleagues evaluated the impact of the Behavioural Skills Training Programme (Wurtele, 1986) which covered the curriculum set out in Table 9.1 and was taught using behavioural training methods including instruction, modelling, role-play, rehearsal and social reinforcement (Sarno & Wurtele, 1997; Wurtele, 1990; Wurtele & Sarno-Owens, 1997).

In all four studies the 'What If' Situations Test (WIST, Wurtele, 1986) was used to evaluate self-protective skills. The WIST evaluates children's ability to recognize and respond to hypothetical abusive situations. Effect sizes based on post-programme WIST scores ranged from 1.1 to 2.7 with a mean of 1.6, indicating that the average child who participated in these behavioural skills training programmes had better developed self-protection skills than 95% of children in control groups who received no training. Nemerofsky et al. (1986) found that older children gained more self-protective skills, as assessed by the WIST, than younger children.

In the three studies conducted by Wurtele's group, the Personal Safety Questionnaire (PSQ, Wurtele, 1986) was used to evaluate children's knowledge and attitudes concerning sexual abuse (Sarno & Wurtele, 1997; Wurtele, 1990; Wurtele & Sarno-Owens., 1997). Effect sizes based on PSQ post-test scores ranged from 0.3 to 0.8, with a mean of 0.5, indicating that the average child who completed the programme had more advanced knowledge about sexual abuse than 69% of youngsters in the control group.

In Wurtele's 1990 study, children were assessed again at one-month follow-up. Effect sizes of 1.0 for WIST and 0.9 for PSQ were obtained, indicating that the average child who completed the programme had better self-protective skills and knowledge about sexual abuse than 82% of controls one month after participation. In this study, side effects of participation were also measured using the Teachers' Perception Questionnaire (TPQ; Wurtele, 1989a) and the Parents' Perception Questionnaire (PPQ; Wurtele, 1989b). Teachers and parents reported no increases in negative behaviours and 74% of parents rated the programmes as producing positive effects.

From the four studies reviewed in this section it may be concluded that behavioural skills training programmes improve children's safety skills and knowledge about sexual abuse. Preschoolers as young as three and primary school age children up to the age of twelve can benefit from these pro-grammes. Greater gains are made by older children. The benefits of these programmes are enduring and gains made persist over time and include mak-ing disclosures of sexual abuse. Behavioural skills training programmes do not lead to increased sexualized behaviour, anxiety or other significant adjustment difficulties.

Studies comparing interventions

Wurtele et al. (1989) compared the effectiveness of their behavioural skills training programme mentioned in the previous section and a feelings-based programme in which children were taught to distinguish between good and bad touches (Anderson, 1986). A placebo control group was also included in the design of the study.

Effect sizes based on comparisons of post-programme WIST scores with those of the control group were 0.7 for the behavioural skills training pro-gramme and 0.5 for the feelings-based programme. This indicates that the average child in the behavioural skills training programme had greater self-protective skill scores than 76% of controls and the average child in the feelings-based programme had greater self-protective skill scores than 69% of controls. At one-month follow-up effect sizes for the behavioural skills train-ing programme and the feelings-based programme were 0.6 and 0.2 respect-ively. Thus, one month after programme completion, the average child in the behavioural skills training programme had greater self-protective skill scores than 73% of controls and the average child in the feelings-based programme had greater self-protective skill scores than 58% of controls. Parents and teachers reported no negative side-effects for either programme. From the results of this comparative study it may be concluded that both behavioural skills training programmes and feelings-based programmes lead to increases in self-protective skills, and the durability of these skills may be greater for the behavioural skills training programme.

Studies comparing instructors

In a series of two studies Wurtele's group compared the impact of different instructors and settings on the effectiveness of their behavioural safety skills training programme for preschool children (Wurtele et al., 1992a, 1992b). In the first study the effects of a parent-taught, home-based programme were compared with those of teacher-taught school-based programme (Wurtele et al., 1992a). In the second study, the effects of their behavioural skills training programme taught by teachers only, parents only and both parents and teachers were compared (Wurtele et al., 1992b). Control groups were included in both studies. In each study teachers and parents reported that the programme led to no negative side-effects and a majority of parents in each study rated the programme as having a positive effect on their children.

However, there were differences in comparative results of the two studies, with the first indicating little difference between parent- and teacher-taught programmes and the second suggesting the superiority of parent-taught programmes or programmes taught by both parents and teachers.

In the first study (Wurtele et al., 1992a), compared with the control group, programmes taught by teachers and parents both led to significant improvements in self-protective knowledge and skills as assessed by the PSQ and WIST and these gains were maintained at two-month follow-up. However, there were no significant differences in the gains made by children from the teacher- and parent-taught programmes. For the school-based programme, in the first study, post-programme effect sizes of 1.0 were found for both the WIST and the PSQ, and two months later effect sizes of 0.7 and 0.8 were obtained for the WIST and PSQ respectively. Thus at two-month follow-up, the average child in the teacher-taught programme demonstrated better safety skills and knowledge than 76% and 79% of controls. Similarly, for the home-based programme, post-training effect sizes of 1.4 and 1.2 were found for the WIST and the PSQ respectively, and two months later effect sizes of 1.0 for the WIST and 0.7 for the PSQ were obtained. Thus, at two-month follow-up, the average child in the parent-taught programme demonstrated better safety skills and knowledge than 84% and 76% of controls.

In the second study (Wurtele et al., 1992b), compared with the control group, programmes taught by teachers, parents, and both teachers and parents led to significant improvements in self-protective knowledge and skills as assessed by the PSQ and WIST and these gains were maintained at five-month follow-up. The average effect size across both measures and the three different training programme formats was 1.0 following training and 0.8 at five-month follow-up. This indicates that the average child participating in training had better safety knowledge and skills than 84% of controls after the programme and 79% of controls five months later. However, children who were taught by their parents or by both parents and teachers made greater gains in safety skills assessed by the WIST than those taught by their teachers only. Post-training effect sizes based on the WIST were 0.8 for the teacher-led programme and 1.3 and 1.4 for the programmes led by parents alone and by combined teacher and parent teams respectively. Thus the average child who participated in a programme in which their parents were involved in teaching had better safety knowledge and skills than 92% of controls after the programme, whereas the average child who participated in an exclusively teacher-led programme after training had better safety knowledge and skills than only 79% of controls.

From these two studies it may be concluded that behavioural skills training programmes for preschoolers led by teachers and parents are effective in helping children develop safety skills and knowledge and these gains persist over time once they have been learned. It may also be concluded that programme effectiveness may be enhanced by involving parents in the training process. Finally, it may be concluded that behavioural skills training programmes do not lead to negative side effects and are positively evaluated by parents.

Multimodal programmes

In five studies programmes that included multimodal training techniques were evaluated (Conte, 1985; Fryer et al., 1987a, 1987b; Harvey, 1988; Saslawsky & Wurtele, 1986; Tutty, 1997).

In two of these studies, multimodal training programmes which included both behavioural skills training procedures and traditional group instruction and discussion were assessed (Conte, 1985; Fryer et al., 1987a, 1987b). In Conte's (1985) study, younger (4–5 years) and older (6–10 years) children's acquisition of knowledge and skills was evaluated using a questionnaire that yielded scores for a set of questions that involved abstract reasoning and a set of questions that evaluated less sophisticated explicit knowledge. The average effect size (across types of knowledge and age groups) was 1.0, indicating that the average child who participated in the programme had better-developed safety skills and knowledge after training than 84% of untreated controls. However, older children learned more than younger children, and all children, but particularly the younger children, found explicit self-protective concepts easier to learn than safety concepts involving abstract reasoning. Fryer et al., (1987a), using a multimodal programme designed to help children develop safety skills required to prevent abduction and sexual abuse by strangers, obtained an effect size of 0.6 based on researcher ratings of children's behavioural responses under simulated abduction conditions. This indicates that the average child who completed their training programme had better safety skills than 73% of controls. These skills were maintained at six-month follow-up (Fryer et al., 1987b).

Three studies evaluated multimodal programmes which included video modelling of safety skills along with behavioural skills training procedures or traditional group instruction or both (Harvey, 1988; Saslawsky & Wurtele, 1986; Tutty, 1997). Harvey (1988) used a customized safety knowledge and skills questionnaire to evaluate the *Good Touch–Bad Touch* programme for preschool children which included behavioural skills training, video modelling and instructional teaching using a story book. Saslawsky and Wurtele (1986) used the WIST and PSQ to evaluate a programme which combined video modelling using the film *Touch* (Anderson et al., 1990) and guided discussion. Tutty (1997) used the Revised Children's Knowledge of Abuse Questionnaire (Tutty, 1995) to evaluate the *Who Do you Tell Programme* (Calgary Communities Against Sexual Assault, 1995). The curricula for all of these programmes covered topics listed in Table 9.1.

After training, the average effect size (across knowledge and skills domains) for these three programmes was 0.6, indicating that the average child who completed these complex multimodal programmes had better-developed safety knowledge and skills than 73% of controls. The average effect size (across knowledge and skills domains) based on Saslawsky and Wurtele's (1986) three-month follow-up data and Harvey's (1988) two-month follow-up data was also 0.6, indicating that gains made in safety skills and knowledge persisted for two to six months after programme completion.

From these five studies it may be concluded that multimodal programmes that include some combination of behavioural skills training, didactic instruction and discussion, and video modelling are effective in helping both preschool and primary school aged children develop safety skills and knowledge and these gains persist over time once they have been learned. Primary school aged children learn more than preschool children, and all children, but particularly preschool aged children, find explicit self-protective concepts easier to learn than safety concepts involving abstract reasoning.

Multimodal-multisystemic programmes

In three studies multimodal-multisystemic programmes were evaluated in which multimodal training techniques were used and multiple members of children's social systems were targeted (Hazzard et al., 1991; Kolko et al., 1987; MacIntyre & Carr, 2000).

Hazzard et al. (1991) in a study of eight- and nine-year-olds evaluated the impact of a multimodal-multisystemic programme which targeted both children and teachers. Children in this study completed *The Feeling Yes–Feeling No Programme* (National Film Board of Canada, 1985) which involved video modelling, behavioural skills training, didactic instruction and discussion, and also read the *Spiderman Power Pack* comic book on sexual abuse (Marvel Comics, 1984). Teachers in this programme participated in video-modelling-based training. The child and teacher training modules of the programme were delivered by trained mental health professionals. Effect sizes for self-protective knowledge based on scores from the *What I Know About Touching Scale* (Hazzard, 1999) were 1.0 after training and 0.7 at six-week follow-up, indicating that after training the average participant had more self-protective knowledge than 84% of controls and better knowledge than 76% of controls six weeks later. However, on a videotaped measure of safety skills acquisition, gains made by programme participants were less impressive. Both after training and at follow-up the effect size for safety skills acquisition was only 0.1, indicating that after training the average child had better safety skill than only 55% of controls. The programme was evaluated positively by 69% of parents and there was also no evidence that participation in the programme led to increased anxiety among participating children.

Two studies evaluated comprehensive multisystemic-multimodal programmes targeting teachers, parents and children and used video modelling, skills training and routine instructional training techniques (Kolko et al., 1987; MacIntyre & Carr, 2000).

Kolko et al. (1987) evaluated the *Red Flag – Green Flag Programme* (Williams, 1980), which includes children's workbooks and materials for teachers and parents. This was supplemented with video modelling for children based on the film *Better Safe than Sorry II* (Film Fair Communications, 1979) and in addition school staff received intensive instruction on child protection and CSA. MacIntyre and Carr (2000) evaluated the *Stay Safe Programme* (MacIntyre & Lawlor, 1991), a multisystemic-multimodal programme in which parents, teachers and children received multimodal training involving video modelling, didactic instruction and discussion and in the case of the children, behavioural skills training. Workbooks for children and manuals for parents and teachers are included in the programme along with a video in which safety skills are modelled. The programme is developmentally staged with separate curricula for younger (seven and eight years) and older (ten and eleven years) children. The average post-training effect size across measures of children's safety knowledge and skills for these two comprehensive multimodal multisystemic programmes was 1.4. This indicates that the average child who completed these programmes had better safety knowledge and skills than 92% of controls. MacIntyre and Carr (2000) found that these gains were maintained at three-month follow-up and Kolko et al. (1987) found considerable maintenance of training effects at six-month follow-up and also that 7% of children who participated in the training programme made sexual abuse disclosures. MacIntyre and Carr (2000) found that the greatest gains in safety knowledge and skills were made by seven-year-olds, who also showed a significant increase in self-esteem, which was maintained three months later. This may be attributable to the fact that the programme had a developmentally staged curriculum. Both parents and teachers showed improvements in knowledge and attitudes to child protection. These gains were also maintained at follow-up.

From the three studies reviewed in this section it can be concluded that complex multimodal-multisystemic programmes in which multimodal training techniques are used and multiple members of children's social systems are targeted are particularly effective in teaching children safety skills and self-protective knowledge; in improving parents' and teachers' child protection knowledge and attitudes; and in creating enduring change in safety of the child's social system.

Conclusions

Child sexual abuse is a problem of significant proportions in most industrialized cultures, requiring urgent preventative action. From the studies reviewed here a number of conclusions may be drawn which have implications for policy, best practice and future research. First, child abuse prevention programmes which cover the curriculum set out in Table 9.1 can lead to significant gains in children's safety knowledge and skills. Preschoolers as young as three and primary school age children up to the age of twelve can benefit from these programmes. Rates of sexual abuse disclosure may increase as a result of programme participation. Disclosure data were reported in only five of the seventeen studies reviewed here and disclosure rates ranged from 0.6 to 7%. Nevertheless, these studies do provide preliminary evidence that primary prevention programmes can also have a secondary prevention effect by helping precipitate or facilitate the revelation of sexual victimization for some children.

Second, a range of preschool- and school-based child-focused programmes may be effective in reducing the risk of CSA. Behavioural safety-skills training programmes, observing a play that models self-protective skills and discussing its implications, and feelings-based programmes that teach the difference between good and bad touch are all effective in improving children's safety skills and knowledge about sexual abuse. Of these three types of child-focused programmes, the evidence suggests that behavioural skills training which involves modelling, role-play rehearsal and social reinforcement of safety skills may be marginally more effective than other child-focused interventions.

Third, the effectiveness of behavioural skills training programmes may be improved by using multimodal training techniques including video modelling, didactic instruction and discussion, as well as routine skills training techniques.

Fourth, in most standard programmes, primary school aged children learn more than preschool children and all children, but particularly preschool aged children, find explicit self-protective concepts easier to learn than safety concepts involving abstract reasoning. However, in developmentally staged programmes, younger children learn more than older children.

Fifth, complex multimodal-multisystemic programmes in which multimodal training techniques are used and multiple members of children's social systems are targeted are particularly effective in teaching children safety skills and self-protective knowledge; in improving parents and teachers child protection knowledge and attitudes; and creating enduring change in the safety of the child's social system. Complex multimodal-multisystemic programmes are probably more effective in fostering the development of children's safety skills than programmes which focus exclusively on children, and this may be because parents and teachers extend the teaching beyond the confines of the classroom. The benefits of multimodal-multisystemic programmes are enduring and gains made persist over time.

Sixth, the curriculum of the parents' and teachers' training components in effective multisystemic programmes includes an overview of child abuse and child protection issues, a preview of the children's programme lesson plans, and information on local child protection procedures and the roles of parents and teachers in these procedures.

Seventh, while there was no definitive evidence concerning the optimum duration of programmes, it is probably best practice to opt for longer rather than shorter programmes.

Eighth, training is probably important for effective programme delivery and a range of personnel may be effective instructors. Thus parents, teachers, mental health professionals and law enforcement officers may all take the role of instructors in child abuse prevention programmes provided they are adequately trained. The effectiveness of behavioural skills training programmes for preschoolers may be enhanced by involving parents in the training process.

Ninth, CSA prevention programmes do not lead to increased sexualized behaviour, anxiety or other significant adjustment difficulties.

Implications for policy and practice

This review has clear implications for policy and practice. Primary prevention programmes which equip preadolescent children with the skills necessary for preventing CSA should be routinely included in primary school curricula. These programmes should cover the topics listed in Table 9.1; be developmentally staged with different programme materials for younger and older children; be of relatively long duration spanning a school term; be taught using multimedia materials and active skills training methods; and be multisystemic. Programmes should include components which target not only children but also parents, teachers and members of the local health, social and law enforcement services.

Implications for research

Studies that evaluate the impact of prevention programmes on disclosure rates over follow-up periods that span years rather than months should be a research priority since disclosure rate is the most valid outcome index. As primary preventative interventions, safety skills programmes should lead to increased rates of disclosures of threatened abuse. As secondary preventative interventions, they should increase rates of disclosures of previous abuse.

Future evaluation studies should include assessments of programme integrity. In such studies, training sessions are recorded and blind raters use programme integrity checklists to evaluate the degree to which sessions approximate manualized training curricula. Such integrity checks allow researchers to say with confidence the degree to which a pure and potent version of their programme has been evaluated.

Studies that examine the impact of design features that may make programmes more effective are required. For example, in our prevention programme we used broad developmentally tailored curricula, of longer duration, which were integrated on a cross-curricular basis into children's overall learning programme. We also included local child protection and child health personnel in our parent and teacher training components (MacIntyre & Carr, 2000). The contribution of these programme design features to overall effectiveness of training is an important area for research.

Studies are required which investigate the mechanisms and processes that underpin programme effectiveness. It is clear that there is wide variability in children's responses to safety skills training programmes. Following training, some children thwart threats or assaults with safety skills they learned on the programme. Others use their own unique self-protective strategies which the programme gave them the confidence to employ (Finkelhor & Dziuba-Leatherman, 1995). The determinants of these different outcomes of safety skills training require careful investigation.

There is a need to design and evaluate programmes for children who have been shown to be particularly vulnerable to sexual abuse, such as those with intellectual and physical disabilities. These programmes must involve training methods that maximize knowledge and skills gains by taking account of participants' disabilities and unique instructional requirements.

Not all children respond equally to safety skills training. There is a need to design and evaluate programmes for children who are vulnerable to not recognizing or reporting sexual abuse, particularly boys.

Future research might focus on whether certain types of children respond better to different types of programmes and examine whether those that do not learn the concepts taught can be identified and targeted with alternative interventions. Researchers should evaluate knowledge and skills gains of children, parents, teachers and child protection services, in order to assess fully the effectiveness of prevention programmes.

Assessment resources

Hazzard, A. (1999). *What I Know about Touching Scale*. Atlanta, GA: Grady Memorial Hospital. (Available from Dr Ann Hazzard, Box 26065, Grady Memorial Hospital, 80 Butler Street, S.E., Atlanta, GA 30335.)

Tutty, L. (1995). The Revised Children's Knowledge of Abuse Questionnaire: Development of a measure of children's understanding of sexual abuse prevention concepts. *Social Work Research, 19*, 2, 112–120.

Wurtele, S. (1988a). *"What If" Situations Test* (WIST). Austin, CO: Department of Psychology, University of Colorado. (Dr Sandy Wurtele, Department of Psychology, University of Colorado at Colorado Springs, 1420 Austin Bluffs Parkway, Colorado Springs, CO 80933–7150.)

Wurtele, S. (1988b). *Personal Safety Questionnaire* (PSQ). Austin, CO: Department of Psychology, University of Colorado. (Dr Sandy Wurtele, Department of Psychology, University of Colorado at Colorado Springs, 1420 Austin Bluffs Parkway, Colorado Springs, CO 80933–7150.)

Wurtele, S. (1989a). *Teachers' Perceptions Questionnaire*. Austin, CO: Department of Psychology, University of Colorado. (Dr Sandy Wurtele, Department of Psychology, University of Colorado at Colorado Springs, 1420 Austin Bluffs Parkway, Colorado Springs, CO 80933–7150.)

Wurtele, S. (1989b). *Parents' Perceptions Questionnaire*. Austin, CO: Department of Psychology, University of Colorado. (Dr Sandy Wurtele, Department of Psychology, University of Colorado at Colorado Springs, 1420 Austin Bluffs Parkway, Colorado Springs, CO 80933–7150.)

Programme resources

Anderson, C. (1986). A history of the Touch Continuum. In M. Nelson & K. Clark (Eds.), *The Educator's Guide To Preventing Child Sexual Abuse* (pp. 15–25). Santa Cruz, CA: Network Publications.

Anderson, C., Morris, B. & Robins, M. (1990). *Touch*. Minneapolis, MN: Illusion Theatre.

Anderson, C., Venier, M. & Roderiquez, J. (1992). *Touch Discussion Guide*. Minneapolis, MN: Illusion Theatre.

Calgary Communities Against Sexual Assault (1995). *Who Do you Tell Programme*. Calgary, Alberta, Canada: Author. (Phone: Canada 403–237–6905.)

Committee for Children (1983). *Talking About Touching: A Personal Safety Curriculum*. (Available from Committee for Children, PO Box 15190, Seattle, WA98115.)

Film Fair Communications (1979). *Better Safe than Sorry II*. Ventura, CA. Author. (Available from Film Fair Communications, 900 Ventura Blvd, Box 1278, Studio, CA, 91604.)

Kraizer, S. (1981). *Children Need to Know Personal training Programme*. New York, NY: Health Education Systems.

MacIntyre, D. & Lawlor, M. (1991). *The Stay Safe Programme*. Dublin: Department of Health, Child Abuse Prevention Programme.

Marvel Comics (1984) *Spiderman & Power Pack Comic Book on sexual abuse*. (Available from: National Committee for the Prevention of Child Abuse, PO Box 94283, Chicago, IL 60990.)

National Film Board of Canada (1985). *Feeling Yes–Feeling No Programme*. Canada: National Film Board of Canada.

Nemerofsky, A.G., Sanford, H.J., Baer, B., Cage, M. & Wood, D. (1986). *The Children's Primary Prevention Training Programme*. Baltimore, MD: Authors.

Riestenberg, N. (1993). *Trust: Teaching Reaching Using Students & Theatre: A Manual To Train Child Sexual Abuse Prevention Peer Educators*. Minneapolis, MN: Illusion Theatre.

Williams, J. (1980). *Red Flag – Green Flag People*. Fargo, ND: Rape and Abuse Crisis Center.

Wurtele, S.K. (1986). *Teaching Young Children Personal Body Safety: The Behavioural Skills Training Program*. Colorado Springs, CO: Author.

Resources for parents

Anderson, C. & Baumann, A. (1988). *A Parents Guide To Sexual Abuse And The Touch Video*. Minneapolis, MN: Illusion Theatre.

Corcoran, C. (1987). *Take Care. Preventing Child Sexual Abuse – A Handbook For Parents*. Dublin: Poolbeg Press.

10 Prevention of bullying

Orna McCarthy and Alan Carr

Bullying at school is a problem of significant proportions, a problem requiring urgent preventative action. While there has been a proliferation of anti-bullying programmes, the effectiveness of many of these remains untested. The aim of this chapter is to review methodologically robust research studies on the effectiveness of bullying prevention programmes, draw reliable conclusions about the effectiveness of these, and outline the implications of these conclusions for policy and practice.

A person is being bullied in school when they are repeatedly exposed to the negative actions of one or more other students. Negative actions include physical violence, verbal abuse, abusive gestures, extortion, spreading reputation-damaging rumours and intentional exclusion from peer-group activities (Olweus, 1997). A major difficulty in defining bullying is knowing where teasing or playful behaviour ends and bullying begins. Olweus (1997) argues that bullying, unlike teasing or playful behaviour, is characterized by an imbalance in power between the bully and the victim. The imbalance of power may be either real or perceived. This imbalance can be physical or intellectual in nature. The victim can be outnumbered or unable to identify the reason for the bullying. This is the case where a youngster is excluded from peer-group activities because bullies have spread reputation-damaging rumours without the victim being aware of the rumours. With bullying, victimization is unprovoked and bullies are usually aware that it is unpleasant for the victim. Pain is caused not only as a direct result of the bullying, but also by the threat or fear of future victimization. A variety of victimization strategies may be used in the bullying process. Tattum (1997) distinguishes between gesture bullying, verbal bullying, physical bullying, extortion bullying and exclusion bullying. Olweus (1997) on the other hand differentiates between direct and indirect bullying. Direct bullying takes the form of open attacks on the victim, whereas indirect bullying takes the form of exclusion and spreading malicious rumours.

Epidemiology

From Table 10.1 it may be seen that estimates for the prevalence of being bullied frequently (once a week or more) vary from 4 to 13%. Estimates of engaging in frequent bullying range from 1 to 7%. However, when once-off or occasional bullying is assessed, up to 35% of children have been found to be bullied and up to 26% have been found to bully others. The process of frequent bullying or being frequently bullied is relatively stable over time.

Epidemiological studies have found that a variety of variables are associated with the bullying process (Mooij, 1993; O'Moore et al., 1997; Olweus, 1997; Perry et al., 1988; Rigby, 1997; Smith, 1997). The majority of bullying is carried out in the playground, particularly in primary schools. For secondary pupils, being bullied in the classroom or school corridors is also common. Being bullied going to or from school is less common than being bullied in school. Younger children and boys are more likely to be bullied. Boys are bullied almost entirely by boys, while girls are bullied by both sexes. Direct bullying, particularly bullying by violent physical means, is more common among males, while females use more indirect bullying techniques such as exclusion from peer-group activities. Bullying may be more prevalent in large secondary schools and in schools in socially disadvantaged areas. Victims develop significant adjustment problems following bullying, notably internalizing behaviour problems, lowered self-esteem, academic difficulties and relationship problems.

Table 10.1 Epidemiological studies of bullying

		Been bullied		Bullied others	
		Frequently	*Infrequently*	*Frequently*	*Infrequently*
		Once a week or more	*Once or occasionally*	*Once a week or more*	*Once or occasionally*
O'Moore et al. (1997)	Ireland	4	27	1	26
Mooij (1993)	Holland	5	13	6	16
Smith (1997)	UK	7	19	3	9
Pepler et al. (1994)	Canada	8	—	—	—
Olweus (1997)	Norway	9	—	7	—
Perry et al. (1988)	USA	10	—	—	—
Rigby (1997)	Australia	13	35	4	24

Note
All values are percentages.

Aetiology

A variety of factors contribute to the bullying process, including personal characteristics of bullies and victims, characteristics of the families of bullies and victims, and features of the school environment and ethos (Olweus, 1993). Victims of bullying have personal characteristics that signal to others that they feel vulnerable and will not retaliate if attacked, while bullies commonly use aggression as way of relating to others and resolving conflict. Victims tend to come from supportive families while there is a tendency for bullies to come from disorganized families characterized by harsh or punitive parent–child relationships. Bullying is more likely to occur in schools where supervision is less than optimal due to poor staffing levels, the structure of the physical environment, and the overall organization, ethos and values of the school.

Victims

Olweus (1993) distinguishes between passive and provocative victims. Both passive and provocative victims are distinguished by personal characteristics that signal to others that they feel vulnerable and will not retaliate effectively if attacked. Passive victims are typically submissive youngsters who respond to bullying with further submission. Provocative victims are typically over-active or aggressive youngsters who respond to bullying with increased ineffective aggression. Passive victims may have some or all of the following characteristics: being physically weaker than peers; being fearful of being hurt; having poor physical co-ordination; being ineffective in physical sports and rough play; becoming tearful in the face of threats; being submissive, unassertive, shy, anxious or sensitive; and having low self-esteem. Provocative victims, in contrast, may be distinguished by some or all of the following attributes: being ineffectually aggressive and hot-tempered when threatened; being hyperactive and restless; being immature and having irritating habits. While passive victims typically have positive relationships with parents, teachers and other adults, the relationships between provocative victims and significant adults in their social systems tend to be somewhat conflictual.

Bullies

Most of the research on bullying has focused on male bullies (Olweus, 1993, 1997). The profiles of male bullies differ from those of victims. Bullies commonly use aggression as a way of relating to others and resolving conflict. They may be physically stronger than their classmates; physically effective in sports and physical activities; have a strong need to dominate others; and be easily angered. They are not insecure, do not have low self-esteem, and show little empathy for their victims. Their relationships with adults are marked by conflict. Olweus (1993, 1997) argues that bullies are motivated by three clusters of factors. First, the process of bullying meets the bully's need for power and dominance. Second, bullies benefit from victimizing others. It may bring them material benefits such as money, sweets, toys or cigarettes on the one hand and prestige among their peers on the other. Third, bullies may displace anger and aggression towards their parents (who often adopt a harsh and punitive parenting style) onto their victims. Thus bullying provides an outlet for aggression which has its roots in unsatisfactory family relationships.

Social contexts supportive of bullying

Specific school contexts may promote bullying (Farrington, 1993; Clarke & Kiselica, 1997) Bullying is more likely to occur in schools where supervision of pupils during both instructional and recreational periods is less than optimal. Non-optimal supervision may reflect inadequate staffing. It may also occur where the physical structure of the school prevents teachers from routinely observing pupils' movements, particularly during recreation periods or while moving from one class to another. Non-optimal supervision may also reflect organizational difficulties within schools where inadequate staff or parental supervision routines and rosters are in place. Finally, non-optimal supervision may reflect a school ethos underpinned by values supportive of violence, humiliation and victimization as appropriate ways of managing hierarchical relationships and solving interpersonal problems. For example, in schools where physical or verbal abuse, humiliation and victimization are used by teachers in their relationships with pupils, it is more likely that pupils will use violence and bullying in their relationships with each other.

Previous reviews

Clarke and Kiselica (1997) outlined a series of elements that have characterized the development of the field of bullying prevention, research and practice. First, there has been a shift in attitudes about bullying and a clear recognition that it is distinct and separate from playful behaviour. The second important development has been the integration of education about bullying into school curricula. A third development has been the recognition of the need for consistency in rules and procedures for dealing with bullying. A fourth critical factor has been a recognition that supervision is central to the prevention of bullying at school. A fifth development is the recognition that the primary prevention of bullying must take account of research findings on the bullying process. That is, the attributes of bullies and victims, the familial precursors of these and the social context within which bullying occurs. A sixth development has been the use of questionnaires to assess levels of bullying in schools and also to monitor the effectiveness of bullying prevention programmes. A final development has been the introduction of counselling and training programmes to help victims recover from the sequelae of bullying and protect themselves from revictimization.

Farrington (1993) in an extensive literature review concluded that approaches to bullying prevention may be classified as those that focus on the victim, those that focus on the bully, and those that focus on the social context within which bullying occurs. Strategies for bullying prevention which focus on bullies include:

- punishing bullies
- encouraging disapproval of bullies' actions by peers, teachers and parents
- providing feedback to bullies on the amount of distress they cause to victims by their actions and so help them to develop empathy for their victims
- holding conjoint conflict-resolution meetings between bullies and victims to promote reconciliation
- providing opportunities for bullies to behave positively towards their victims and rewarding this prosocial behaviour

Strategies for bullying prevention which focus on victims include:

- warning the victim about the possibility of being bullied
- coaching victims to avoid being in situations where they can be bullied
- using drama to teach children how to deal with being bullied
- encouraging children to 'shadow' each other and report bullying to teachers if it occurs
- improving victims' social skills, self-confidence and self-esteem
- developing of support groups for victims
- holding workshops for parents to educate them about bullying

Bullying prevention strategies which focus on the environment include:

- increasing supervision at school
- establishment of *bully courts* which are forums in which students elected by their peers hear cases of bullying and set punishments for the bully
- taking a *whole-school approach* to bullying

The whole-school approach to bullying incorporates all of the strategies listed above but within the context of an overall school policy in which the administration of the school, including the board of management, the headteacher, teachers and other staff along with the pupils, take responsibility for preventing bullying (Olweus, 1991, 1992, 1993; Olweus & Alaskar, 1991). They do this by developing an anti-bullying school policy which is given the highest priority and which is backed up with specific prevention strategies. Strategies are developed for implementation at school, class and individual levels. Examples of such strategies along with statements of the goals and policy principles of whole-school anti-bullying programmes are given in Table 10.2.

These reviews have been useful in highlighting major developments within the field of bullying research but they have drawn few conclusions about evidence for the effectiveness of bullying prevention pogrammes, a concern central to this chapter.

Method

The aim of the present review was to identify effective bullying prevention programmes. A PsychLit database search of English language journals for the years 1977 to 2000 was conducted to identify studies in which bullying prevention programmes were evaluated. The term *bullying* was combined with terms that define psychological intervention such as *prevention* and *intervention*. A manual search of bibliographies of recent review articles on bullying was also carried out. The Anti-bullying Centre in Trinity College was contacted for bibliographical assistance also. Studies were selected for review if they involved repeated measures over control and intervention periods or included a control group, included more than four schools, and included reliable and valid outcome measures. Single case designs and studies reported in dissertations or convention papers were not included in the review. Using these rigorous inclusion and exclusion criteria, only four studies were identified and selected for review.

Characteristics of the studies

All four studies were published between 1989 and 1997. Two were carried out in Norway, one was conducted in the UK and one in Canada. They all examined the effectiveness of a whole-school approach to bullying (Olweus, 1991, 1992, 1993, 1997; Olweus & Alaskar, 1991). Although only four studies were identified for inclusion in this review, in total, 110 schools containing over 19,507 pupils were involved in these four studies. Pupils in the schools ranged in age from seven to sixteen years, were from various socioeconomic backgrounds and were representative of the general school-going population of the three countries in which the studies were conducted.

Methodological features

Methodological features of the four studies are given in Table 10.3. Only one of the four studies included a control group and here schools were not randomly assigned to groups. In the other three studies conclusions about programme effectiveness were based on time-lagged contrasts between age-equivalent groups, i.e. data from Time 1 were used as a baseline against which data from Time 2, and in some instances Time 3, could be compared. In all four studies groups of schools contained relatively homogeneous groups of

Table 10.2 Components of whole-school bullying prevention programmes

Goals	• To increase awareness and knowledge of bully–victim problems • To achieve active involvement on the part of parents and teachers • To develop clear rules against bullying • To provide support and protection for victims
Policy principles	• Parents and teachers co-operate in engaging in authoritative adult–child relationships with pupils • Firm limits to unacceptable behaviour • Non-physical sanctions consistently applied for rule violations
School strategies	• Develop joint long-term action plan for the school • Regular meetings of teachers together; parents together; and parents and teachers together, to develop anti-bullying social milieu of the school • Provide supervision of children during recess and lunchtime • Teachers to be contactable by children and parents in confidence
Class strategies	• Regular class meetings • Teachers and pupils jointly establish class rules and sanctions against bullying • Teachers praise pupils for pro-social behaviour • Teachers consistently apply sanctions for bullying • Teachers promote co-operative learning through group projects and activities where participation and effort are encouraged • Teachers use role-playing, rehearsal, and discussion of bullying-related videos and literature to support anti-bullying social milieu
Individual strategies	• Teachers talk with bullies and victims and their parents about bullying incidents as soon as incidents come to light • These meetings continue until the bullying is resolved • Parents and teachers co-operate in applying sanctions for bullying consistently • Parents and teachers support both victims and bullies as they move on from the bullying incident • Neutral pupils may be involved to aid this support process • Where the incident cannot be resolved within a class, the bully not the victim may be moved to another class • Assertiveness training for victims • Peer counselling where pupils run a helpline for victims • Bully courts in which peers hear both sides of the story
Materials	• Booklet for schools (37-page booklet in Olweus pack) • Booklet for parents (4-page booklet in the Olweus pack) • Bullying questionnaire • Video of bullying events for classroom discussion (25 minutes on events in lives of victims in the Olweus pack)

Table 10.3 Methodological features of bullying prevention programmes

Feature	Study number			
	S1	*S2*	*S3*	*S4*
Time-lagged comparison	1	1	1	1
Control group	0	0	0	1
Random assignment	0	0	0	0
Diagnostic homogeneity	1	1	1	1
Demographic similarity	1	1	1	1
Pre-programme assessment	1	1	1	1
Post-programme assessment	1	1	1	1
3-month follow-up assessment	1	0	0	1
Chilldren's self-report	1	1	1	1
Parents' ratings	1	1	1	1
Teachers' ratings	0	0	0	0
Trainers' ratings	0	0	0	0
Researcher ratings	0	0	0	0
Deterioration assessed	1	1	1	1
Drop-out assessed	1	1	1	1
Clinical significance of change assessed	0	0	0	0
Experienced therapists or trainers used	1	0	1	1
Programmes were equally valued	0	0	0	0
Programmes were manualized	1	1	0	0
Supervision was provided	1	1	1	1
Programme integrity checked	1	1	1	0
Data on concurrent intervention given	0	0	0	0
Data on subsequent intervention given	0	0	0	0
Total	14	11	12	13

Notes
S = study. 1 = design feature was present. 0 = design feature was absent

students. In all four studies pre-programme and post-programme assessments were conducted and in two studies long-term follow-up data were collected at eighteen months in one study and three years in another. Quite appropriately, children's self-reports were the main type of data recorded in all four studies. Levels of bullying were assessed using the Olweus Bully–Victim questionnaire (Olweus, 1989) or an adaptation of it. In addition to this, all four studies carried out a dose–response analysis of the interventions based on information provided by teachers or members of the research team. Deterioration and drop-out were assessed in all four studies. The clinical significance of change was not assessed in any of the four studies. Experienced trainers were involved in three of the four studies and in these school-staff training, consultation and supervision was provided. In all four studies programmes were manualized, although in two studies variations on the manual were optionally available to some schools. Programme integrity was checked in three of the four studies. Data on concurrent or subsequent interventions were not given for any of the studies. Overall, it is clear that these were four methodologically robust studies.

Substantive findings

A summary of the main findings of the studies is contained in Table 10.4.

Olweus's Norwegian study

As part of a nation-wide campaign against bullying in Norway instigated by the Ministry of Education, Olweus conducted a study to evaluate the effectiveness of his whole-school bullying prevention programme (Olweus, 1991, 1992, 1993; Olweus & Alaskar, 1991). The programme was introduced in forty-two schools in Bergen. Staff and parents received booklets and a video about programme implementation, while students completed the Bully–Victim questionnaire. This questionnaire is designed to obtain information about different aspects of bully–victim problems in a school, including the frequency of bully–victim incidents and the readiness of teachers and students to address such problems. Thereafter, staff in each of the participating schools were offered detailed individualized feedback for their school on Time 1 Bully–Victim questionnaire results and the implications of this for programme implementation. This feedback, consultation and training process was of two hours' duration for each school. Data were collected from approximately 2,500 students in the forty-two participating schools. These students were in grades four to seven and were aged eleven to fourteen years at the start of the project. Data were collected, using the Bully–Victim questionnaire, before the introduction of the programme in May 1981 (Time 1); in May 1982 (Time 2) eight months after the introduction of the programme; and twenty months after the introduction of the programme in May 1983 (Time 3).

The programme was effective in reducing reports of both bullying and being bullied. In the short term (after eight months) there was a 26% reduction in bullying (21% for males and 31% for females), while in the long term (after twenty months) there was a 53% reduction in bullying (35% for males and 71% for females). For reports of being bullied, in the short term (after eight months) there was a 53% reduction (49% for males and 57% for females) while in the long term (after twenty months) there was a 62% reduction in reports of being bullied (56% for males and 67% for females).

On a multi-item scale of antisocial behaviour compared with Time 1, at Time 2 there was 34% decrease in antisocial behaviour (31% for males and 36% for females). On the same scale at Time 3 (compared with Time 1) there was a 22% decrease in antisocial behaviour (19% for males and 24% for females).

Effect sizes based on Time 1 and Time 2 data were 1.42 for being exposed to direct and indirect bullying and 1.12 for the score on the multi-item scale of antisocial behaviour (Olweus, 1997). Thus, eight months after the introduction of the programme the average pupil reported being bullied less often than 92% of pupils before the introduction of the programme. Also, eight

Table 10.4 Overview and main findings from bullying prevention programmes

Authors	Year	Country	N schools	N pupils	Age	Interventions	Key findings
Olweus	1991	Norway	IG = 42	IG = 2,500	11–14 y	ST + C MIP Video	• The overall results showed the programme was effective • After 8 months there was a 26% reduction in bullying (21% for males and 31% for females) • After 20 months there was a 53% reduction in bullying (35% for males and 71% for females) • After 8 months there was a 53% reduction in being bullied (49% for males and 57% for females) • After 20 months there was a 62% reduction in being bullied (56% for males and 67% for females) • On a multi-item scale of antisocial behaviour compared with Time 1, at Time 2 there was 34% decrease in antisocial behaviour (31% for males and 36% for females). At Time 3 (compared with Time 1) there was a 22% decrease in antisocial behaviour (19% for males and 24% for females) • Effect size based on Time 1 and Time 2 data was 1.42 for being exposed to direct and indirect bullying • Effect size based on Time 1 and Time 2 data was 1.12 for the score on the multi-item scale of antisocial behaviour • The programme was most effective when it was implemented fully following implementation guidelines
Roland	1989 a, b	Norway	IG = 37	IG = 7,800	7–16 y	MIP Video	• The overall results showed that the programme was ineffective • After 3 years there was a 20% increase in overall levels of bullying (24% increase for males and 14% reduction for females) • After 3 years there was a 14% increase in the level of being bullied (a 44% increase for males and a 13% reduction for females) • The programme was most effective when it was implemented fully following implementation guidelines • Overall the programme had a marginally positive effect on girls but may in fact have led to deterioration in boys

Author	Year	Country			Age	Intervention	Results
Smith & Sharp	1994	England	IG = 23 CG = 4	IG = 6,468 CG = 1841	8–16 y	ST + C WM Video	• The programme was effective in reducing reports of both bullying and being bullied • After 2 years there was a 12% reduction in bullying in both primary and secondary schools in the intervention group compared with a 14% increase in the control group • After 2 years there was an 11% reduction in the overall level of being bullied in schools in the intervention group compared with a 3% increase in the control group • Interim monitoring data from a sample of students who completed a short questionnaire about bullying for periods of five days at a specified time each term showed that levels of bullying on this very sensitive measure decreased by approximately 46% over two years • Overall there was an increase in pupils' willingness to tell someone they are being bullied • The programme was most effective when it was implemented fully following implementation guidelines
Pepler et al.	1993	Canada	IG = 4	IG = 898	9–14 y	ST + C WM	• The overall results showed that the programme was ineffective in the short and long term but children were reactive to anticipated assessment of programme effectiveness • In the short term there was an 8% increase in being bullied over the school term and then a 31% reduction in the week prior to assessment • In the long term there was a 20% increase in being bullied over the school term and then an 18% reduction in the week prior to assessment • In the long term there was a 33% increase in bullying over the school term and then a 24% reduction in the week prior to assessment

Notes

IG = intervention group. CG = control group. ST + C = staff training and consultation; MIP = manualized Intervention Programme. WM = written material. y = year.

months after the introduction of the programme the average pupil reported less antisocial behaviour occurring within the school than 86% of pupils before the introduction of the programme.

The degree to which the integrity of the bullying prevention programme was preserved, and the degree to which the programme was implemented in full, affected its effectiveness. Compared with schools where the programme was not fully implemented in accordance with programme guidelines, there was a larger reduction in levels of bullying in schools which had correctly implemented three essential components of the whole bullying prevention programme (introducing class rules against bullying; having regular class meetings about bully–victim problems; and having training sessions involving bully–victim role-playing).

Overall these results indicate that the whole-school bullying prevention programme led to a marked reduction in bully–victim problems at eight and twenty months following its introduction for both males and females. The effects of the intervention programme on bullying and being bullied were greater after eight than twenty months. The programme was most effective when it was implemented fully and in accordance with programme guidelines.

Roland's Janus Project

The Janus Project was carried out by Roland (1989a, 1989b; Munthe, 1989) to evaluate the effectiveness of a modified version of Olweus's whole-school bullying prevention programme in 37 schools in Rogaland in Norway. In the Janus Project, the manuals, video material and assessment instruments for Olweus's programme were used, but staff in participating schools were not offered consultation and training to help them introduce the programme into their schools. That is, unlike schools in Olweus's project, staff in the Janus Project did not receive two hours of consultation and training in which individualized feedback for their school was given on the implications of a synopsis of Time 1 Bully–Victim questionnaire data for programme implementation.

Data were collected from approximately 7,800 students in the thirty-seven participating schools. These students were in grades one to nine and were aged seven to nineteen years at the start of the project. Data were collected, using the Bully–Victim questionnaire, before the introduction of the programme in May 1983 (Time 1) and in October 1986 (Time 2) three years after the introduction of the programme.

The overall results showed that the programme was ineffective. Three years after the introduction of the programme there was a 20% increase in overall levels of bullying (from 2.4% to 2.9%), with a 24% increase for males (from 4.1% to 5.1%) and 14% decrease for females (from 0.8% to 0.7%). Three years after the introduction of the programme there was a 14% increase in the level of being bullied (from 3.8% to 4.4%), with a 44% increase for males (from 3.6% to 5.2%) and a 13% reduction for females (from 4.0% to 3.5%). These results are from Munthe's (1989) report in which the criterion of once a week or more often was used to define bullying and being bullied. The programme was most effective when it was implemented fully following implementation guidelines and least effective where there was incomplete or incorrect implementation.

The negative results of the Janus Project, when considered in light of Olweus's findings, show that the overall effectiveness of whole-school bullying prevention programmes depends not only upon the provision of programme materials (manuals and video training packs) but also on consultation, training and support from professionals outside of the school (Roland & Munthe, 1997). Consultation, training and support is essential for helping schools implement programmes fully and in accordance with programme guidelines. That is, consultation and training are vital to programme integrity. It is also noteworthy that the programme had a marginally positive effect on girls but may in fact have led to deterioration in boys.

The Sheffield study

In the Sheffield study, which was funded by the UK Department of Education, Peter Smith evaluated a whole-school bullying prevention programme (Smith, 1997; Smith & Sharp, 1994). As with the programme developed by Olweus, the Sheffield programme involved participating schools developing a whole-school policy on bullying, creating a document which clearly laid out what was meant by bullying; what steps should be taken when it occurs; and how the effectiveness of the programme should be monitored. The programme was also individually tailored to meet the unique needs of each school. In addition to the features given in Table 10.2, the Sheffield bullying prevention programme included additional preventative strategies at the school, class and individual levels. At the school level, the playground environments were redesigned to facilitate supervision where appropriate. At the class level, stories, videos and drama were used as media for fostering an anti-bullying ethos and quality circles were instituted as a forum to encourage pupils to develop their own solutions to bullying. *Only Playing, Miss* by the Neti Neti Theatre Company and *Sticks and Stones* produced by Central Television were the videos used. The *Heartstone Odyssey* by Arvan Kumar was the novel used in the programme. At the individual level, assertiveness training was offered for victims in small safe support groups. For bullies Pikas's (1989) *Method of Shared Concern* was used to encourage tolerance. Throughout the programme, the research team offered training and consultation on demand, to help schools implement the bullying prevention programme.

Data were collected from approximately 8,380 students in the twenty-seven participating schools. There were seven primary schools and twenty secondary schools. Of the twenty-seven schools, twenty-three schools containing 6,468 pupils were in the intervention group and four schools containing 1841 pupils were in the control group (one primary school and three secondary schools). These students were aged eight to sixteen years at the start of the project. For schools in the intervention group, data were collected, using an adapted version of the Olweus Bully-Victim questionnaire (Ahmad et al., 1991) before the introduction of the programme in November 1990 (Time 1) and in November 1992 (Time 2) two years after the introduction of the programme. Data from control group schools were collected at two time points separated by a two-year period, but these data collection periods did not exactly coincide with Time 1 and Time 2 of the intervention group. A wide variety of process variables concerning the degree of implementation of the programme and changes over the course of the two-year period between Time 1 and Time 2 were also assessed.

The programme was effective in reducing reports of both bullying and being bullied. After two years there was a 12% reduction in bullying in both primary and secondary schools. In control group schools there was a 14% increase in bullying during the same period. In schools where the programme was implemented, there was an 11% reduction in the overall level of being bullied after two years, with a 14% reduction in primary schools and a 7% reduction in secondary schools. In the control group there was a 3% increase in being bullied during the same period.

Interim monitoring was carried out on a sample of students who completed a short questionnaire about bullying for periods of five days at a specified time each term. Results from this highly sensitive monitoring process showed that levels of bullying decreased by approximately 46% over two years in schools where the programme was implemented. Overall there was an increase in pupils' willingness to tell someone they are being bullied. The programme was most effective when it was implemented fully following implementation guidelines.

Toronto study

The Toronto Project was carried out by Pepler et al. (1993, 1994) to evaluate the effectiveness of a modified version of Olweus's whole-school bullying prevention programme in four schools in Toronto, Canada. For the Toronto Project, the elements of the whole-school approach set out in Table 10.2 were supplemented with a number of additional strategies, particularly at the class level. Drama and literature were used as a basis for learning about managing bullying, and learning circles which allowed pupils to talk in a safe, structured way were also established. Both of these features were similar to elements of the programme evaluated in the Sheffield study. A mentoring system with small groups of children and a teacher was implemented in the higher grades. A peer-conflict mediation programme was also introduced which trained children to intervene in playground conflicts (Roderick, 1988).

Data were collected from 898 students, aged nine to fourteen years in four participating schools, three of which contained pupils aged five to fourteen and one of which contained pupils aged twelve to fourteen. Data were collected, using an adapted version of the Olweus Bully–Victim questionnaire (Ziegler et al., 1992) in October (Time 1) and May (Time 2) of a single academic year and follow-up data were collected in May of the next academic year (Time 3).

After eight months there was a decrease of 31% (from 13% to 9%) in those stating that they had been bullied in the five days prior to completing the questionnaire. At eighteen-month follow-up there was a further decrease of 18%. There was also a decrease in exclusion bullying as indicated by the reduction in those stating that they had spent break-time alone. At eight months this had decreased by 27%, while at follow-up the decrease was 30%. Finally there was a decrease in those who claimed that their teacher stopped bullying from occurring. After eight months there was a 32% decrease (from 11% to 8%) in reports of teachers stopping bullying and at follow-up a 15% decrease occurred. This indicates that teachers were taking greater action against bullying.

Conclusions

From this review it may be concluded that whole-school bullying prevention programmes effectively reduce both reports of bullying and reports of being bullied in the short term (over periods of an academic year) but also in the longer term over periods of up to three years. Whole-school programmes comprehensively address bullying by specifying how anti-bullying policies can be developed to guide bullying prevention strategies at school, class and individual levels.

The effectiveness of whole-school bullying prevention programmes is determined by the degree to which programme integrity is maintained. Where programmes are implemented completely, consistently and in accordance with programme guidelines, they are highly effective. Where programmes are implemented inconsistently and programme integrity is not maintained over time, they are ineffective and may even lead to an increase in bullying.

External training, consultancy and support are essential to ensuring proper implementation of whole-school bullying prevention programmes. Without such external support, programme integrity is not maintained and programmes are ineffective.

Implications for policy and practice

This review has implications for policy and practice. To prevent bullying, the whole-school approach to bullying should be routinely introduced into primary and secondary schools. Particular care should be taken to implement such programmes fully and consistently in accordance with programme guidelines. School staff should be provided with periodic training and consultancy to help them implement programmes effectively.

Implications for research

Future research should focus on clarifying the degree to which different design features of the whole-school approach contribute to its effectiveness. We already know that the intensity and consistency with which programmes are implemented affects their effectiveness. However, other factors such as strategies used at the individual, class and school level may also be important. Studies are also required which investigate the interpersonal and organizational processes which underpin programme effectiveness.

There is a need to design and evaluate programmes for schools known to be particularly vulnerable to bullying problems, such as those in low SES and high crime areas. These programmes must involve design features, staff training, and consultancy processes which address the unique vulnerabilities of these schools.

Assessment resources

Ahmad, Y., Whitney, I. & Smith, P.K. (1991). A survey service for schools on bully/victim problems. In P.K. Smith & D.A. Thomson (Eds.), *Practical Approaches to Bullying* (pp. 50–61). London: David Fulton.

Olweus, D. & Smith, P.K. (in press). *Manual for the Olweus Bully/Victim Questionnaire*. Oxford: Blackwell.

Olweus, D. (1989). *Questionnaire for Students* (Junior and senior versions). Unpublished manuscript.

Programme resources

Besag, V. (1992). *We don't have Bullies Here!*. 57 Manor House Road, Jesmond, Newcastle upon Tyne, NE2 2LY.

Central Television (1990). *Sticks and Stones*. Community Unit, Central Television, Broad Street, Birmingham.

Department of Education (1994). *Don't Suffer in Silence. An Anti-bullying Pack for Schools*. London: HMSO. (Resource pack and video based on the Sheffield Project Available from the Department of Education, London, UK.)

Elliott, M. (1994). *Bullying: A Practical Guide to Coping for Schools*. Harlow: Longman.

Johnstone, M., Munn, P. & Edwards, L. (1991). *Action Against Bullying: A Support Pack for Schools*. Edinburgh: SCRE.

Munn, P. (1993). *Schools Action Against Bullying: Involving Parents and Non Teaching Staff*. Edinburgh: SCRE.

Olweus, D. (1993). *Bullying in Schools: What We Know and What We Can Do*. Oxford: Blackwell.

Sharp, S. & Smith, P. (1994). *Tackling Bullying in Your School: A Practical Handbook for Teachers*. London: Routledge.

Smith, P. & Thompson, D. (1991). *Practical Approaches to Bullying*. London: David Fulton.

Sullivan, K. (2000). *The Anti-Bullying Handbook*. Oxford: Oxford University Press.

Tattum, D. & Herbert, G. (1993). *Countering Bullying*. Stoke on Trent: Trentham Books (book of case studies).

Tattum, D., Tattum, E. & Herbert, G. (1993). *Cycle of Violence*. Cardiff: Drake Educational Associates. (Video)

Resources for clients

Elliott, M. (1994). *Bullying: A Practical Guide for Coping in Schools*. London: Longman.

Kidscape: *Stop Bullying*, booklet available through the International Society for the Prevention of Cruelty to Children (ISPCC).

Mellor, A. (1993). *Bullying and How to Fight it: A Guide for Families*. Edinburgh: SCRE.

Murray, M. & Keane, C. (1998). *The ABC of Bullying*. Dublin: Mercier.

Olweus, D. (1993). *Bullying In Schools: What We Know and What We Can Do*. Oxford: Blackwell.

Rigby, K. (1996). *Bullying In Australia Schools – And What to Do About it*. Melbourne: ACER.

Roland, E. & Munthe E. (1989). *Bullying: An International Perspective*. London: David Fulton.

Sharp, S. & Smith, P.K. (1994). *Tackling Bullying in Your School: A Practical Handbook for Teachers*. London: Routledge.

Tattum, D.P. (1993). *Understanding and Managing Bullying*. Oxford: Heinemann Educational Books.

11 Prevention of adjustment problems in children with asthma

Aoife Brinkley, Ruth Catherine Cullen and Alan Carr

Asthma is the most common chronic illness of childhood. It affects all areas of a child's life. It can lead to sleep disturbances, restrictions in daily activity, absences from school, repeated hospitalization during severe attacks, hypoxia, seizures, brain damage and, if left untreated, asthma is potentially fatal (Eggleston, 1999; Creer & Levstek, 1997). Asthma is a disease of the respiratory system characterized by reversible airway obstruction, airway inflammation, and airway hyperresponsiveness to a variety of stimuli. It results in attacks characterized by breathing distress. The course of asthma is determined by the interaction between abnormal respiratory system physiological processes to which some youngsters have a predisposition, physical environmental triggers (such as allergens and viral infections of the respiratory system), and psychological processes, particularly stress. Psychological interventions for children with asthma and their families aim to help them understand the condition, adhere to medication regimes, reduce exposure to environmental triggers, and manage stress. The aim of the present review was to draw reliable conclusions about the efficacy of psychological intervention programmes that attempt to increase adjustment and decrease morbidity among children with asthma and outline the implications of these conclusions for policy and practice.

Epidemiology

The prevalence of asthma is between 2% and 10% among children (Eggleston, 1999; Murphy, 1994). The prevalence rate of asthma in the USA and UK has increased by more than 40% in the past 20 years. There are important demographic differences in the prevalence and morbidity of asthma. Prevalence, hospitalization and mortality rates are higher for boys, and children in poverty. In the USA, a disproportionate burden of asthma morbidity and mortality occurs among racial or ethnic minorities who are poor and live in urban environments. The long-term prognosis for children with asthma is a major concern. Between 30% and 60% of children continue to suffer from the condition in adulthood. There has also been a sharp increase in deaths from asthma over the past twenty years.

Aetiology

The central feature of an asthma attack is bronchial constriction (Eggleston, 1999). Asthma attacks begin when the immune system produces antibodies that cause the bronchial tubes to release histamine. Histamine causes the smooth muscles in the walls of the smaller air passages of the lungs (bronchi and bronchioles) which are controlled by the autonomic nervous system to become inflamed, contract and produce mucus. These secretions in the air passages of the lungs accumulate and the walls of the air passages swell. Tissue damage may occur as a result of this swelling and make future attacks more likely. The child has difficulty breathing and coughing up the secretions. The lungs tend to become overfilled with air and the chest cavity becomes over-expanded. As the attack continues, the child has more and more difficulty breathing. Wheezing occurs and less oxygen is taken in. If the attack persists without treatment, the child becomes unconscious, develops seizures due to lack of oxygen and may suffer brain damage due to hypoxia; severe attacks of asthma may result in death. The fatalities due to asthma, which have increased in recent years, are associated with hypoxic seizures, previous respiratory arrest, non-adherence to medication regime, poor self-care and family dysfunction.

Both physiological and psychosocial predisposing factors have been identified for asthma (Miller & Wood, 1991). At physiological level, children may be genetically predisposed to developing asthma. Immunoglobulin E (IgE) plays a central role in the mechanism underpinning symptom expression in asthma and the regulation of IgE antibody level is under genetic control. A history of viral respiratory infections in infancy may also predispose youngsters to developing asthma. Such infections may damage the respiratory system, rendering it sensitive to certain triggering conditions. At a psychological level, parental beliefs about asthma may lead them to interact with their children and other family members in stressful anxiety-provoking ways. High levels of family anxiety may predispose youngsters, particularly those with a genetic vulnerability, to developing asthma. Suggestibility may also be a predisposing factor since there is clear evidence that bronchodilation and constriction may be influenced by suggestion, particularly in suggestible youngsters (Isenberg et al., 1992).

Asthma attacks may be precipitated by allergy, infection, physical exercise and cold air or psychological factors that lead to autonomic arousal. Common allergens that cause asthma attacks are dust, pollen, cat and dog hair, air pollution and house mites. Psychological factors which may lead to hyper-arousal and precipitate an asthma attack include stresses within the family, school or peer group that pose an immediate threat to the person's perceived safety or security and so cause anger or anxiety. These stresses include rigid repetitive family interaction patterns characterized by enmeshment or overinvolvement with a highly anxious parent; triangulation where the child is required, usually covertly, to take sides with one or other parent in a conflict;

or a chaotic family environment where parents institute no clear rules and routines for children's daily activities or medication regime when asthma attacks are likely to occur.

The child's breathing difficulties during an attack may be extremely distressing both for the child and for the parents. The distressing nature of the respiratory symptoms, and the fact that asthma may be fatal, may lead some children and their parents to respond to asthma with considerable anxiety, which in turn may exacerbate or maintain the symptoms. Alternatively, where parents view asthma as a sign of weakness or attention seeking, the child's anticipation of the parent's punitive response to the attacks may exacerbate or maintain the attacks. There is also considerable variability in the ways in which family physicians and paediatricians respond to asthma. Some intervene early with aggressive treatment while others intervene later with a less intensive approach. Such variability may be confusing for parents, who themselves are uncertain how to proceed when an attack begins. This confusion fuels parental anxiety, which in turn increases the child's arousal level and exacerbates or maintains the condition.

Intervention

Routine paediatric treatment of asthma includes prevention of known triggers, long-term prophylactic therapy (inhaled or oral steroid-based medication), and use of bronchodilator drugs during acute attacks. Thus, treatment goals are the prevention and reduction of the likelihood of asthma attacks, and managing attacks appropriately when they occur. Psychological interventions for youngsters with asthma complement routine paediatric treatment. They include psychoeducation to help youngsters and their families understand the condition; relaxation training to help youngsters reduce physiological arousal levels; skills training to increase adherence to asthma management programmes and promote optimal crisis management; and family therapy to empower family members to work together to manage asthma effectively (Bernard-Bonnin et al., 1995; Campbell & Patterson, 1995; Showland et al., 1988; Klingelhofer & Gershwin, 1988; McQuaid & Nassau, 1999).

Psychoeducation

In psychoeducational programmes, the symptoms of asthma and the biological, psychological and environmental predisposing, precipitating and maintaining factors that may underpin the condition are explained. Information is given about avoiding triggers which precipitate attacks and on self-monitoring of respiratory functioning using a peak flow meter to assess exacerbations in asthma. This information may be used as a guide in taking medication or seeking medical care.

Relaxation

In relaxation skills training, youngsters are trained in how to use progressive muscle relaxation, breathing exercises, visualization or biofeedback to reduce physiological arousal and so reduce asthma symptoms.

Behavioural skills training

In behavioural skills training, modelling, role-play, rehearsal and reinforcement are used to train youngsters and their families in the skills required to manage asthma on a day-to-day basis and during crises. Day-to-day asthma management skills include self-monitoring of medication use and symptomatology; managing the home, school and recreational environments so as to avoid asthma triggers; modulating the level of exercise taken to avoid asthma attacks; taking extra precautions when viral respiratory infections occur, and using medication appropriately. Families are shown how to use reward programmes to reinforce adherence to such regimes. Central to such systems is the gradual transition from parent-directed reward programmes to self-directed reward programmes, so youngsters as they move into adolescence develop relatively autonomous control of their condition. In skills training for coping with crises, families learn how to use cognitive coping skills and decision-making skills during asthma attacks. Cognitive coping skills involve using self-instructions to reduce catastrophizing and other anxiety-provoking thinking styles that increase arousal and exacerbate asthma symptoms. Decision-making skills involve using information from the peak flow meter, the youngster's sense of well-being, and the rate and effectiveness of recent medication usage to make decisions about whether an attack can safely be managed with or without medical intervention.

Family therapy

Family intervention aims to empower families to manage asthma effectively and to disrupt interaction patterns that maintain symptoms. These fall broadly speaking into two categories. First, there are those interaction patterns that increase autonomic arousal which in turn lead to bronchial constriction and eventually to asthma attacks. Second, there are interaction patterns which do not facilitate adherence to the medication regime and the avoidance of environments that contain allergens that precipitate asthma attacks. Intense, intrusive emotional interactions between an overinvolved parent and an asthmatic child may increase arousal. Such interactions often occur as part of a pattern of triangulation, where the child is involved in an intense relationship with one parent and a distant relationship with another and the parents have a weak interparental alliance (Minuchin et al. 1975). Interaction patterns that do not facilitate adherence to the medication regime and the avoidance of environments that contain allergens which precipitate asthma attacks tend to occur in disorganized families. Family therapy sessions provide a forum where alternatives to these symptom-maintaining patterns of interaction may be negotiated.

Previous reviews

From previous reviews of the literature a number of conclusions may be drawn about the efficacy of psychological interventions in the management of childhood asthma (Bernard-Bonnin et al. 1995; Campbell & Patterson, 1995; Showland et al., 1988; Klingelhofer & Gershwin, 1988; McQuaid & Nassau, 1999). First, psychological interventions in the short and long term can improve the adjustment of children with asthma. Second, there is some evidence to support the effectiveness of psychoeducational interventions; biofeedback and relaxation skills training programmes; multimodal multi-systemic interventions which include psychoeducation, relaxation and behavioural skills training for children and their parents; and family therapy. Third, family-based multimodal-multisystemic interventions may be more effective than individually based approaches. Fourth, psychological interventions can directly affect both physiological and self-reported indices of respiratory functioning in children with asthma. Fifth, psychological interventions can also improve adherence to medication and asthma-management regimes, reduce the frequency of emergency medical care, and reduce school absences due to illness. Sixth, children with moderate or severe asthma benefit most from psychological intervention programmes. Seventh, the mechanisms underpinning effective programmes are not fully understood, but such programmes may reduce symptomatology by helping children and families remove triggers from the environment; increase adherence; increase self-efficacy beliefs about asthma control; reduce asthma-related anxiety; and disrupt stressful or symptom-maintaining patterns of interaction within children's social systems. All reviewers expressed concerns about methodological inadequacies of some studies included in their reviews.

Method

The aim of the present review was to identify effective programmes for preventing adjustment problems in children with asthma. PsychLit and Medline database searches of English language journals for the years 1977 to 2000 were conducted to identify studies in which such programmes were evaluated. The term *asthma* was combined with general terms such as *prevention*, *intervention*, *family therapy*, *relaxation* and *behaviour therapy*. This search was complemented by a manual search of the bibliographies of review articles and indices of relevant journals. Studies were selected for review if they included a treatment group and a control group, if they included homogeneous groups of cases, if there were at least five participants in each group, and if pre- and post-treatment measures were included. Single case studies and studies reported in dissertations or convention papers were not included in the review. Twenty studies were selected for review.

Characteristics of the studies

The characteristics of the twenty studies selected for review are given in Table 11.1. All of the studies were conducted between 1978 and 1999, with the majority being conducted in the 1990s. Seven studies evaluated child-focused programmes, two of which involved relaxation or biofeedback (Kostes et al., 1978; Kohen, 1996), three of which were psychoeducational (Rakos et al., 1985; Holzheimer et al., 1998; Parcel et al., 1980), and two of which involved psychoeducation along with relaxation and behavioural skills training (Colland, 1993; Dahl et al., 1990). The remaining thirteen studies evaluated family-based multisystemic programmes. In four studies family psychoeducational programmes were assessed (Fireman et al., 1981; Kubly & McClellan, 1984; Tal et al. 1990; Hughes et al., 1991); in three, programmes that combined family psychoeducation and relaxation training were evaluated (Whitman et al., 1985; Gebert et al., 1998; Castes et al., 1999); and four studies evaluated programmes which included family psychoeducation, relaxation and behavioural skills training (Perrin et al., 1992; Perez et al., 1999; Lewis et al., 1984; Vazquez & Buceta, 1993). In two studies the impact of family therapy on children's adjustment to asthma was evaluated (Lask & Matthew, 1979; Gustaffson et al., 1986). Nine of the studies were conducted in the USA, two in Venezuala, two in Sweden and one each in the UK, Australia, the Netherlands, Israel, Canada, Spain and Germany. All of the studies were tertiary prevention studies involving comparative group designs. All children had a diagnosis of asthma, although the way in which this was ascertained and the severity of asthma, where reported, varied considerably from study to study. Altogether across the twenty studies there were 946 children of whom 506 participated in psychological intervention programmes and 440 were assigned to control or comparison groups. Treatment and control group sizes ranged from seven to fifty-three. Participants' ages ranged from two to sixteen years, with a mean age of nine years, while 60% of cases were male and 40% were female. Cases were predominantly from middle-class backgrounds. In eight studies, the intervention took place in a clinic setting with additional sessions in the home. Two studies involved home-based interventions, while in one study intervention took place in either the home or school. One study involved school-based intervention and one involved residential camp-based intervention. The duration of interventions ranged from two weeks to one year, while intensity ranged from two to 180 sessions (mean = 17 sessions over 12 weeks).

Table 11.1 Characteristics of studies of intervention programmes for children with asthma

Study no.	Study type	Authors	Year	Country	N per group	Mean age and range	Gender	Family characteristics	Programme setting	Programme duration
1	R	Kotses et al.	1978	USA	1. R-FBF = 10 2. R-BBF = 10 3. C1 = 10 4. C2 = 10	11 y	M 70% F 30%	—	Camp	9 sess over 3 w
2	R	Kohen	1996	USA	1. R-SH = 7 2. R-WS = 7 3. P = 7 4. C = 7	7–12 y	M 70% F 30%	—	Clinic	5 sess over 2 y
3	PE-SA	Rakos et al.	1985	USA	1. PE-SA = 20 2. C = 23	10 y 7–12 y	M 63% F 37%	—	Home	
4	PE-SA	Holzheimer et al.	1998	Australia	1. PE-SA-B + V = 20 2. PE-SA-B = 20 3. PE-SA-V = 20 4. C = 20	4 y 2–6 y		—	Home	3 sess over 4 m
5	PE-C	Parcel et al.	1980	USA	1. PE-G-C = 53 2. C = 51	9 y 5–11 y	M 41% F 63%	Low SES 47%	School	24 sess over 24 w
6	PE-C	Colland	1993	Netherlands	1. PE-G-C + R + BST = 48 2. P = 34 3. C = 30	10 y 8–12 y	M 61% F 39%	Mixed SES		10 h over 10 w
7	PE-C	Dahl et al.	1990	Sweden	1. PE-I-C + R + BST = 10 2. C = 10				Home School	4 sess over 4 w
8	PE-F	Fireman et al.	1981	USA	1. PE-I-G-F = 13 2. C = 13	7 y 2–14 y	M 81% F 19%	Low SES 8%	Clinic	4 h over 8–16 m 4 h group sess telephone contact
9	PE-F	Kubly & McClellan	1984	USA	1. PE-G-F = 13 2. C = 15	8 y	M 25% F 75%	Non-white 12%	School	4 sess over 3/4 w
10	PE-F	Tal et al.	1990	Israel	1. PE-G-F = 18 2. C = 10	8–12 y		—	Clinic	2 h over 6 w

	Treatment	Author	Year	Country	Groups (n)	Age	Gender	SES/Other	Setting	Duration
11	PE-F	Hughes et al.	1991	Canada	1. PE-I-F = 44 2. C = 45	10 y 6–16 y	M 63% F 37%	—	Clinic and home	4 sess over 1 y 2 home visits
12	PE-F + R	Whitman et al.	1985	USA	1. PE-G-F + R = 19 2. C = 19	9 y 6–14 y	M 65% F 35%	—		8 sess over 4 w
13	PE-F + R	Gebert et al.	1998	Germany	1. PE-G-F + R = 29 2. PE-G-F + R + BS = 27 3. C = 25	9 y 7–14 y		—	Clinic Home	5 d + 6 BS over 6 m
14	PE-F + R	Castes et al.	1999	Venezuela	1. PE-G-F + R + SE = 19 2. C = 16	11 y 6–15 y	M 39% F 61%	Low SES		180 sess over 6 m
15	PE-F + R + BST	Perrin et al.	1992	USA	1. PE-G-F + R + BST = 29 2. C = 27	9 y 6–14 y	M 59% F 41%	Non-white 15% Mixed SES		2 h over 4 w
16	PE-F + R + BST	Perez et al.	1999	Venezuela	1. PE-G-F + R + BST = 17 2. C = 12	6–14 y	M 55% F 45%		Clinic	P- 2 sess over 2 w C-6 h
17	PE-F + R + BST	Lewis et al.	1984	USA	1. PE-G-F + R + BST = 48 2. P = 28	10 y 8–12 y	M 77% F 23%	SPF 20%	Clinic	5 h over 5 w
18	PE-F + R + BST	Vazquez & Buceta	1993	Spain	1. PE-I-F + R + BST = 9 2. PE-I-F + BST = 9 3. C = 9	11 y 8–13 y	M 70% F 30%	—		6 h over 6 w
19	FT	Lask & Matthew	1979	UK	1. FT = 18 2. C = 11	4–14 y		—	Clinic	6 h over 4 m
20	FT	Gustaffson et al.	1986	Sweden	1. FT = 9 2. C = 8	9 y 6–15 y		—		8 sess

Notes

R = relaxation. PE-SA = self-administered psychoeducation. PE-C = psychoeducation. PE-F = psychoeducation for children. PE-F = psychoeducation for families. PE-F + R = psychoeducation for families with relaxation skills training. PE-F + R + BST = psychoeducation for families with relaxation and behavioural skills training. FT = family therapy. R-FBF = relaxation through frontalis biofeedback. R-BBF = relaxation through brachioradialis biofeedback. R-SH = relaxation by self-hypnosis. R-WS = relaxation by waking suggestion. PE-SA-B + V = self-administered psychoeducation programme using book and video. PE-SA-V = self-administered psychoeducation programme using video. PE-SA-B = self-administered psychoeducation programme using book. PE-G-C = group psychoeducation for children. PE-G-C + R + BST = group psychoeducation for children with relaxation and behavioural skills training. PE-I-C + R + BST = individual psychoeducation for children with relaxation and behavioural skills training. PE-I-G-F = individual and group psychoeducation for families. PE-I-F = individual psychoeducation for families. PE-G-F = group psychoeducation for families. PE-I-F + BST = individual psychoeducation for families with behavioural skills training. PE-G-F + R = group psychoeducation for families with relaxation skills training. PE-G-F + R + BS = group psychoeducation for families with relaxation skills training and booster sessions. PE-G-F + R + SE = group psychoeducation for families with relaxation skills training and self-esteem work. PE-G-F + R + BST = group psychoeducation for families with relaxation and behavioural skills training. C = control group. P = attention placebo control group. SES = socioeconomic status. SPF = single parent family. h = hour. d = day. w = week. m = month. y = year. sess = sessions.

Methodological features

Methodological features of the twenty studies are given in Table 11.2. All of the studies were comparative group outcome studies and in fifteen of the twenty studies cases were randomly assigned to treatment or control groups. While all of the studies involved cases that were diagnostically homogeneous, only fifteen out of twenty studies involved cases that were demographically similar. While all of the studies involved pre- and post-treatment assessment, a follow-up assessment was conducted in only twelve of the twenty studies. The most common types of outcome measure were parent ratings, which were included in eighteen of the twenty studies, followed by children's self-reports, which were included in fifteen studies. Physicians' ratings or information abstracted from medical records were used in ten studies. In six studies teachers' ratings or information abstracted from school records were used. Clinicians' ratings were used in only three studies. Physiological measures were used in nine studies. Deterioration was assessed in fifteen studies and drop-out rates were reported in eighteen studies. Only four studies offered data on the clinical significance of treatment gains. While eleven studies gave information on concurrent treatment, none reported information on subsequent treatment. None of the studies evaluated manualized programmes or included integrity checks for treatment fidelity. None of the studies reported that therapists received supervision. However, experienced trainers or therapists were used in twelve of the twenty studies. From a methodological viewpoint, it may be concluded that the studies reviewed here are sufficiently well designed to allow relatively reliable conclusions to be drawn from a review of their findings.

Substantive findings

Effect sizes and improvement rates for the twenty studies are given in Table 11.3. A narrative summary of key findings from all of the studies is presented in Table 11.4.

Relaxation through self-hypnosis and biofeedback training

Two studies evaluated the effects of relaxation training, involving self-hypnosis and biofeedback, on the adjustment of children with asthma (Kotses et al., 1978; Kohen, 1996). Kotses et al. (1978) found that electromyographic (EMG) frontalis biofeedback was more effective than brachioradialis biofeedback in leading to reduced muscle tension as indexed by EMG level and improved peak flow meter ratings. The efficacy of each type of biofeedback was evaluated by comparing the status of children receiving accurate information on their muscle activity level with that of a non-contingent group who received inaccurate muscle feedback. The effect

Table 11.2 Methodological features of studies of intervention programmes for children with asthma

Study number

Feature	S1	S2	S3	S4	S5	S6	S7	S8	S9	S10	S11	S12	S13	S14	S15	S16	S17	S18	S19	S20
Control or comparison group	1	1	1	1	1	1	1	0	1	1	1	1	1	1	1	1	1	1	1	1
Random assignment	1	1	1	1	0	1	1	0	0	0	1	1	1	0	1	1	0	1	1	1
Diagnostic homogeneity	1	1	0	1	1	1	0	1	1	1	1	1	1	1	1	1	1	1	1	1
Demographic similarity	1	1	1	0	1	1	0	1	0	0	1	1	1	1	0	1	1	1	1	0
Pre-treatment assessment	1	1	1	1	1	1	1	1	1	1	1	1	1	1	1	1	1	1	1	1
Post-treatment assessment	1	1	1	1	1	1	1	1	1	1	1	1	1	1	1	1	1	1	1	1
3-month follow-up assessment	0	1	1	0	0	1	1	0	0	1	1	1	0	0	0	1	1	1	1	1
Children's self-report	0	1	0	1	1	1	1	1	1	0	1	1	1	1	1	1	1	1	1	0
Parents' ratings	0	1	1	1	1	1	1	1	0	1	1	0	1	0	1	0	1	0	1	1
Teachers' ratings/school records	0	0	1	0	0	1	0	1	0	0	0	0	0	0	0	0	0	0	0	0
Therapist or trainer ratings	0	0	0	0	0	0	0	0	0	1	1	1	1	0	1	0	0	1	0	0
Physician ratings/medical records	0	1	1	0	0	1	0	1	0	0	0	0	0	1	0	1	1	0	0	1
Physiological measures	1	1	0	0	0	0	0	0	0	0	0	1	1	1	0	0	0	0	0	1
Deterioration assessed	0	1	1	1	0	1	1	0	0	1	0	0	1	1	1	1	1	1	1	1
Drop-out assessed	1	1	1	1	1	1	1	1	1	1	0	1	1	1	1	0	1	1	1	1
Clinical significance of change assessed	0	0	1	0	0	0	1	0	0	1	0	0	0	0	0	0	0	1	0	0
Experienced therapists or trainers used	0	0	0	1	0	1	0	1	1	1	1	1	1	0	0	1	1	0	1	0
Programmes were equally valued	0	0	0	0	0	0	0	0	0	0	0	0	0	0	0	1	0	0	0	0
Programmes were manualized	0	0	0	0	0	0	0	0	0	0	0	0	0	0	0	0	0	0	0	0
Supervision was provided	0	0	0	0	0	0	0	0	0	0	0	0	0	0	0	0	0	0	0	0
Programme integrity checked	0	0	0	0	0	0	0	0	0	1	0	0	0	1	0	0	0	0	0	0
Data on concurrent treatment given	1	1	0	1	0	0	0	1	0	0	0	1	1	1	1	1	0	0	1	1
Data on subsequent treatment given	0	0	0	0	0	0	0	0	0	0	0	0	0	0	0	0	0	0	0	0
Total	9	14	14	11	8	14	13	11	10	10	15	12	14	10	11	13	13	13	15	13

Notes
S = study. 1 = design feature was present. 0 = design feature was absent.

Table 11.3 Summary of results of treatment effects and outcome rates of studies of intervention programmes for children with asthma

Variable	Child-focused relaxation skills training — Study 1 R-FBF v C	Study 2 R-BBF v C	Study 2 R-SH v R-WS	Study 2 R-SH v C	Study 2 R-SH v C	Study 2 R-SH v P	Child-focused psychoeducation — Study 3 PE-SA v C	Study 4 PE-SA-B+V v C	Study 4 PE-SA-B v C	Study 4 PE-SA-V v C	Study 5 PE-G-C v C	Child-focused psychoeducation with relaxation and behavioural skills training — Study 6 PE-G-C+R+BST v P	Study 7 PE-G-C+R+BST v C	Study 7 PE-I-C+R+BST v C
Improvement after programme														
Children's knowledge	—	—	—	—	—	—	0.0	0.9	0.4	0.7	0.4	0.8	0.8	—
Health locus of control	—	—	—	—	—	—	0.5	—	—	—	0.4	—	—	—
Self-management	—	—	—	—	—	—	0	0.5	0.0	0.0	—	—	—	—
ER/physician visits	—	—	0.0	1.2	0	—	0.5	—	—	—	—	0.5	0.5	—
School absences	—	—	2.3	2.3	0	—	0.0	—	—	—	—	—	—	—
Symptoms	—	—	2.3	1.4	1.4	1.4	—	0.0	0.0	0.0	—	—	—	1.1
Physiological measures	1.2	0.0	0.0	0.0	0.0	0.0	—	0.0	0.0	0.0	—	0.0	0.0	0.0
Improvement at follow-up														
Children's knowledge	—	—	—	—	—	—	—	—	—	—	—	0.8	—	—
Health locus of control	—	—	—	—	—	—	—	—	—	—	—	—	—	—
Self-management	—	—	—	—	—	—	—	—	—	—	—	—	—	—
ER/physician visits	—	—	—	—	—	—	—	—	—	—	—	0.5	—	—
School absences	—	—	—	—	—	—	—	—	—	—	—	0.5	—	—
Symptoms	—	—	—	—	—	—	—	—	—	—	—	0.5	—	—
Physiological measures	—	—	—	—	—	—	—	—	—	—	—	0.0	—	—
Positive clinical outcomes														
% improved after treatment	—	—	—	52%	—	—	—	—	—	—	—	50%	50%	50%
% improved at follow-up	—	—	—	35%	—	—	—	—	—	—	—	23%	33%	12%

Negative clinical outcomes

% Deterioration	—	—	14%	—	—	—	—	—	—	—	—	—
			v									
			0									
% Drop-out	—	—	15%	—	—	—	—	—	—	0%	—	—

Notes
R-FBF = relaxation through frontalis biofeedback. R-BBF = relaxation through brachioradialis biofeedback. R-SH = relaxation by self-hypnosis. R-WS = relaxation by waking suggestion. PE-SA-B + V = self-administered psychoeducation programme using book and video. PE-SA-V = self-administered psychoeducation programme using video. PE-SA-B = self-administered psychoeducation programme using book. PE-G-C = group psychoeducation for children. PE-G-C + R + BST = group psychoeducation for children with relaxation and behavioural skills training. PE-I-C + R + BST = individual psychoeducation for children with relaxation and behavioural skills training. PE-I-G-F = individual and group psychoeducation for families. PE-I-F = individual psychoeducation for families. PE-G-F = group psychoeducation for families. PE-I-F + BST = individual psychoeducation for families with behavioural skills training. PE-G-F + R = group psychoeducation for families with relaxation skills training. PE-G-F + R + BS = group psychoeducation for families with relaxation skills training and booster sessions. PE-G-F + R + SE = group psychoeducation for families with relaxation skills training and self-esteem work. PE-G-F + R + BST = group psychoeducation for families with relaxation and behavioural skills training. FT = Family therapy. C = control group. P = attention placebo control group.

Table 11.3 (continued) Summary of results of treatment effects and outcome rates of studies of intervention programmes for children with asthma

	Study number and condition													
	Family psychoeducation				Family psychoeducation with relaxation skills training				Family psychoeducation with relaxation and behavioural skills training				Family therapy	
	Study 8	Study 9	Study 10	Study 11	Study 12	Study 13		Study 14	Study 15	Study 16	Study 17	Study 18	Study 19	Study 20
Variable	PE-I-G-F v C	PE-G-F v C	PE-G-F v C	PE-I-F v C	PE-G-F + R v C	PE-G-F + R v C	PE-G-F+ R+BS v C	PE-G-F + R + SE v C	PE-G-F + R + BST v C	PE-G-F + R + BST v C	PE-G-F + R + BST v C	PE-G-F + R + BST v C	FT v C	FT v C
Improvement after programme														
Children's knowledge	—	—	—	—	1.1	—	—	—	0.6	1.4	0.0	—	—	—
Health locus of control	—	0.8	—	—	—	—	—	—	—	—	—	0.0	—	—
Self-management	—	0.0	0.8	0.7	1.1	1.2	1.4	—	—	1.7	0.5	2.3	—	—
ER/physician visits	0.8	—	—	0.4	—	—	—	0.0	—	—	0.4	—	—	0.8
School absences	—	—	—	0.5	—	0.0	0.0	—	0.0	—	—	0.0	—	—
Symptoms	1.1	—	—	0.7	0.6	0.6	0.5	0.7	—	0.8	—	0.0	1.3	1.4
Physiological measures	—	—	—	0.7	—	—	—	—	—	—	—	0.0	0.9	0.0
Improvement at follow-up														
Children's knowledge	—	—	—	—	—	—	—	—	—	—	—	—	—	—
Health locus of control	—	—	—	—	0.8	—	—	—	—	—	—	—	—	—
Self-management	—	—	0.9	0.6	0.9	—	—	—	—	—	—	—	—	—
ER/physician visits	—	—	—	0.5	—	—	—	—	—	—	—	—	—	—
School absences	—	—	—	0.0	0.6	—	—	—	—	—	—	—	—	—
Symptoms	—	—	—	—	—	—	—	—	—	—	—	—	—	—
Physiological measures	—	—	—	0.0	—	—	—	—	—	—	—	—	—	—
Positive clinical outcomes														
% improved after treatment	61% v	75% v	85% v	29% v	—	—	—	—	—	—	16% v	—	66% v	—
% improved at follow-up	38%	25%	25%	11%	—	—	—	—	—	—	11%	—	13%	—

Negative clinical outcomes

% Deterioration	—	—	0 v 25%	11% v 29%	—	—	—	—	—	—	11% v 50%
% Drop-out	58%	—	0	6%	0%	3%	31%	33%	34%	22%	10%

Notes

R-FBF = relaxation through frontalis biofeedback. R-BBF = relaxation through brachioradialis biofeedback. R-SH = relaxation by self-hypnosis. R-WS = relaxation by waking suggestion. PE-SA-B + V = self-administered psychoeducation programme using book and video. PE-SA-V = self-administered psychoeducation programme using video. PE-SA-B = self-administered psychoeducation programme using book. PE-G-C = group psychoeducation for children. PE-G-C + R + BST = group psychoeducation for children with relaxation and behavioural skills training. PE-I-C + R + BST = individual psychoeducation for children with relaxation and behavioural skills training. PE-I-G-F = individual and group psychoeducation for families. PE-I-F = individual psychoeducation for families. PE-G-F = group psychoeducation for families. PE-I-F + BST = individual psychoeducation for families with behavioural skills training. PE-G-F + R = group psychoeducation for families with relaxation skills training. PE-G-F + R + BS = group psychoeducation for families with relaxation skills training and booster sessions. PE-G-F + R + SE = group psychoeducation for families with relaxation skills training and self-esteem work. PE-G-F + R + BST = group psychoeducation for families with relaxation and behavioural skills training. FT = family therapy. C = control group. P = attention placebo control group.

Table 11.4 Summary of key findings of studies of intervention programmes for children with asthma

Study no.	Authors	Year	N per group	No. of sessions	Group differences	Key findings
1	Kotses et al.	1978	1. R-FBF = 10 2. R-BBF = 10 3. C1 = 10 4. C2 = 10	9 sess over 3 w	Morbidity 1 > 3, 2 = 4	• Following participation in an operant frontalis relaxation training programme, children in the treatment group improved significantly in EMG levels and peak expiratory flow rate, compared to control group • Children trained in brachioradialis muscle relaxation did not improve significantly on physiological indices, compared to the control group
2	Kohen	1996	1. R-SH = 7 2. R-WS = 7 3. P = 7 4. C = 7	5 sess over 2 y	Morbidity 1 > 2 = 3 = 4 Functionality 1 = 3 > 2 = 4	• Following participation in a self-hypnosis training programme, children in the treatment group had significantly fewer emergency room visits and school absences and showed significant improvements on measures of asthma severity, compared to the control group • Children in the self-hypnosis group improved significantly on measures of school absenteeism and asthma severity compared to a group receiving waking suggestion only
3	Rakos et al.	1985	1. PE-SA = 20 2. C = 23		Morbidity 1 = 2 Functionality 1 > 2 Attitudes 1 = 2	• Following participation in a self-administered psychoeducation programme, children in the treatment group improved significantly in asthma self-control, progression of asthma and school attendance, compared to control group • There were no significant differences between the groups in self-esteem, health locus of control, medical contact, severity of disease and average asthma attack
4	Holzheimer et al.	1998	1. PE-SA-B + V = 20 2. PE-SA-B = 20 3. PE-SA-V = 20 4. C = 20	3 sess (10 min) over 4 m	Morbidity 1 = 2 = 3 = 4 Functionality 1 > 2 = 3 = 4 Knowledge 1 > 3 > 2 > 4	• Following treatment, children in all three psychoeducational groups improved significantly on measures of asthma knowledge compared to the control group • The group who were exposed to both a video and a book showed the greatest improvements. • Children who were exposed to both a video and a book resource had significantly fewer physician contacts than children in the control group • Following intervention, no significant differences were found between the treatment groups and control groups on measures of compliance and health
5	Parcel et al.	1980	1. PE-G-C = 53 2. C = 51	24 sess over 24 w	Attitudes/ knowledge 1 > 2	• Following participation in a group psychoeducation programme, children in the treatment group improved significantly on measures of knowledge, health locus of control, and anxiety associated with illness. • No significant changes were observed among children in the control group

No.	Author	Year	Groups	Duration	Outcomes	Findings
6	Colland	1993	1. PE-G-C + R + BST = 48 2. P = 34 3. C = 30	10 h over 10 w	Morbidity 1 = 2 = 3 Functionality 1 > 2 = 3 Knowledge 1 > 2 = 3	• Following participation in a group programme which incorporated psychoeducation, relaxation and behaviour skills training, children in the treatment group improved significantly on measures of knowledge and self-management, compared to both the placebo and control group • These gains were maintained at follow-up • Children in treatment group had significantly fewer physician visits and school absenteeism than the placebo or control group
7	Dahl et al.	1990	1. PE-I-C + R + BST = 10 2. C = 10	4 h over 4 w	Morbidity 1 = 2 Functionality 1 > 2	• Following participation in an individual programme which incorporated psychoeducation, relaxation and behaviour skills training, children in the treatment group significantly reduced their use of medication without increasing asthma symptoms and had significantly fewer days of school absence, compared to the control group
8	Fireman et al.	1981	1. PE-I-G-F = 13 2. C = 13	4 h over 8–16 m 4 h group sess telephone contact	Morbidity 1 > 2 Functionality 1 > 2	• Following participation, with their parents, in a psychoeducation programme which incorporated individual and group sessions, children in the treatment group had significantly fewer asthma attacks and school absences compared to the control group • During the study period children in the treatment group had no hospitalizations compared to four (31%) hospitalizations among the comparison group
9	Kubly & McClellan	1984	1. PE-G-F = 13 2. C = 15	4 sess over 3/4 w	Functionality 1 = 2 Attitudes 1 > 2	• Following a family group psychoeducation programme, children in the treatment group improved significantly on measures of health locus of control, compared to a control group who received only factual information about asthma • There were no significant differences between the treatment and control groups in asthma self-care activities
10	Tal et al.	1990	1. PE-G-F = 18 2. C = 10	2 h over 6 w	Functionality 1 > 2	• Following intervention, children who participated in a family group psychoeducation programme improved significantly in self-management and there was a significant increase in the encouragement of independence in the intervention group families, compared to the control group
11	Hughes et al.	1991	1. PE-I-F = 44 2. C = 45	4 sess over 1 y 2 home visits	Morbidity 1 > 2 Functionality 1 > 2	• Following participation in a family psychoeducation programme that focused on ambulatory and home care, children in the treatment group had improved significantly on measures of pulmonary function, asthma severity, aerosol technique and school absenteeism compared to the control group • At one-year follow-up, improvements in self-management were maintained, and the treatment group had significantly fewer visits to physicians than control group

Table 11.4 continued

Study no.	Authors	Year	N per group	No. of sessions	Group differences	Key findings
12	Whitman et al.	1985	1. PE-G-F + R = 19 2. C = 19	8 sess over 4 w	Functionality 1 > 2 Knowledge 1 > 2	• In the 3 months following intervention, children who had participated in a family group psychoeducation and relaxation programme had significantly fewer asthma episodes and days of severe asthma than the control group • Children in the intervention group improved significantly in knowledge of asthma and management skills compared to the control group, both immediately following the intervention and at 3-month follow-up
13	Gebert et al.	1998	1. PE-G-F + R = 29 2. PE-G-F + R + BS = 27 3. C = 25	5 d follow-up = 6 sess over 6 m	Morbidity 1 + 2 > 3 Functionality 1 = 2 > 3	• Following participation with their parents in a group programme that incorporated psychoeducation and relaxation, children in the treatment groups significantly improved on measures of self-management and morbidity compared to the control group • Children who received follow-up meetings showed greater improvements in asthma self-management than children receiving training programme but no follow-up
14	Castes et al.	1999	1. PE-G-F + R + SE = 19 2. C = 16	180 sess over 6 m	Morbidity 1 > 2 Functionality 1 = 2	• Following participation in a family group psychoeducation and relaxation programme which also included work on self-esteem, children in the treatment group showed significant improvement on a number of physiological measures compared to control group • The results suggest that psychosocial intervention induces immunological alterations that are responsible for the clinical and physiological improvements observed in the intervention group
15	Perrin et al.	1992	1. PE-G-F + R + BST = 29 2. C = 27	2 h over 4 w	Functionality 1 = 2 Knowledge 1 > 2	• Following participation in a family group programme that incorporated psychoeducation, relaxation, and behaviour skills training, children in the treatment group improved significantly on the total behaviour problems score and internalizing scale of the CBCL and on measures of asthma knowledge, and a significant increase in daily chores compared to control group • Children in the intervention group increased significantly in measures of asthma knowledge. • Results indicate that the intervention may have had a buffering effect on the children's response to negative life events

	Author	Year	Groups (N)	Duration	Outcomes	Findings
16	Perez et al.	1999	1. PE-G-F + R + BST = 17 2. C = 12	P: 2 sess over 2 w C: 6 h	Functionality 1 > 2 Knowledge 1 > 2	• Following treatment and at follow-up, children who participated in a family-based programme that incorporated psychoeducation, relaxation, and behaviour skills training had improved significantly on measures of children's and parents' asthma knowledge and self-management skills compared to control group • Younger children benefited from the programme more than older children, independently of their asthmatic condition
17	Lewis et al.	1984	1. PE-G-F + R + BST = 48 2. P = 28	5 h over 5 w	Functionality 1 > 2 Knowledge 1 = 2	• Following participation in a family group programme that incorporated psychoeducation, relaxation, and behaviour skills training, children in the treatment group had significantly fewer emergency room visits and days of hospitalization compared to the control group • Self reported compliance behaviour significantly improved among children in the treatment group, but not among children in the control group • There were no significant differences between the groups in knowledge about asthma and beliefs
18	Vazquez & Buceta	1993	1. PE-I-F + R + BST = 9 2. PE-I-F + BST = 9 3. C = 9	6 h over 6 w	Morbidity 1 = 2 = 3 Functionality 1 = 2 > 3 Attitudes 1 = 2 = 3	• Following participation with a family-based programme that incorporated psychoeducation and behaviour skills training, with or without relaxation, children in the treatment groups improved significantly on measures of self-management compared to the control group • Patients with poor pre-training asthma self-care benefited most from the programme • Relaxation training did not specifically contribute to the changes observed following intervention
19	Lask & Matthew	1979	1. FT = 18 2. C = 11	6 h over 4 m	Morbidity 1 > 2	• Following treatment, the group receiving family therapy showed significant improvements in asthma morbidity and thoracic gas volume, compared to the control group • There was no significant difference between the groups on peak expiratory flow rate, forced expiratory volume and levels of activity
20	Gustaffson et al.	1986	1. FT = 9 2. C = 8	2–21 sess (mean = 8)	Morbidity 1 > 2 Functionality 1 > 2	• Following treatment, the group receiving family therapy showed significant improvements in number of functionally impaired days and general paediatric assessment compared to the control group

Notes

R = relaxation. PE-SA = self-administered psychoeducation. PE-C = psychoeducation for children. PE-F = psychoeducation. PE-C = psychoeducation for children. PE-F = family therapy. FT = family therapy. R-FBF = relaxation through frontalis biofeedback. R-BBF = relaxation through brachioradialis biofeedback. R-SH = relaxation by self-hypnosis. R-WS = relaxation by waking suggestion. PE-SA-B + V = self-administered psychoeducation programme using book and video. PE-SA-V = self-administered psychoeducation programme using video. PE-SA-B = self-administered psychoeducation programme using book. PE-G-C = group psychoeducation for children. PE-I-C + R + BST = group psychoeducation for children with relaxation and behavioural skills training. PE-I-C + R + BST = individual psychoeducation for children with relaxation and behavioural skills training. PE-I-G-F = individual and group psychoeducation for families. PE-I-F = individual psychoeducation for families. PE-G-F = group psychoeducation for families. PE-I-F + BST = individual psychoeducation for families with behavioural skills training. PE-G-F + R = group psychoeducation for families with relaxation skills training. PE-G-F + R + BS = group psychoeducation for families with relaxation skills training and booster sessions. PE-G-F + R + SE = group psychoeducation for families with relaxation skills training and self-esteem work. PE-G-F + R + BST = group psychoeducation for families with relaxation and behavioural skills training. C = control group. P = attention placebo control group. h = hour. d = day. w = week. m = month. y = year. sess = sessions.

size for the EMG frontalis biofeedback group was 1.2, indicating that the average treated case fared better than 88% of controls.

Compared with controls and children who received waking suggestion, Kohen (1996) found that children who trained in self-hypnotic relaxation showed greater improvement. Effect sizes based on comparison with controls were 0.0 for pulmonary functioning, 1.4 for self-reported symptoms, 2.3 for school absences and 1.2 for emergency hospital visits. Averaging across these domains the mean effect size was 1.6, so the average treated case fared better than 95% of untreated controls.

In summary, the studies reviewed in this section show that both self-hypnosis training and biofeedback involving the frontalis muscles are effective in improving adjustment among children with asthma.

Child-focused psychoeducational programmes

In three studies child-focused psychoeducational programmes were evaluated, two of which involved self-administered psychoeducational information packs (Rakos et al., 1985; Holzheimer et al., 1998) and one of which was a group training programme (Parcel et al., 1980). Rakos et al. (1985) found that compared with controls youngsters who received *Superstuff* (Weiss, 1981), a psychoeducational information pack, improved significantly in asthma self-control, progression of asthma and school attendance. Holzheimer et al. (1998) found that compared with controls youngsters who received a psycho-educational pack containing either a video – *Young Children Managing Asthma* (Mohay & Masters, 1993) – or a book – *What's that Noise?* (Holzheimer, 1993) – or both showed improved knowledge of asthma and children who received the pack containing both the video and book had significantly fewer medical emergency visits than children in the control group. Parcel et al. (1980) found that compared with controls, youngsters who participated in a group psychoeducation programme based on the book *Teaching Myself about Asthma* (Parcel et al., 1979) showed greater improvement on measures of asthma knowledge, health locus of control, and asthma-related anxiety.

From these three studies it may be concluded that child-focused psycho-educational programmes can improve adjustment to asthma in specific ways. First, effect sizes for knowledge about asthma ranged from 0.4 to 0.9 with a mean of 0.6, indicating that the average programme participant showed greater knowledge about asthma and its management than 73% of untreated controls. Second, effect sizes for adherence and self-management of asthma ranged from 0 to 0.5 with a mean of 0.3, indicating that the average programme participant showed better adherence than 62% of untreated controls. Third, in the single study where school absence was assessed the effect size was 0.5, indicating that the average programme participant showed better school attendance than 69% of untreated controls. Fourth, in the single study where health locus of control was assessed the effect size was 0.4, indicating that the average programme participant showed a more internal health locus of control than 66% of untreated controls. Fifth, effect sizes for self-reported symptoms and emergency medical visits were 0, indicating that psychoeducational programmes had no effect on morbidity. In summary, psychoeducation programmes were found to have a significant impact on knowledge, adherence, school absenteeism and health locus of control, but no impact on emergency medical service use and morbidity.

Child-focused psychoeducational programmes with combined relaxation and behavioural skills training

In two studies child-focused psychoeducational programmes with combined relaxation and behavioural skills training were evaluated (Colland, 1993; Dahl et al., 1990). Colland (1993) found that compared with controls and children in an attention placebo group, children who participated in a group-based programme which combined psychoeducation with relaxation and behavioural skills training showed improved adjustment which was maintained at one-year follow-up. Effect sizes after treatment and at follow-up were 0.8 for increased knowledge about asthma and 0.5 for fewer emergency medical visits. For a reduction in school absenteeism at follow-up, the effect size was 0.5. However, the programme has no effect on self-reported symptoms. Averaging across these domains and assessment periods the mean effect size was 0.4, indicating that the average programme participant fared better than 66% of controls.

Dahl et al. (1990) found that compared with controls, children who participated in an individually based programme involving psychoeducation, relaxation and behaviour skills training showed a reduction in use of medication without increasing asthma symptoms and a reduction in school absenteeism. The mean effect size for school absence was 1.1 and there was no effect size for symptom reduction.

From these two studies it may be concluded that child-focused psychoeducational programmes with combined relaxation and behavioural skills training improved knowledge, school absenteeism and emergency medical service use but not morbidity.

Family psychoeducation programmes

In four studies family psychoeducational programmes were evaluated, two of which used a group family format (Kubly & McClellan, 1984; Tal et al., 1990), one of which used a format where families were seen on an individual basis (Hughes et al., 1991), and one of which combined group family sessions with individual family sessions (Fireman et al., 1981). Kubly and McClellan (1984) found that, compared with controls, youngsters whose families participated in a group psychoeducation programme, showed improvements on measures of health locus of control but not adherence. Tal et al. (1990) found that compared with controls, in families who participated in a group psychoeducation programme, parents encouraged their asthmatic youngsters to be more autonomous in their management of asthma and children showed improvements in self-management and adherence. Hughes et al. (1991) found that compared with controls, children whose families participated in a programme where families were seen individually showed improvement in pulmonary functioning, asthma severity, aerosol technique and a reduction in school absenteeism. Improvements in self-management were maintained at one-year follow-up and fewer emergency medical service visits were made by programme participants. Fireman et al. (1981) found that compared with controls, youngsters whose families participated in a psychoeducational programme which incorporated both individual and group family sessions had fewer asthma attacks and school absences. During the study period children in the treatment group had no hospitalizations compared to four (31%) hospitalizations among children in the comparison group.

From these three studies it may be concluded that family-oriented psychoeducational programmes can improve adjustment to asthma in specific ways. First, effect sizes for self-management ranged from 0.0 to 0.9 with a mean of 0.5 after treatment and 0.8 at follow-up, indicating that the average programme participant showed greater adherence than 69% of untreated controls after treatment and 79% of controls at follow-up. Second, in the single study where emergency medical visits were used, the effect size was 0.5 at follow-up, indicating that the average programme participant made fewer emergency medical visits than 69% of untreated controls during the follow-up period. Third, effect sizes for school absenteeism ranged from 0.0 to 0.8 with a mean of 0.6 after treatment and 0 at follow-up, indicating that the average programme participant showed better school attendance than 73% of untreated controls after treatment but the groups did not differ at follow-up. Fourth, effect sizes for self-reported symptoms ranged from 0.5 to 1.1 with a mean of 0.8, indicating that the average programme participant reported less severe symptoms than 79% of untreated controls after treatment. Fifth, in the single study where physiological indices of respiratory functioning were used the effect size was 0.7 after treatment and 0 at follow-up, indicating that the average programme participant showed better functioning than 76% of untreated controls after treatment and the groups did not differ at follow-up. Sixth, in the single study where health locus of control was assessed the effect size was 0.8, indicating that the average programme participant showed a more internal health locus of control than 79% of untreated controls. In summary, family psychoeducational programmes were found to have a significant impact on adherence, symptom severity, school absenteeism, emergency medical service use, and health locus of control. While improvements in physiological measures of respiratory functioning and school absenteeism were not maintained in the long term, improvements in adherence and emergency medical service use were maintained.

Family psychoeducation programmes with relaxation training

In three studies family psychoeducation programmes which also included relaxation skills training were evaluated (Whitman et al., 1985; Gebert et al., 1998; Castes et al., 1999). Whitman et al. (1985) found that compared with controls, children whose families participated in a family group psychoeducation and relaxation programme reported fewer asthma episodes and fewer days of severe asthma in the three months following the programme. These children also showed greater gains in knowledge of asthma and self-management skills compared to the control group, both immediately following the programme and at three-month follow-up. Gebert et al. (1998) found that compared with controls, children whose families participated in a five-day family group psychoeducation and relaxation programme run by a multidisciplinary team showed greater improvement in adherence and morbidity. Children who received follow-up booster sessions showed greater improvements in asthma self-management than children who did not. Castes et al. (1999) found that, compared with controls, children whose families participated in a family group psychoeducation and relaxation programme that also included activities to enhance self-esteem showed greater improvement on physiological measures of respiratory system functioning.

From these three studies it may be concluded that family-oriented psychoeducational programmes which also include relaxation skills training can improve adjustment to asthma in specific ways. First, effect sizes for self-management ranged from 0.9 to 1.4 with a mean of 1.2 after treatment and a single effect size of 0.9 at follow-up, indicating that the average programme participant showed greater adherence than 88% of untreated controls after treatment and 82% of controls at follow-up. Second, effect sizes for self-reported symptoms ranged from 0.5 to 0.6 with a mean of 0.6 after treatment and a single effect size of 0.6 at follow-up, indicating that the average programme participant reported less severe symptoms than 73% of untreated controls after treatment and at follow-up. Third, in the single study where physiological indices of respiratory functioning were used the effect size was 0.7 after treatment, indicating that the average programme participant showed better functioning than 76% of untreated controls after treatment. Fourth, in the single study where knowledge of asthma was assessed the effect size was 1.1 after treatment and 0.8 at follow-up, indicating that the average programme participant showed greater knowledge than 86% of untreated controls after treatment and 79% of controls at follow-up. Fifth, effect sizes for reductions in school absenteeism and visits to emergency medical services were 0. In summary, family psychoeducation programmes that incorporated relaxation training led to significant improvements in knowledge, adherence and symptoms but had no impact on use of emergency health care services and school absenteeism.

Family psychoeducation programmes with relaxation and behaviour skills training

In four studies family psychoeducation programmes that incorporated both relaxation and behaviour skills training were evaluated, of which three used a group family format (Perrin et al., 1992; Perez et al., 1999; Lewis et al., 1984) and one involved individual family sessions (Vazquez & Buceta, 1993). Perrin et al. (1992) found that, compared with controls, children from families who participated in a group psychoeducational programme that included both relaxation and behavioural skills training showed an increase in knowledge about asthma, improvement on the total behaviour problems scale and the internalizing scale of the Child Behaviour Checklist (Achenbach, 1991), and an increase in rates of completion of daily chores. Perez et al. (1999) found that, compared with controls, children and parents from families who participated in a group psychoeducational programme that included both relaxation and behavioural skills training showed an increase in knowledge about asthma and the children showed increased adherence. Younger children benefited from the programme more than older children. Lewis et al. (1984) found that, compared with controls, children from families who participated in group psychoeducational programmes that included both relaxation and behavioural skills training showed an increase in knowledge about asthma, increased adherence, fewer emergency medical service visits, and fewer days of hospitalization. Vazquez and Buceta (1993) found that, compared with controls, children from families who participated in psychoeducational programmes that included both relaxation and behavioural skills training showed improved self-management and adherence. Patients who showed poor initial adherence benefited most from the programme. The study included a second treatment group which received all elements of the programme with the exception of relaxation training, and this group fared as well as the group that received the total programme, indicating that relaxation skills training added little to the overall effectiveness of this programme.

From these four studies it may be concluded that family-oriented psychoeducational programmes which also include relaxation and behavioural skills training can improve adjustment to asthma in specific ways. First, effect sizes for knowledge of asthma ranged from 0 to 1.4 with a mean of 0.7 after treatment, indicating that the average programme participant showed greater knowledge gains than 76% of untreated controls. Second, effect sizes for self-management ranged from 0.5 to 2.3 with a mean of 1.5, indicating that the average programme participant showed greater adherence than 93% of untreated controls. Third, effect sizes for self-reported symptoms ranged from 0 to 0.8 with a mean of 0.4, indicating that the average programme participant reported less severe symptoms than 66% of untreated controls. Fourth, in the single study where use of emergency services was assessed the effect size was 0.4, indicating that the average programme participant used emergency medical services less than 66% of untreated controls. Fifth, effect sizes for health locus of control, reductions in school absenteeism and physio-logical indices of respiratory system functioning were 0. In summary, family psychoeducational programmes which included relaxation and behavioural skills training were found to have a significant impact on knowledge, adher-ence, self-reported symptom severity, and use of emergency health services but not health locus of control, school absenteeism or physiological indices of respiratory system functioning.

Family therapy

In two studies the effectiveness of family therapy for asthma-related adjust-ment problems was evaluated (Lask & Matthew, 1979; Gustaffson et al., 1986). Lask and Matthew (1979) found that compared with controls, children from families who participated in family therapy showed significant improve-ments in self-reported symptom severity (day-wheeze score, effect size = 1.3) and a physiological index of respiratory system functioning (thoracic gas volume, effect size = 0.9). The average effect size across these two domains was 1.1, indicating that the average child whose family received family ther-apy fared better afterwards than 86% of controls. There was no significant difference between the groups on peak expiratory flow rate, forced expiratory volume and levels of activity. Gustaffson et al. (1986) found that compared with controls, children from families who participated in family therapy showed significant improvement on a general paediatric assessment (effect size = 1.4) and the number of functionally impaired days (effect size = 0.8). The average effect size across these two domains was 1.1, indicating that the average child whose family received family therapy fared better afterwards than 86% of controls. There was no significant difference between the groups on peak expiratory flow rate or medication usage. In summary, family therapy led to significant improvement in symptom severity and adjustment.

Conclusions

Asthma is one of the most common chronic diseases with a prevalence rate of about 10% among children. Its effects are pervasive and can lead to restric-tions in daily activity, absences from school, repeated hospitalization during severe attacks, hypoxia, seizures and brain damage; and, if left untreated, asthma is potentially fatal. The course of asthma is determined by the inter-action between abnormal respiratory, system physiological processes to which some youngsters have a predisposition, physical environmental trig-gers, and psychological processes. Psychological interventions for paediatric asthma include psychoeducation to improve understanding of the condition; relaxation training to help reduce physiological arousal; skills training to increase adherence to asthma management programmes; and family therapy to empower family members to work together to manage asthma effectively. From the present review it may be concluded that psychological intervention programmes involving one or more of these components can effectively prevent adjustment problems in children with asthma. From Table 11.5 it may be seen that overall family-based programmes are more effective than child-focused programmes and that the most effective programmes involve relaxation training (using frontalis biofeedback or self-hypnosis) and family therapy. The effectiveness of psychoeducational interventions may be enhanced by combining them with relaxation and behavioural skills training in multisystemic family-oriented programmes. Psychological intervention programmes have greatest impact on cognitive variables such as asthma-related attitudes and knowledge; a lesser impact on behavioural variables such as adherence, school absenteeism and health service use; and least impact on symptom severity.

Implications for policy and practice

These conclusions have implications for clinical practice and service development. First, they highlight the need to provide psychological interventions in conjunction with routine paediatric management of asthma, particularly where children have severe symptoms, repeated hospitalizations and/or adherence problems. Multisystemic family-based, psychoeducational programmes which include relaxation and behavioural skills training should be provided. These should typically be clinic based and involve approximately about six to eight sessions. Where service demands greatly outweigh available resources, self-administered psychoeducation should be provided as a preliminary measure but this should ideally be followed up with further intervention, particularly where youngsters have severe symptoms or adherence problems. If resources permit and particularly when parents cannot engage in

Table 11.5 Summary of results of treatment effects of studies of intervention programmes for children with asthma

Programme target	Programme components	Mean post-intervention effect size
Child focused	Relaxation skills training	1.2
	Psychoeducation	0.3
	Psychoeducation + relaxation + behavioural skills training	0.5
	All child focused	0.7
Family focused	Psychoeducation	0.7
	Psychoeducation + relaxation	0.6
	Psychoeducation + relaxation + behavioural skills training	0.7
	Family therapy	1.1
	All family focused	0.8

treatment, relaxation training and biofeedback techniques should be made available within the context of child-focused programmes. For children with severe asthma that is not well controlled with conventional treatment methods, family therapy (rather than multiple family group psychoeducation) should be provided.

Implications for research

Studies that examine the impact of design features that may make programmes more effective in particular circumstances are required. For example, comparative studies are required to assess if multisystemic family-oriented programmes which include family therapy, psychoeducation, relaxation skills training and behavioural skills training are more effective than any of these interventions alone or individually based psychoeducational or skills training programmes. Furthermore, such studies need to be carried out with patient groups who have different illness-related and demographic profiles. For example, studies are required that examine the effectiveness of programmes with different design features on youngsters with severe and moderate levels of symptom severity; or groups of youngsters from low and middle socioeconomic groups. These studies are important because morbidity and mortality rates have been found to be higher among those with severe symptom profiles from lower socioeconomic groups.

Programme integrity was not evaluated in any of the studies reviewed in this chapter. Future evaluation studies should include assessments of programme integrity. In such studies, training sessions are recorded and blind raters use programme integrity checklists to evaluate the degree to which sessions approximate manualized training protocols.

Studies are required which investigate the mechanisms and processes which underpin programme effectiveness. For example, studies are required to assess whether decreases in symptom severity, increases in pulmonary functioning, reduction in school absences and emergency service usage arise from improvements in avoidance of triggers, better use of medication, reductions in anxiety, increases in self-efficacy beliefs or alterations in patterns of family functioning.

Finally, future research should increase efforts to follow up participants after interventions so that long-term effects can be determined. Although the reversibility and variability of asthma contribute to high drop-out rates in longitudinal studies, various measures can be taken to overcome this, such as increasing initial sample size or giving participants incentives to co-operate with repeated assessments.

Assessment resources

Colland, V. & Fournier, E. (1990) The Asthma Coping Test. *Gedrag Gezondheid*, 18, 68–77.

Creer, T.L., Marion, R.J. & Creer, P.P. (1983). Asthma problem behavior checklist: Parental perceptions of the behavior of asthmatic children. *Journal of Asthma*, 20(2), 97–104.

Parcel. G.S. & Meyer, M.P. (1978). Development of an instrument to measure children's health locus of control. *Health Education Monograph*, 6, 149.

Spielberger, C.H.D. (1973). *State Trait Anxiety Inventory For Children*. Palo Alto: Consulting Psychologist.

Standardisation of lung function testing in children (1980). Proceedings and recommendations of the GAP conference committee, Cystic Fibrosis Foundation. *Journal of Pediatrics*, 97, 668–678.

Treatment manuals and resources

Bernstein, D.A. & Borkovec, T.D. (1973). *Progressive Relaxation Training: A Manual for the Helping Professions*. Champaign: Research Press.

Holzheimer, L. (1993). *What's That Noise?* Brisbane: Queensland University of Technology.

McDaniel, S.H., Hepworth, J. & Doherty, W. (1992). *Medical Family Therapy*. New York: Basic Books.

Mohay, H. & Masters, B. (1993). *Young Children Managing Asthma* [Video recording]. Brisbane: TSNII.

Parcel, G.G., Tiernan, K. & Nadar, R.R. (1979). *Teaching Myself about Asthma*. St Louis: CV Mosby.

Weiss, J.B. (1981). *Superstuff. In Self Management Educational Programs for Childhood Asthma* (Vol. 2., pp. 273–294). Bethesda, MD: National Institute of Allergic and Infectious Diseases.

12 Prevention of adjustment problems in children with diabetes

Eimear Farrell, Ruth Catherine Cullen and Alan Carr

Type 1 or insulin-dependent diabetes mellitus (IDDM) is an endocrine disorder typically diagnosed in childhood, characterized by complete pancreatic failure (Cox & Gonder-Frederick, 1992). It is distinguished from Type 2 or non-insulin-dependent diabetes mellitus (NIDDM), an adult onset disorder in which the pancreas continues to produce some insulin and which can often be managed by weight reduction and attention to diet. In this chapter, the focus is exclusively on IDDM. Poor adherence to the medical regime for IDDM and poor metabolic control occur quite frequently among diabetic children, with serious consequences. The purpose of this review was to examine the effectiveness of psychological interventions conducted with diabetic children and adolescents experiencing poor metabolic control.

Epidemiology

IDDM is one of the most chronic systemic disorders that affects children (Plotnick, 1999). The prevalence rate is approximately 1.2–1.9 cases per 1,000 children under the age of twenty. The onset of IDDM occurs most commonly in middle childhood. The long-term outcome of IDDM is associated with devastating complications in some cases, particularly those where there has been poor regime adherence. About 30–40% of IDDM cases develop endstage renal disease requiring dialysis or kidney transplantation; 5–10% of IDDM patients become blind due to retinopathy; and a proportion develop peripheral vascular disease leading to gangrene necessitating lower limb amputation.

Management of diabetes

The main treatment goal for children and adolescents with diabetes is the achievement of blood glucose levels as close as possible to the range for non-diabetics (Plotnick, 1999). This is achieved through a combination of insulin injections, balanced diet, exercise and self-monitoring of blood glucose (SMBG). Insulin injections are usually given twice a day, twenty minutes before meals. Consequently, meals must be carefully timed to coincide with injections. In addition, the glucose content of food has to be carefully titrated with the amount and strength of insulin injected. Exercise plays an important role in diabetes management because it improves glucose utilization and sensitivity to insulin, which results in greater glucose tolerance, more stable glucose levels and a reduction in the amount of insulin required. Self-monitoring of blood glucose (SMBG) also plays a key role in diabetes management, as it provides information on insulin levels which is used to adjust insulin dosage, diet and exercise as required. Diabetic children and adolescents are required to self-monitor their blood glucose several times a day.

Consequences of poor metabolic control

IDDM is associated with many short- and long-term complications that create a psychological burden for patients and their families (Plotnick, 1999). Short-term complications are caused by variability in insulin dosage, dietary intake, activity level and psychological stress which can result in hypoglycaemia and hyperglycaemia. Hypoglycaemia occurs when little is eaten given the available supply of insulin whereas hyperglycaemia occurs when too much is eaten given the available supply of insulin. If left untreated, hyperglycaemia can lead to ketoacidosis, coma and ultimately death. Long-term complications associated with IDDM include heart disease, peripheral vascular disease, neuropathy, retinopathy (leading to impaired vision), renal disease, and infections. The onset and progression of these complications can, however, be delayed by strict regimen adherence. Precise metabolic control over 4–9 years may lead to a 50% reduction in retinopathy among adolescents (DCCT, 1994).

Because the serious complications and consequences of diabetes can only be minimized through daily adherence to a strict, complex and demanding regimen, enhancing adherence is central to most psychological interventions for diabetic youngsters (McQuaid & Nassau, 1999). Unfortunately non-adherence and poor metabolic control affects 20–30% of youngsters with IDDM, particularly during adolescence (Ryden et al., 1994). The demands of the diabetic regimen coupled with physiological and psychological factors associated with adolescence contribute to poor metabolic control and non-adherence during the teenage years. Hormonal upheaval and increased physical growth are the main physiological factors affecting metabolic control. Psychological factors, such as the need to be like peers and to gain peer acceptance (leading to denial of the diabetes) and the need for increased autonomy from parental control (leading to conflict over parental demands for adherence), can have an adverse impact on adherence and metabolic control. A small group of adolescents with 'brittle diabetes' have particularly poor metabolic control and require frequent hospitalization due to recurrent episodes of either hypoglycaemia or ketoacidosis (Moran et al., 1991; Fonagy & Moran, 1990).

Previous reviews

From previous literature reviews and meta-analyses of studies of the effectiveness of psychological interventions for children with diabetes a number of conclusions may be drawn (Campbell & Patterson, 1995; Grey et al., 1999; Kibby et al., 1998; Padgett et al., 1988; Rubin & Peyrot, 1992). First, for diabetic youngsters psychoeducational interventions lead to increased knowledge but not increased adherence or metabolic control. Second, behavioural interventions which focus on enhancing skills necessary for adhering to diabetic regimes lead to increased adherence. Effective behavioural programmes involve goal setting, use of contingency contracts, modelling, feedback, reinforcement and skills practice. Behavioural programmes may be family-based or child-focused. Third, family interventions may improve adherence and diabetic control. Family interventions may affect adherence by reducing parent–child conflict about regimen-related issues and improving family communication and problem-solving so that discussions between parents and youngsters about regime adherence are more productive. Family interventions may directly affect metabolic control by reducing the levels of stress and increasing the levels of support experienced by diabetic youngsters and so reducing the release of adrenaline and other stress-related hormones. Fourth, coping skills training programmes in which youngsters learn stress management or social skills may enhance metabolic control by reducing psychosocial stress. Such stress reduction may improve metabolic control directly by reducing the release of adrenaline and other stress-related hormones, and indirectly by empowering youngsters to cope effectively with interpersonal situations that might otherwise compromise adherence. For example, managing social pressure to violate diabetic dietary restrictions. Fifth, the intensity of intervention required to optimize metabolic control may depend on the severity of the diabetic symptoms. For severe disturbances in metabolic control, intensive individual and family therapy on an inpatient basis may be required, whereas moderate problems with adherence and metabolic control may be treated effectively on an outpatient basis.

Method

The aim of the present review was to identify effective psychological intervention programmes for preventing poor metabolic control, regimen non-compliance and psychosocial adjustment difficulties in children and adolescents with IDDM. A PsychLit database search of English language journals for the years 1977 to 2000 was conducted to identify studies in which such prevention programmes were evaluated. Terms that defined diabetes including *diabetes*, *diabetes mellitus*, *juvenile diabetes* and *insulin-dependent diabetes mellitus* were combined with terms that defined interventions such as *social skills training*, *self-instruction training*, *stress management training*, *treatment*, *therapy*, *behavioural programmes* and *family therapy*. A manual search through the bibliographies of recent reviews and relevant journals was also conducted. Studies were selected for review if they included a treatment and control or comparison group with at least nine cases in each group and if sufficient data were reported to allow the calculation of effect sizes. In total eleven studies were selected for review.

Characteristics of the studies

A summary of the main characteristics of the eleven studies is given in Table 12.1. In seven studies family-oriented interventions were evaluated and in four studies the efficacy of child-focused interventions was assessed. Within this broad classification five main approaches were identified over the eleven studies. Four studies involved behaviourally oriented family interventions which focused on key aspects of diabetes management (Delamater et al., 1990; Anderson et al., 1989; McNabb et al., 1994; Mendez & Belendez, 1997). In two studies the efficacy of family communication and problem-solving programmes was assessed (Satin et al., 1989; Wysocki et al., 2000). One study involved a multimodal crisis intervention programme (Galatzer et al., 1982). In three studies child-focused coping skills training programmes were evaluated (Kaplan et al., 1985; Grey et al., 1998, 2000; Boardway et al., 1993) while one investigated the effects of individual psychoanalytical therapy on brittle diabetes (Moran et al., 1991). Eight of the eleven studies were conducted in the USA, and the three others were conducted in Spain, Israel and the UK. All were published between 1982 and 2000. A total of 662 cases were included in the eleven studies. Mean ages of participants ranged from nine to fifteen years. Seven of the eleven studies were conducted with adolescents. Overall, 55% of participants were female and 45% were male. Ten of the eleven studies provided pre- and post-intervention measures of metabolic control. In nine of these ten studies, the measure used was HbA_{1c} levels. In one study, mg/dl was used as a measure of metabolic control (Mendez & Belendez, 1997). Cases in all studies where HbA_{1c} information was provided had a mean HbA_{1c} level of at least 9%, which is indicative of poor metabolic control. In four of the eleven studies reviewed, baseline HbA_{1c} levels were 12% or more, indicating that participants in these studies had metabolic control levels that were in the clinically problematic range (Satin et al., 1989; Boardway et al., 1993, Kaplan et al., 1985; Moran et al., 1991). Information on duration of diabetes was provided in ten of the eleven studies. Apart from two studies which focused on newly diagnosed diabetics, all other studies involved youngsters who had diabetes for at least four years. In one study, youngsters had had diabetes for a mean of eight years (Grey et al., 1998, 2000). Treatment intensity ranged from five sessions over eighteen months (Anderson et al., 1989) to three or four sessions per week over four months (Moran et al., 1991).

Table 12.1 Characteristics of studies of intervention programmes for youngsters with diabetes

Study no.	Study type	Authors	Year	Country	N per group	Mean age and range	Gender	Baseline metabolic control HbA1c > 9 poor > 12 Clin prob	Duration of diabetes	Programme duration
1	F-BP	Delamater et al.	1990	USA	1. F-BP = 12 2. SC = 12 3. C = 12	9 y 5–13 y	F 47% M 53%	11	Poor	Newly diagnosed	1 h × 7 over 16 w + BS @ 6 and 12 m later
2	F-BP	McNabb et al.	1994	USA	1. F-BP = 10 2. C = 12	10 y	F 46% M 54%	12	Poor	Under 3 m	1 h × 6 over 6 w
3	F-BP	Anderson et al.	1989	USA	1. F-BP = 30 2. C = 30	13 y	F 53% M 47%	10	Poor	5 y	1.5 h × 5 over 18 m
4	F-BP	Mendez & Belendez	1997	Spain	1. F-BP = 18 2. C = 19	14 y 12–16 y	F 52% M 48%	161 (mg/dl)	—	4 y	2 h × 12 over 12 w
5	F-CPS	Satin et al.	1989	USA	1. F-CPS = 11 2. F-CPS + S = 12 3. C = 9	15 y 12–18 y	F 61% M 39%	13	Clinical problem	6 y	1.5 h × 6 over 6 w
6	F-CPS	Wysocki et al.	2000	USA	1. F-CPS = 35 2. PE = 39 3. C = 41	14 y 13–15 y	F 50% M 50%	12	Poor	5 y	1.5 h × 10 over 10 w
7	F-CI	Galatzer et al.	1982	Israel	1. F-CI = 107 2. C = 116	15 y	F 50% M 50%	—	—	Newly diagnosed	1 h × 5 for 1 w + 1 h × 6 for 3 w + 1 h × 2 for 8 w
8	C-CST	Kaplan et al.	1985	USA	1. C-CST = 11 2. PE = 10	14 y 12–16 y	F 50% M 50%	13	Clinical problem	6 y	3 h × 15 for 3 w
9	C-CST	Grey et al.	1998 2000	USA	1. C-CST = 41 2. C = 34	14 y 12–16 y	F 58% M 42%	9	Poor	9 y	1.5 h × 6 over 6 w + 1.5 h × 12 over 12 m
10	C-CST	Boardway et al.	1993	USA	1. C-CST = 9 2. C = 10	15 y 14–16 y	F 73% M 27%	15	Clinical problem	6 y	1 h × 10 over 12 w + 1 h × 3 over 3 m
11	C-PS	Moran et al.	1991	UK	1. I-PS = 11 2. C = 11	14 y 10–18 y	F 64% M 36%	14	Clinical problem	6 y	45 min × 60 over 15 w

Note

F-BP = family-based behavioural programme. F-CPS = family-based communication and problem-solving skills training. F-CPS + S = family-based communication and parental simulation of diabetes management for 1 w. F-CI = family-based crisis intervention. C-CST = individual coping skills training. I-PS = individual psychoanalytic psychotherapy. C = control. PE = psychoeducation. SC = supportive counselling. BS = booster sessions. min = minutes. h = hour. w = week. m = month. y = year. Metabolic control refers to HbA1c level over 6 to 10 weeks for which 7–8% is normal. 9–11% indicates poor glycaemic control, and 12% + indicates chronic hyperglycaemia and is a definite clinical problem.

Methodological features

A summary of the methodological features of the eleven studies is provided in Table 12.2. All eleven studies included a control or comparison group. In eight of the eleven studies, cases were randomly assigned to groups. All studies had diagnostically homogeneous treatment and comparison groups and in all but one study, the control and intervention groups were demographically similar. The exception – Wysocki et al.'s (2000) study – had fewer intact families and higher levels of conflict in one of the intervention groups. Pre- and post-intervention assessment occurred in all studies apart from the one retrospective study (Galatzer et al., 1982). Six studies incorporated a follow-up period. In two studies data were collected at six-month follow-up (Satin et al., 1989; Grey et al., 2000) while in four studies, twelve-month follow-up data were collected (Delamater et al., 1990; Mendez & Belendez, 1997; Grey et al., 1998, 2000; Moran et al., 1991). Delamater et al. (1990) also conducted a two-year follow-up. Drop-out was assessed in almost half (45%) of the eleven studies. The clinical significance of treatment gains was reported in only two

Table 12.2 Methodological features of studies of intervention programmes for youngsters with diabetes

Feature	Study number										
	S1	S2	S3	S4	S5	S6	S7	S8	S9	S10	S11
Control or comparison group	1	1	1	1	1	1	1	1	1	1	1
Random assignment	1	1	1	0	1	1	0	1	1	1	0
Diagnostic homogeneity	1	1	1	1	1	1	1	1	1	1	1
Demographic similarity	1	1	1	1	1	0	1	1	1	1	1
Pre-treatment assessment	1	1	1	1	1	1	0	1	1	1	1
Post-treatment assessment (>6 months)	1	1	1	1	1	1	0	1	1	1	1
6-month follow-up assessment	0	0	0	0	1	0	0	0	1	0	0
12-month follow-up assessment	1	0	0	1	0	0	0	0	1	0	1
24-month follow-up assessment	1	0	0	0	0	0	0	0	0	0	0
Drop-out assessed	0	1	1	1	0	0	0	1	1	0	0
Clinical significance of change assessed	0	0	1	0	0	0	0	0	0	0	1
Experienced therapists or trainers used	0	0	0	0	0	1	1	0	1	0	1
Programmes were manualized	0	1	0	0	0	1	0	0	0	0	0
Programme integrity checked	0	0	0	0	0	1	0	0	1	0	1
Metabolic control assessed	1	1	1	1	1	1	0	1	1	1	1
Regimen adherence/self-care assessed	1	1	1	1	1	1	1	0	0	1	0
Psychosocial adjustment to diabetes assessed	0	1	0	1	0	1	1	0	1	1	0
Total	10	11	10	10	9	11	6	8	13	9	10

Notes
S = study. 1 = design feature was present. 0 = design feature was absent.

studies. Experienced therapists were used in only one-third of the studies and manualized programmes were used in only two studies. Programme integrity was checked in three studies and supervision was provided in only one study (Moran et al., 1991). Metabolic control was the main outcome variable assessed and post-treatment indicators of metabolic control were provided in all studies with the exception of the one retrospective study (Galatzer et al., 1982). Eight of the eleven studies included some measure of adherence or diabetic self-care. Five studies investigated some aspect of psychosocial adjustment to diabetes. A wide variety of different measures were employed across studies to investigate adherence and psychosocial adjustment, some of which are listed at the end of this chapter in the 'Assessment Resources' section. Overall, the studies selected were sufficiently well designed to allow valid and reliable conclusions to be drawn about the effectiveness of the interventions evaluated.

Substantive findings

Effect sizes and outcome rates for the eleven studies are presented in Table 12.3. A narrative account of the main findings from the studies is presented in Table 12.4.

Family-based behavioural programmes

In four studies, family-based behavioural programmes which focused directly on improving adherence were evaluated (Delamater et al., 1990; Anderson et al., 1989; McNabb et al., 1994; Mendez & Belendez, 1997). In these programmes the principal aim was to help youngsters develop and practise skills such as self-monitoring of blood glucose, administering insulin injections, dietary management, exercise management, and diabetes-related problem-solving. This type of problem-solving involves using general information about diabetes and specific information from self-monitoring of blood glucose levels to make decisions about insulin injections, diet, and exercise. In all of these programmes skills were modelled and rehearsed, corrective feedback was given and appropriate skill performance was reinforced. Skills learned during therapeutic sessions were practised at home. Parents and other family members were involved in monitoring youngsters' use of these skills, prompting them to use their skills in appropriate situations, and reinforcing them for doing so correctly. Gradually, parental prompting and reinforcement was faded out and youngsters took increasing responsibility for self-management of their diabetes regime. There were some differences between studies in programme format and content and participant characteristics. Delamater et al. (1990) used a conjoint family session format, while a parallel parent and child session format was used in the other three programmes (Anderson et al., 1989; McNabb et al., 1994; Mendez & Belendez, 1997). Additional stress management and social skills training sessions were incorporated into the

Table 12.3 Summary of results of treatment effects and outcome rates from studies of intervention programmes for youngsters with diabetes

Variable	Family-based behavioural programmes				Family communication and problem-solving skills programmes		Family crisis intervention	Individual coping skills training programmes			Psychodynamic therapy
	Study 1	Study 2	Study 3	Study 4	Study 5	Study 6	Study 7	Study 8	Study 9	Study 10	Study 11
	F-BP v C	F-BP v C	F-BP v C	F-BP v C	F-CPS + S v C	F-CPS v C	F-CI v C	C-CST v PE	C-CST v C	C-CST v C	C-PS v C
Improvement after programme											
Metabolic control	—	0.9	0.4	0.9	3.3	0.2	—	1.5	0.5	0.2	0.8
Regimen adherence and diabetes self-care	—	0.5	0.6	0.2	1.1*	0.3	—	—	—	-0.2	—
Psychosocial adjustment to diabetes	—	1.0	—	0.7	—	0.1	—	—	0.2	0.4	—
Improvement at 6 months											
Metabolic control	—	—	—	—	4.8*	—	—	—	0.5	—	—
Improvement at 12 months											
Metabolic control	0.7	—	—	0.1	—	—	—	—	0.7	0.3	0.8
Diabetes self-care and regimen adherence	1.1	—	—	0.0	—	—	—	—	—	-0.1	—
Psychosocial adjustment to diabetes	—	—	—	0.9	—	—	—	—	0.5	1.0	—
Improvement at 24 months											
Metabolic control	0.7	—	—	—	—	—	0.6	—	—	—	—
Regimen adherence and diabetes self-care	—	—	—	—	—	—	0.5	—	—	—	—
Psychosocial adjustment to diabetes	—	—	—	—	—	—	—	—	—	—	—
% Improved after treatment	—	—	76% v 50%	—	—	—	—	—	—	—	91% v 27%
Negative clinical outcomes											
% Drop-out	—	29%	14%	32% v 22%	—	—	—	—	3%	8%	—

Notes

F-BP = family-based behavioural programme. F-CPS = family-based communication and problem-solving skills training. F-CPS + S = family-based communication and problem-solving skills training and parental simulation of diabetes management for 1 w. F-CI = family-based crisis intervention. C-CST = individual coping skills training. C-PS = individual psychoanalytic psychotherapy. C = control. PE = psychoeducation.

*Effect sizes calculated excluding first cycle of the programme.

Table 12.4 Summary of key findings from studies of intervention programmes for youngsters with diabetes

Study no.	Authors	Year	N per group	Programme duration	Group differences	Key findings
1	Delamater et al.	1990	1. F-BP = 12 2. SC = 12 3. C = 12	1 h × 7 over 16 w + BS @ 6 and 12 m later	Metabolic control 1 = 2 > 3	• Compared with controls, patients who participated in a family-based behavioural programme following diagnosis had significantly greater metabolic control at 1 and 2 years follow-up
2	McNabb et al.	1994	1. F-BP = 10 2. C = 12	1 h × 6 over 6 w	Adherence 1 > 2	• Compared with controls, patients who participated in a family-based behavioural programme took more responsibility for their diabetes self-care without compromising their levels of diabetic self-care or metabolic control • There was no difference between the 2 groups in levels of metabolic control
3	Anderson et al.	1989	1. F-BP = 30 2. C = 30	1.5 h × 5 over 18 m	Metabolic control Adherence 1 > 2	• Compared with controls, patients who participated in a family-based behavioural programme had significantly greater metabolic control and better self-care in the area of physical exercise patterns
4	Mendez & Belendez	1997	1. F-BP = 18 2. C = 19	2 h × 12 over 12 w	Metabolic control Adherence 1 > 2	• Compared with controls, patients who participated in a family-based behavioural programme had significantly greater metabolic control and better self-care in the areas of blood glucose testing and frequency of glycemic analysis • Improvements in self-care were maintained at 13-month follow-up
5	Satin et al.	1989	1. F-CPS = 11 2. F-CPS + S = 12 3. C = 9	1.5 h × 6 over 6 w	Metabolic control 1 = 2 > 3	• Compared with controls, patients who participated in a family-based communication and problem-solving skills programme had significantly greater metabolic control at post-treatment which was not maintained at 6-month follow-up • Compared with controls, participants in the second and subsequent cycles of the programme showed clinically significant improvements in metabolic control and regimen adherence which were maintained at 6-month follow-up
6	Wysocki et al.	2000	1. F-CPS = 35 2. PE = 39 3. C = 41	1.5 h × 10 over 10 w	Family conflict 1 > 2 = 3	• Compared with controls, participants in a family-based communication and problem-solving skills programme reported a significant reduction in diabetes-related conflict and improvements in adolescent–parent relationships • Younger girls who participated in the programme showed improvements in psychological adjustment and diabetic control

Table 12.4 continued

Study no.	Authors	Year	N per group	Programme duration	Group differences	Key findings
7	Galatzer et al.	1982	1. F-CI = 107 2. C = 116	1 h × 5 for 1 w + 1 h × 6 for 3 w + 1 h × 2 for 8 w	Adherence Adjustment 1 > 2	• Compared with controls, participants in a family-based crisis intervention programme for newly diagnosed diabetic children showed better adherence, social and family adjustment between 3 and 15 years later • Controls who had not participated in the programme who were rated as 'well adjusted' at follow-up required almost triple the amount of psychosocial intervention as cases who receive early crisis intervention to achieve this status • There were no differences between groups in school achievement and work performance • Low SES cases from both groups had the poorest overall outcome at follow-up
8	Kaplan et al.	1985	1. C-CST = 11 2. PE = 10	3 h × 15 for 3 w	Metabolic control 1 > 2	• Compared with controls who received psychoeducation only, participants in a social skills training group had better metabolic control at 4-month follow-up • Self-reported adherence and metabolic control were strongly correlated
9	Grey et al.	1998 2000	1. C-CST = 41 2. C = 34	1.5 h × 6 over 6 w + 1.5 h × 12 over 12 m	Metabolic control Adjustment 1 > 2	• Compared with controls, following treatment and a year later participants in a coping skills programme showed better metabolic control and reported better diabetes self-efficacy and less impact of diabetes on their quality of life • Compared with female controls, fewer females in the coping skills programme showed severe hypoglycaemia or significant weight gain
10	Boardway et al.	1993	1. C-CST = 9 2. C = 10	1 h × 10 over 12 w + 1 h × 3 over 3 m	Diabetes stress reduction 1 > 2	• Compared with controls, participants in the self-management training programme reported a reduction in diabetes-related stress after the programme and at 3-month follow-up • The groups did not differ in metabolic control, adherence, coping styles or diabetes self-efficacy
11	Moran et al.	1991	1. I-PS = 11 2. C = 11	45 min × 60 over 15 w	Metabolic control 1 > 2	• Compared with controls, youngsters with brittle diabetes who received prolonged hospitalization coupled with intensive psychodynamic psychotherapy showed significant improvements in metabolic control after treatment and at 1-year follow-up

Notes

F-BP = family-based behavioural programme. F-CPS = family communication and problem-solving skills training. F-CPS + S = family-based communication and problem-solving skills training and parental simulation of diabetes management for 1 w. F-CI = family-based crisis intervention. I-CST = individual coping skills training. I-PS = individual psychoanalytic psychotherapy. C = control. PE = psychoeducation. SC = supportive counselling. BS = booster sessions. min = minutes. h = hour. w = week. m = month. y = year.

programme evaluated by Mendez and Belendez (1997). Youngsters in these studies ranged from newly diagnosed children (Delamater et al., 1990), to preadolescents (McNabb et al., 1994), to adolescents (Anderson et al., 1989; Mendez & Belendez, 1997).

From the results of these four studies summarized in Tables 12.3 and 12.4, the following conclusions may be drawn. First, these family-based behavioural programmes had a substantial positive effect on the well-being of youngsters with diabetes.

Second, family-based behavioural programmes led to short- and long-term improvements in metabolic control. Averaging across the three studies for which data on metabolic control were reported, the effect size after programme completion was 0.7, indicating that the average youngster who participated in these programmes fared better immediately afterwards than 76% of controls. At one-year follow-up, averaging across the two studies for which data on metabolic control were reported, the effect size was 0.4, indicating that the average youngster who participated in these programmes fared better than 66% of controls a year after programme completion. In the single study where two-year follow-up data were reported, the effect size was 0.7, indicating that the average youngster who participated in this programme fared better after two years than 76% of controls.

Third, family-based behavioural programmes led to short- and long-term improvements in adherence. Averaging across the three studies for which data on adherence were reported, the effect size after programme completion was 0.4, indicating that the average youngster who participated in these programmes showed better adherence immediately afterwards than 66% of controls. At one-year follow-up, averaging across the two studies for which data on adherence were reported, the effect size was 0.6, indicating that the average youngster who participated in these programmes showed better adherence than 73% of controls a year after programme completion. However, there was considerable variability in the one-year follow-up adherence data. One study in which a parallel parent and child session format was used with adolescents showed no effect (Mendez & Belendez, 1997) while the other in which a conjoint family session format was used with newly diagnosed children yielded an effect size of 1.1 (Delamater et al., 1990).

Fourth, family-based behavioural programmes led to short- and long-term improvements in psychosocial adjustment. Averaging across the two studies for which data on psychosocial adjustment were reported, the effect size after programme completion was 0.9, indicating that the average youngster who participated in these programmes showed better psychosocial adjustment immediately afterwards than 82% of controls. In the single study where one-year follow-up data were reported, the effect size was 0.9, indicating that the average youngster who participated in this programme showed better psychosocial adjustment after a year than 82% of controls.

Fifth, drop-out rates ranged from 14 to 32% with a mean of 24%, indicating that about a quarter of families dropped out of these family-based behavioural programmes.

Finally, of the four studies, Delamater et al.'s (1990) intervention with newly diagnosed patients appears to have been the most effective, with gains maintained at two-year follow-up. Thus, it appears that family-based behavioural diabetes management programmes are more effective at diagnosis than either during middle childhood or in adolescence.

Family communication and problem-solving programmes

In two studies family communication and problem-solving programmes were evaluated (Satin et al., 1989; Wysocki et al., 2000). Communication skills include both message sending skills and active listening skills. For training in active listening skills family members are coached in how to listen without interruption, summarize key points, check that the message has been understood accurately, before offering a reply. For training in message sending skills family members are coached in deciding on specific key points to include in their message, organizing them logically, saying them clearly, checking that the other person has understood the message and allowing space for a reply. During communication skills training, family members learn to set aside adequate time and remove distractions before attempting to practise skills; to avoid negative mind-reading, blaming, sulking or abusing; to take turns fairly; and to make congruent *I statements*. That is, to make statements like 'I would like you to tell me when you are coming home tonight' rather than 'You never tell me when you'll be home.' For training in problem-solving skills family members are coached in how to break big, vague, unsolvable problems down into small specific solvable problems; tackle one small specific problem at a time; brainstorm possible solutions; explore the pros and cons of these; agree on a joint action plan; implement the plan; review progress; revise the original plan in light of feedback for the review process; and celebrate success. During problem-solving skills training family members learn to focus on how problems (not people) make them feel distressed and to acknowledge their own share of the responsibility for resolving the problem.

There were some differences between the programmes evaluated in these studies. In the programme evaluated by Satin et al. (1989) a group of families attended sessions together and the focus was exclusively on diabetes management issues whereas in the programme evaluated by Wysocki et al. (2000), each family was offered a series of sessions with a behavioural family therapist and within these sessions the focus was on both diabetes-specific problems and other family difficulties.

From the results of these two studies summarized in Tables 12.3 and 12.4, the following conclusions may be drawn. First, these family-based communication and problem-solving skills programmes had a substantial positive effect on the well-being of youngsters with diabetes.

Second, family-based based communication and problem-solving skills programmes led to short- and long-term improvements in metabolic control. Averaging across the two studies for which data on metabolic control were reported, the effect size after programme completion was 1.8, indicating that the average youngster who participated in these programmes fared better immediately afterwards than 96% of controls. In the single study where one-year follow-up data were reported, the effect size was 4.8, indicating that the average youngster who participated in this programme fared better after a year than 99% of controls.

Third, family-based based communication and problem-solving skills programmes led to short-term improvements in adherence. Averaging across the two studies for which data on adherence were reported, the effect size after programme completion was 0.7, indicating that the average youngster who participated in these programmes showed better adherence immediately afterwards than 76% of controls.

Fourth, family-based behavioural programmes led to minimal short-term improvements in psychosocial adjustment. In the single study where post-intervention data were reported, the effect size was 0.1, indicating that the average youngster who participated in this programme showed better psychosocial adjustment afterwards than only 54% of controls.

Finally, of the two programmes, that which involved a group format and concentrated on diabetes-specific issues was the most effective (Satin et al., 1989). An interesting feature of this programme was the use of a parent simulation exercise. In these exercises parents were invited to complete diabetes management tasks for seven days and during this time their adolescents acted as their 'coaches'. These exercises may have helped them to empathize with the challenges faced by their youngsters and created a context particularly facilitative of joint problem-solving.

Family crisis intervention

Galatzer et al. (1982) found that compared with controls, youngsters who participated in a family crisis intervention programme for newly diagnosed diabetic children showed better adherence and psychosocial adjustment at three to fifteen years' follow-up. In this programme individualized treatment plans were offered by a multidisciplinary team to each family. Treatment plans included psychoeducation, supportive family counselling, school liaison meetings, home visiting, and peer counselling for newly diagnosed patients from youngsters with experience in managing diabetes. At three to fifteen years' follow-up, effect sizes for independent ratings of adherence and psychosocial adjustment were 0.6 and 0.5 respectively. Thus the average participant fared better at follow-up than 73% of controls in terms of adherence, and 69% of controls in terms of psychosocial adjustment. These results suggest that providing intensive multidisciplinary crisis intervention at diagnosis can have long-term benefits in terms of regimen adherence and psychosocial adjustment.

Child-focused coping skills training

In three studies coping skills training programmes which focused on enhancing stress management skills or social skills were evaluated (Kaplan et al., 1985; Grey et al., 1998, 2000; Boardway et al., 1993). These programmes were child-focused rather than family oriented and used a group-based teaching format. In addition to routine psychoeducation about self-management of the diabetes regime, these programmes facilitated the development of social problem-solving skills to cope with social stresses commonly encountered by diabetic youngsters. Typical social situations involving peer pressure to violate the diabetes regime were identified and participants were helped to develop skills to manage these situations and the stress entailed by them. Active teaching methods including modelling, rehearsal, giving corrective feedback, and reinforcement were used to facilitate skill development.

From the results of these three studies summarized in Tables 12.3 and 12.4, the following conclusions may be drawn. First, these coping skills training programmes had a substantial positive effect on the well-being of youngsters with diabetes.

Second, coping skills training programmes led to short- and long-term improvements in metabolic control. Averaging across the three studies, the effect size after programme completion was 0.7, indicating that the average youngster who participated in these programmes fared better immediately afterwards than 76% of controls. In the single study where six-month follow-up data were reported, the effect size was 0.5 and at one-year follow-up, averaging across the two studies for which data on metabolic control were reported, the effect size was also 0.5. Thus, the average youngster who participated in these programmes fared better than 69% of controls at six months and a year after programme completion.

Third, in the single study in which adherence was assessed, coping skills training did not lead to improvements in adherence either after treatment or at follow-up.

Fourth, coping skills training programmes led to short- and long-term improvements in psychosocial adjustment. Averaging across the two studies for which data on psychosocial adjustment were reported, the effect size after programme completion and at one-year follow-up was 0.3, indicating that the average youngster who participated in these programmes showed better psychosocial adjustment immediately afterwards and a year later than 62% of controls.

Fifth, drop-out rates ranged from 3 to 8% with a mean of 6%, indicating that less than one in ten cases dropped out of these coping skills training programmes.

Finally, of the three studies, Grey et al.'s (2000) intervention was the most effective with large post-programme gains which were maintained at one-year follow-up. This programme included monthly booster sessions over a one-year period in addition to the initial intensive coping skills training programme.

Psychoanalytic psychotherapy

Moran et al. (1991) found that compared with controls who received intensive inpatient medical care, youngsters with brittle diabetes who engaged in intensive inpatient psychoanalytic psychotherapy with three to five sessions per week for fifteen weeks showed greater improvement after treatment and a year later. The psychoanalytic psychotherapy was based in each case on an individualized formulation which explained how both biological and psychological factors contributed to poor metabolic control. The psychotherapy aimed to help youngsters gain insight into the unconscious psychological function of their non-adherence and/or lack of metabolic control. Non-adherence and lack of metabolic control were found in this group of patients to serve a variety of functions including expressing repudiated sexual or aggressive wishes; expressing feelings of guilt and self-punishment; expressing unconscious anxiety about bodily damage; expressing separation anxiety and anger about dependency on parents; and distracting attention from painful intrapsychic conflicts or distressing interpersonal situations. In addition to providing insight, psychotherapy provided a context within which youngsters could work through the painful feelings associated with the conflict that underpinned their poor metabolic control. This inpatient psychoanalytic psychotherapy was offered in conjunction with brief parental counselling and routine liaison meetings with ward staff. Parents and staff were advised on the management of youngsters, and particularly on the avoidance of strong protective or punitive countertransference reactions which might be elicited by youngsters' (provocative or apparently helpless) non-adherence and lack of metabolic control. After treatment and one year later, an effect size of 0.8 was obtained for metabolic control, indicating that participants in psychoanalytic psychotherapy had better metabolic control than 79% of controls. At one-year follow-up, 91% of the psychotherapy group had experienced a clinically significant improvement in metabolic control, as indicated by a reduction in HbA_{1c} levels, compared to only 27% of controls.

Conclusions

Type 1 or insulin-dependent diabetes mellitus (IDDM) is an endocrine disorder typically diagnosed in childhood, characterized by complete pancreatic failure. The prevalence rate is approximately 1.2–1.9 cases per 1,000 children under the age of twenty. The long-term outcome of IDDM is associated with devastating complications in some cases, including blindness and leg amputation, particularly those where there has been poor regimen adherence. For youngsters with diabetes, blood glucose levels as close as possible to the normal range is achieved through a regime involving a combination of insulin injections, balanced diet, exercise and self-monitoring of blood glucose.

From this review, it may be concluded that for diabetic youngsters five types of psychological intervention programmes can prevent adjustment problems and improve adherence and metabolic control. These are: family-based behavioural programmes, family-based communication and problem-solving skills training programmes, family crisis intervention programmes, child-focused coping skills training programmes, and intensive inpatient psychoanalytic psychotherapy.

Family-based psychological prevention programmes for youngsters newly diagnosed with diabetes are particularly effective in the long term. Family-based behavioural programmes may be more effective with preadolescent children whereas family-based communication and problem-solving skills training programmes are best suited to families with adolescents. Coping skills training programmes are particularly effective for adolescents and regular booster sessions can increase their long-term effectiveness. For adolescents with brittle diabetes, intensive psychoanalytic psychotherapy is effective in the short and long term. Psychological intervention programmes are most effective for diabetic youngsters who have metabolic control levels within the clinically problematic range.

Implications for practice

For newly diagnosed diabetic children, family-based multidisciplinary crisis intervention programmes should be routinely offered. Such programmes should include psychoeducation, supportive family counselling, school liaison meetings, home visiting, and peer counselling for newly diagnosed patients from youngsters with experience in managing diabetes. For youngsters who continue to show poor metabolic control during the preadolescent years family-based behavioural programmes may be offered. In these programmes self-care skills are modelled and rehearsed. Initially parents prompt and reinforce skill use, but gradually youngsters take increasing responsibility for self-management of their diabetes regime. In adolescence, where youngsters show poor metabolic control, family-based communication and problem-solving programmes should be offered. Such programmes should include parent simulation exercises in which parents are invited to complete diabetes management tasks while their adolescents act as their 'coaches'. This exercise helps parents to empathize with the challenges faced by their youngsters and facilitates joint problem-solving. Adolescents with poor metabolic control may also be offered coping skills training programmes to develop the skills to cope with peer pressure to violate their diabetic regimen. Regular booster sessions should be offered after the completion of such programmes. All of the programmes mentioned so far in this section are relatively brief (10–20 sessions). Where brittle diabetes develops intensive inpatient psychoanalytic psychotherapy 3–5 times per week over four months should be offered. The cost of such treatment can be justified in terms of the impact such programmes can have in preventing short-term complications and repeated hospitalizations and in the longer term in delaying the onset and progression of serious complications associated with diabetes.

Implications for research

Most of the studies reviewed here focused on adolescents. Further research on the effectiveness of interventions with younger children and newly diagnosed patients is required, particularly as early intervention seems to be efficient and cost-effective.

Programme integrity was only systematically evaluated in a minority of the studies reviewed in this chapter. Future evaluation studies should include assessments of programme integrity. In such studies, training sessions are recorded and blind raters use programme integrity checklists to evaluate the degree to which sessions approximate manualized training protocols.

Studies that examine the impact of design features that may make programmes more effective in particular circumstances are required. For example, comparative studies are required to assess if multisystemic programmes involving family-based communication and problem-solving skills training and child-focused coping skills training are more effective with adolescents than either intervention alone.

Studies are required which investigate the mechanisms and processes that underpin programme effectiveness. For example, studies are required to assess whether increased metabolic control arises from improvements in adherence, reductions in interpersonal conflict, or reduction in anxiety or some combination of such factors.

Assessment resources

Bradley, C. (1994). *Handbook of Psychology and Diabetes*. Chur, Switzerland: Harwood. (Contains a series of assessment instruments useful in the evaluation of children with diabetes including: Measures of perceived control of diabetes; Barriers to diabetes self-care; The diabetes Quality of life measure; the Diabetes Knowledge Scales; and the ATT39: A measure of psychological adjustment to diabetes.)

Gonen, B., Rubenstein, A., Rochman, H., et al. (1977). Haemoglobin A1: An indicator of the metabolic control of diabetic patients. *Lancet*, ii, 734–737.

Greco, P., La Greca, A.M., Auslander, W.F., Speter, D., Skyler, J.S., Fisher, E. & Santiago, J.V. (1990). Assessing adherence in IDDM: A comparison of two methods. *Diabetes*, 40 (suppl. 3), 108A (abstract). (Contains information on a 14 Item Self-Care Inventory.)

Grossman, H.Y., Brink, S. & Hauser, S.T. (1987). Self-efficacy in adolescent girls and boys with insulin-dependent diabetes mellitus. *Diabetes Care*, 10, 324–329. (Contains a Self Efficacy for Diabetes Scale.)

Johnson, S., Rosenbloom, J., Rosenbloom, A., Carter, R. & Cunningham, W. (1986) Assessing daily management in childhood diabetes. *Health Psychology*, 5, 545–564.

McNabb, W., Quinn, M.T., Murphy, D.M., Thorp, F.K. & Cook, S. (1994). Increasing children's responsibility for diabetes self-care: the In Control Study. *Diabetes Educator*, 20(2), 121–124. (Contains the Children's' Diabetes Inventory.)

Rubin, R., Young-Hyman, D. & Peyrot, M. (1989). Parent-child responsibility and conflict in diabetes care. *Diabetes*, 38 (suppl. 2), 28 A (abstract). (Contains reference to the Diabetes Responsibility and Conflict Scale.)

Schafer, L. (1986). Supportive and non-supportive family behaviours: Relationships to adherence and metabolic control in persons with Type 1 diabetes. *Diabetes*, 9, 179–185. (Contains the Diabetes Family Behaviour Checklist.)

Treatment manuals and resources

American Diabetes Association. (1990). *Diabetes Support Group for Young Adults: Facilitators Manual.* Alexandria, VA: American Diabetes Association.

McNabb, W. (1990). *In Control* (A behaviour-orientated diabetes self-management education program). (W. McNabb, Assistant Professor and Director, Centre for Research in Medical Education and Health Care, Department of Medicine, MC6091, The University of Chicago, 5841 South Maryland Avenue, Chicago, IL 60637.)

Resources for clients

Pirner, C. & Westcott, N. (1994). *Even Little Kids get Diabetes.* New York: Albert Whitman.

13 Prevention of teenage smoking, alcohol use and drug abuse

*Barry J. Coughlan, Mairead Doyle
and Alan Carr*

Adolescent drug abuse, alcohol abuse and smoking are complex public health problems with serious adverse consequences (Botvin, 1999; Hansen & O'Malley, 1996; Newcomb & Bentler, 1988; Pagliaro & Pagliaro, 1996). Distinctions are commonly made between experimental or recreational drug use, harmful drug abuse and drug dependence. Recreational drug use is conceptualized as a normative risk-taking behaviour common to most adolescents. Drug taking that leads to personal harm is referred to as drug abuse and drug dependence refers to those situations where there is a compulsive pattern of use involving the physiological changes that accompany tolerance and withdrawal. Only a proportion of youngsters who engage in recreational drug use progress to drug abuse and develop drug dependence. However, for the proportion that do follow this trajectory the outlook is bleak. Habitual drug abuse may negatively affect mental and physical health, criminal status, educational status, the establishment of psychological autonomy, and the development of long-term intimate relationships. The children of habitual teenage drug abusers may suffer from drug-related problems such as fetal alcohol syndrome, intra-uterine addiction or HIV infection. Even for those youngsters who do not progress to drug abuse, strong links have been established between accidental deaths, such as those due to road traffic accidents, and drug and alcohol use. Four out of five teenagers who smoke more than two cigarettes a day are likely to become regular smokers with an increased risk for major chronic diseases, particularly lung cancer.

Given the serious negative consequences of adolescent drug abuse, it is not surprising that many mass media and school-based prevention programmes have been conducted to address this problem. These programmes have had a number of goals including preventing the onset of recreational drug use, reducing recreational drug use and drug abuse, reducing harm among addicts and habitual drug abusers, and promoting healthier behaviour. In this chapter the focus is exclusively on educational or school-based primary prevention programmes where the aim is to prevent initiation into recreational drug use. The aim of this chapter is to review methodologically robust research studies on the effectiveness of drug abuse prevention programmes, draw reliable conclusions about the effectiveness of these, and outline the implications of these conclusions for policy and practice. Legislation and taxation are other important elements of comprehensive drug abuse prevention policies which go hand in hand with school-based drug abuse prevention programmes. We have reviewed the evidence for effective family-based treatment programmes for regular drug abuses elsewhere (Cormack & Carr, 2000).

Epidemiology

Experimentation with drugs in adolescence is common (Schinke et al., 1991; Farrell & Taylor, 1994). Major US and UK surveys have shown that by 19 years of age approximately 90% of teenagers have drunk alcohol; 60% have tried cigarettes; 50% have used cannabis; and 20% have tried other street drugs such as solvents, stimulants, hallucinogens or opiates. The prevalence of drug abuse and dependence is harder to gauge and varies with the population studied and the definitions used. A conservative estimate based on a review of available surveys is that between 5% and 10% of teenagers under 19 have drug problems serious enough to require clinical intervention. These epidemiological results show that less than half of those youngsters who experiment with street drugs go on to develop serious drug abuse problems.

Aetiology

The normal developmental processes of adolescence increase the likelihood of experimental or recreational drug use (Carr, 1999). During this developmental stage youngsters typically receive decreased supervision from their parents; experience an increased need to conform with peers; and boys in particular experience an increased need for risk taking. If substance use is one of the common risk-taking behaviours endorsed by the peer group, and if parental supervision is relaxed, then the likelihood of recreational drug use increases. Also, the increased capacity for abstract reasoning which develops in adolescence allows youngsters to see the inconsistencies between parental rules prohibiting smoking, alcohol and drug use on the one hand and parental drug-using behaviour on the other. When adolescents become aware of these inconsistencies, it decreases the effectiveness of parental rules in preventing drug use.

In any particular situation the chances that a youngster will drink alcohol, smoke cigarettes or marijuana or take other drugs, according to the social influence model of drug abuse (Hansen & O'Malley, 1996), are determined by social forces acting on the youngster (peers, parents and the media) and the youngster's perception of norms for drug use. According to this model, youngsters whose parents and peers drink, smoke and use drugs; who are exposed to pro-drug messages from the media; and who believe that it is the norm for most youngsters to drink, smoke and use drugs are more likely to use drugs in situations where there are immediate opportunities and immediate social pressure to do so. These actions are mediated by a variety of cognitive factors including beliefs about the consequences of drug use, self-efficacy beliefs about resisting drug use, and intentions and expectation to use drugs. Youngsters are more likely to use drugs if they believe that drug use does not have immediate negative consequences; if they have weak self-efficacy beliefs about resisting drugs; and if they have strong expectations and intentions that they will use drugs. Youngsters are less likely to use drugs if their parents and peers do not do so and if they have the skills to neutralize pro-drug media messages. Youngsters are less likely to use drugs if they believe that it is the norm for youngsters not to smoke, drink or use drugs; if they believe that drug use has immediate negative consequences; if they have strong self-efficacy beliefs about resisting drugs; and if they have weak expectations and intentions for using drugs. The social influence model of drug use and prevention underpins prevention programmes that aim to establish conservative norms for drug use and teach resistance skills.

While not all adolescents who experiment with drugs progress to harmful drug abuse, those who do are more likely to be characterized by one or more risk factors with increased risk being associated with a greater number of factors. The following risk factors, specified in Hawkins et al.'s (1992) social developmental model of drug abuse, are associated with progression from recreational drug use to harmful drug abuse:

- parental alcohol and drug use
- unclear rules, lax supervision and inconsistent discipline
- chronic and severe family conflict
- chronic family disorganization
- early childhood behaviour problems which have persisted into adolescence
- poor academic attainment, learning difficulties, and school problems
- limited social skills and skills required for regulating negative mood states
- membership of a deviant peer group
- family membership of a disorganized, stressful, unsupportive or high crime community in which drugs are readily available

Protective factors that make it more likely that youngsters will avoid harmful drug abuse include good social skills and skills required for emotional self-regulation, membership of a non-deviant peer group and membership of a supportive well-organized family in which there is consistent discipline and moderate levels of supervision based in a supportive community. The social developmental model of drug abuse provides a framework for developing multisystemic drug abuse prevention programmes that include school-based programmes as one element of community-wide intervention.

Previous reviews

A number of conclusions have been drawn in previous reviews of the literature of the effectiveness of drug abuse prevention programmes (Botvin, 1999; Duesenbury & Falco, 1997; Hansen & O'Malley, 1996). Programmes have been developed which focus on (1) psychoeducation; (2) personal growth; (3) resistance skills training; (4) social influence procedures; (5) life skills training; and (6) multisystemic intervention. Psychoeducational programmes rest on the premise that drug use arises from lack of accurate information and so the provision of information alone should prevent drug abuse. With personal growth programmes it is assumed that youngsters who are anxious, depressed, or who have low self-esteem use drugs to improve their mood state. Personal growth programmes (also referred to as affective education programmes) aim to equip youngsters with the psychological skills or therapeutic experiences necessary to improve negative mood states without recourse to drugs. In resistance skills training programmes it is assumed that if youngsters have adequate refusal skills they will not succumb to social or peer pressure to use drugs. In social influence based programmes, it is assumed that youngsters are less likely to use drugs if they believe that the prevalence of drug use is low, and so these programmes help youngsters develop conservative norms for drug use. Life skills training programmes include resistance skills training and procedures to help youngsters develop conservative drug use norms, assertiveness skills, skills for improving self-control and self-esteem, stress management skills, social communication and problem-solving skills, decision-making skills, and skills for developing social alternatives to drug use. These programmes rest on the premise that a range of life skills is required to avoid drug use. Multisystemic programmes include classroom-based life skills training, but in addition, intervention occurs into the significant social systems of which youngsters are members including the peer group, family, school and community. These programmes are based on the assumption that drug use evolves from, and is maintained by, a wide range of factors within the youngster and the youngster's social network, so effective intervention must address not only the youngster, but also his or her social system.

Evaluations of these different types of programmes have not always supported the theoretical assumptions on which they are based. Psychoeducational programmes which offer information on drugs and the short- and long-term effects of drug abuse are not effective in preventing the onset of drug use or reducing drug use, although they may increase knowledge about drugs and strengthen anti-drug attitudes. Fear-based psychoeducational programmes which highlight in an anxiety-provoking way the long-term negative effects of drug abuse are not effective and may reduce the overall effectiveness of multimodal programmes if included in them. This is because fear-based psychoeducation may undermine the credibility of other programme elements. Despite the ineffectiveness of fear-based psychoeducation, many contemporary media campaigns continue to develop drug prevention campaigns using this approach. Personal growth programmes which include activities to enhance self-esteem, develop mood management skills and promote insight into personal developmental issues are not effective in preventing the onset of drug use or reducing drug abuse. There is some evidence to suggest that psychoeducational and personal growth programmes increase experimental drug abuse, possibly by cultivating curiosity.

However, these findings do not imply that psychoeducation should be abandoned as preventative strategy. When psychoeducational components are built into other types of more effective programmes such as life skills and multisystemic interventions, the focus is on giving relevant facts about the immediate physiological, psychological and social effects of drugs and epidemiological information but not extreme anxiety-provoking information about the long-term negative effects of drugs.

Evidence for the effectiveness of resistance skills training is mixed. One argument is that youngsters will only use resistance skills to avoid succumbing to social pressure from peers and the media to smoke, drink and use drugs, if they believe that it is normatively appropriate to do so, that is, if they hold conservative norms for drug use. Thus, resistance skills training is only effective for very young teenagers who believe that they are not old enough yet to begin drug use. Not surprisingly, evidence is stronger for the effectiveness of social influence programmes which combine resistance skills training with procedures for engendering conservative norms for drug use.

There is growing evidence that life skills training programmes which aim to enhance social competence by teaching a broad range of social problem-solving skills and multisystemic programmes which aim to favourably alter the youngster's social network are the most effective types of programmes for preventing drug use.

Certain design features characterize effective programmes. Peer-led programmes are more effective than programmes led by adults such as teachers, mental health professionals or addiction counsellors. Training of programme leaders in manualized procedures is important for programme efficacy. Programmes that use skills training methods such as modelling, rehearsal (during class), and giving corrective feedback and extended practice (outside the classroom) are more effective than those that rely on traditional didactic lectures as the main training method. The most effective programmes are introduced at the transition from primary to secondary school when youngsters are aged 11–13 and include at least five classes per year over two years. Effective programmes are incorporated into existing school curricula. Effective programmes are socially and culturally acceptable to the community in which they are conducted.

Finally, the best classroom-based programmes have greater effects on knowledge about drugs and attitudes to drug use than on drug-using behaviour. That is, increases in knowledge about drugs and their effects and improvements in attitudes towards avoiding drug use are not matched by reduced rates of drug use or initiation of drug use. Unfortunately, the positive effects of most programmes diminished with time, but periodic booster sessions can maintain programme effectiveness.

Method

The aim of the present review was to identify effective classroom-based drug abuse primary prevention programmes. A PsychLit database search of English language journals for the years 1977 to 2000 was conducted to identify studies in which drug abuse prevention programmes were evaluated. Terms such as *smoking, tobacco, alcohol, drinking, drug use, drug abuse, substance use, substance abuse, addiction,* and *drug addiction* limited to the term *adolescent* were combined with terms such as *prevention, programme, drug education, classroom-based, school-based, school interventions, peer, peer-led* and *evaluation.* A manual search through the bibliographies of all recent reviews and relevant journals on drug abuse prevention was also conducted. With respect to programme design, studies were selected for review if they evaluated programmes which focused on more than the prevention of cigarette smoking, involved fairly comprehensive skills training curricula, or were multisystemic in design. Thus, studies which evaluated smoking prevention programmes, psychoeducational programmes and personal growth programmes were excluded from the review. With respect to methodological rigour, studies were selected for review if they had a group design which included an intervention and control or comparison group; if 100 cases were included in each group; and if reliable pre- and post-intervention measures were included. Using these stringent inclusion criteria, nine studies were selected for review.

Characteristics of studies

Characteristics of the nine studies included in the review are given in Table 13.1. In three studies programmes in which resistance skills and normative education were the central focus of the curriculum were evaluated (Schope et al., 1996, 1998; Hansen et al., 1988, 1991; Hansen & Graham, 1991). In three studies the effectiveness of life skills training programmes was assessed (Botvin et al., 1990a, 1990b, 1994, 1995a, 1995b). The efficacy of multisystemic programmes was determined in the remaining three studies (Pentz et al., 1990; Johnson et al., 1990; Chou et al., 1998; Perry et al., 1996, 2000; Williams & Perry, 1998). All studies were published between 1988 and 2000. Overall the studies involved a total of 19,028 participants of whom 13,761 were in prevention programmes and 5,267 were in control groups. There were an equal number of male and female participants and they ranged in age from eleven years to fourteen years when they entered their respective studies. Participants were predominantly from lower to middle socioeconomic groups. In seven studies participants were predominantly Caucasian and two

Table 13.1 Characteristics of drug abuse prevention studies

Study no.	Study type	Authors	Year	N per group	Mean age and range	Gender	Family characteristics	Programme setting	Programme duration
1	RS	Schope et al.	1996 1998	1. RS + NE = 308 2. C = 134	13 y 12–13 y	M 52% F 48%	Middle to lower class	Suburban second level	14 sessions
2	RS	Hansen et al.	1988	1. RS + NE = 852 2. AF = 818 3. C = 1,193	11 y	M 51% F 49%	Black 30% Hispanic 38%	Second level urban school	12 sessions
3	RS	Hansen & Graham Hansen et al.	1991 1991	1. RS + NE = 532 2. RS = 676 3. NE = 553 4. C = 655	14 y	M 52% F 48%	Middle class	Second level school	4–10 sessions
4	LST	Botvin et al.	1990a	1. LST-B-P = 200 2. LST-P = 200 3. LST-B = 200 4. LST = 200 5. C = 200	—	M 49% F 51%	—	Suburban second level	30 sessions
5	LST	Botvin et al. Botvin et al.	1990b 1995a	1. LST = 762 2. LST + T-V = 848 3. C = 1,142	13 y	M 52% F 48%	Middle class	Suburban and rural second level	30 sessions
6	LST	Botvin et al.	1995b	1. LST-CF-P = 252 2. LST = 252 3. C = 252	13 y	M 47% F 53%	Lower class Black 49% Latino 37%	Inner city second level	23 sessions
7	MSP	Pentz et al. Johnson et al.	1990 1990	1. MSP = 1,536 2. MSP-L = 1,536 3. C = 2,304	11–13 y	M 51% F 49%	Ethnic minority 22%	Urban schools	10 sessions for children Parent training Community leader training Mass media coverage
8	MSP	Chou et al.	1998	1. MSP = 557 2. C = 516	11–13 y	M 43% F 57%	Lower class 78% Ethnic minority 20%	Suburban and urban	10 sessions for children Parent training Community leader training Mass media coverage
9	MSP	Perry et al. Perry et al. Williams & Perry	1996 2000 1998	1. MSP = 1,175 2. C = 1,175	11–12 y	—	American Indian 6% White 94%	Suburban and urban	24 sessions for children Parent training Teacher Training Peer Training Community task force training

Notes

RS = resistance skills training. NE = normative education. LST = life skills training. MSP = multisystemic programme. AF = affective education. -P = peer-led. -B = booster sessions. -CF = culturally focused. -L = programme offered with a low level of integrity. C = control or comparison group. T-V = teachers trained by video.

studies included participants who were predominantly from ethnic minorities. The duration of the classroom programmes evaluated in these studies ranged from four to thirty sessions, although the multisystemic programmes involved large amounts of unquantified intervention with peer groups, schools, families and communities.

Methodological features

The methodological features of the nine are given in Table 13.2. In all studies there were control or comparison groups. Cases were randomly assigned to groups in eight of these and in the remaining study an attempt at partial randomization was made. Groups were diagnostically and demographically homogeneous in all fifteen studies. Pre- and post-programme assessments using self-report instruments were conducted in all studies. Assessments based on reports from other informants were conducted in

Table 13.2 Methodological features of drug abuse prevention studies

	Study number								
Feature	*S1*	*S2*	*S3*	*S4*	*S5*	*S6*	*S7*	*S8*	*S9*
Control or comparison group	1	1	1	1	1	1	1	1	1
Random assignment	0	1	1	1	1	1	1	1	1
Diagnostic homogeneity	1	1	1	1	1	1	1	1	1
Demographic similarity	1	1	1	1	1	1	1	1	1
Pre-treatment assessment	1	1	1	1	1	1	1	1	1
Post-treatment assessment	1	1	1	1	1	1	1	1	1
2-year follow-up assessment	1	1	0	1	1	1	1	1	1
Children's self-report	1	1	1	1	1	1	1	1	1
Parents' ratings	0	0	0	0	0	0	0	0	1
Teachers' ratings	0	0	0	0	0	0	1	0	1
Trainer ratings	0	0	0	0	0	0	0	0	1
Researcher ratings	0	0	0	0	0	0	1	0	1
Deterioration assessed	1	1	0	0	0	0	1	1	1
Drop-out assessed	1	1	1	1	1	1	1	1	1
Clinical significance of change assessed	0	1	1	1	1	1	1	1	1
Experienced trainers used	0	0	1	0	1	1	1	1	1
Programmes were equally valued	0	1	1	1	1	1	0	0	0
Programmes were manualized	1	1	1	1	1	1	1	1	1
Staff training or supervision was provided	1	1	1	1	1	1	1	1	1
Programme integrity checked	1	0	0	0	1	1	1	0	1
Data on concurrent treatment given	0	0	0	1	1	0	0	0	0
Data on subsequent treatment given	0	0	0	1	0	0	0	0	0
Total	12	14	13	15	16	15	17	14	19

Notes
S = study. 1 = design feature was present. 0 = design feature was absent.

only two studies. In eight studies post-intervention or follow-up data collected at least two years after the beginning of the programme were reported. Drop-out rates were reported in all studies. In all studies programmes were partially or completely manualized and training and/or supervision of teachers or peers who implemented programmes was given. In five studies programme integrity was checked. This was a methodologically robust group of studies.

Substantive findings

Treatment effect sizes and outcome rates for the nine studies are presented in Table 13.3. A narrative summary of key findings from each study is given in Table 13.4.

Resistance skills training and normative education

In three studies resistance skills and normative education programmes were evaluated (Schope et al., 1996, 1998; Hansen et al., 1988, 1991; Hansen & Graham, 1991). In all three studies, the programmes evaluated aimed to teach participants specific communication and assertiveness skills to resist social and peer pressures to drink alcohol and smoke cigarettes or marijuana and also to establish conservative norms for drug use. Active teaching methods were used for skills training including modelling, rehearsal, role-play, giving corrective feedback and extended practice through homework assignments. Programme curricula covered some or all of the following topics: the impact of social factors, particularly pressure from advertising and peers, on personal drug-using attitudes, beliefs, intentions and behaviour; misconceptions about drug-using norms among peers; the immediate short-term effects of drugs on physiological, psychological and social functioning; enhancing commitment to avoid or reduce drug use; and drug refusal skills training. These programmes focused typically on 'gateway' drugs (smoking, alcohol and marijuana) which can lead on to the use of other drugs. These programmes avoided considering the anxiety-provoking long-term impact of drug abuse and addiction. In all three of the studies in which social influence programmes were evaluated, participants made positive short-term gains, particularly in peer-led programmes.

Schope et al. (1996) evaluated a smoking, alcohol and drug use prevention programme in sixteen schools in Michigan. They found that compared with controls, participants in an adult-led resistance skills and normative education programme of which half the classes were taught in grade six and half in grade seven, immediately after the programme showed reductions in alcohol, nicotine and drug use and an increase in knowledge about the effects of drugs, pressures to use drugs and resistance skills. However, gains were lost at six-year follow-up.

In Project SMART, Hansen et al. (1988) evaluated a resistance skills and

Table 13.3 Summary of results of treatment effects and outcome rates of drug abuse prevention studies

	Study number and condition									
	Resistance skills training			Life skills training				Multisystemic programme		
Variable	Study 1	Study 2	Study 3	Study 4	Study 5	Study 6		Study 7	Study 8	Study 9
	RS + NE	RS + NE	RS + NE	LST-P-B	LST	LST	LST-CF-P	MSP	MSP	MSP
	C	C	C	C	C	C	C	C	C	C
Reduction in use after programme	2 y	1 y	1 y	2 y	1 y			1 y	6 m	3.5 y
Alcohol	0.3	0.2	0.7	0.0	0.1	—	—	0.3*	0.3	0.2
Smoking	0.4	0.2	0.0	0.9	0.1	—	—	0.2*	0.3	0.2
Other drugs	0.2	0.3	0.2	0.6	0.1	—	—	0.4*	0.6	0.1
Improvement in knowledge and attitudes after programme	2 y	—	—	2 y	1 y	4 m	4 m	—	—	3.5 y
Alcohol	0.2	—	—	0.4	0.2	0.3	0.3	—	—	0.1
Smoking	0.2	—	—	0.2	0.1	—	—	—	—	—
Other drugs	0.2	—	—	0.0	0.1	0.0	0.0	—	—	—
Reduction in use at follow-up	5 y	2 y	—	—	6 y	2 y	2 y	3 y	3.5 y	5.5 y
Alcohol	0.0	0.3	—	—	0.1	0.2	0.2	0.2	0.2	0.2
Smoking	0.0	0.3	—	—	0.1	0.5	0.2	0.0	0.2	—
Other drugs	0.0	0.0	—	—	0.1	0.0	0.0	0.3	-0.9	—
Improvement in knowledge and attitudes at follow-up	5 y	—	—	—	—	2 y	2 y	—	—	—
Alcohol	0.0	—	—	—	—	0.4	0.4	—	—	—
Smoking	0.0	—	—	—	—	—	—	—	—	—
Other drugs	0.0	—	—	—	—	—	—	—	—	—

Notes
RS = resistance skills training. NE = normative education. LST = life skills training. MSP = multisystemic programme. -P = peer-led. -B = booster sessions. -CF = culturally focused. C = control or comparison group. y = years. m = months.
*High level of adherence in implementation.

Table 13.4 Summary of key findings of drug abuse prevention studies

Study no.	Study type	Authors	Year	N per group	No. of sessions	Group differences	Key findings
1	RS	Schope et al.	1996 1998	1. RS + NE = 308 2. C = 134	15 sessions over 2 years	1 > 2	• This study evaluated a smoking, alcohol and drug use prevention programme in 16 schools in Michigan • Compared with controls, participants in an adult-led resistance skills training programme of which half the classes were taught in grade 6 and half in grade 7, immediately after the programme showed reductions in alcohol, nicotine and drug use and an increase in knowledge about the effects of drugs, pressures to use drugs and resistance skills • Gains were lost at 6-year follow-up
2	RS	Hansen et al.	1988	1. RS + NE = 852 2. AF = 818 3. C = 1,193	12 sessions	1 > 2 = 3	• This study, Project SMART, evaluated a smoking, alcohol and drug use prevention programme in 8 schools in Los Angeles • Compared with controls and participants in an affectively oriented programme, participants in the resistance skills training programme delayed the onset of their smoking, alcohol and marijuana use and these gains were maintained a year after the programme had ended • A year after the programme participants in the affectively oriented programme were involved in significantly more drug use
3	RS	Hansen & Graham Hansen et al.	1991 1991	1. RS + NE = 532 2. RS = 676 3. NE = 553 4. C = 655	4–10 sessions	1 = 3 > 2 = 4	• This study evaluated a smoking, alcohol and drug use prevention programme, the adolescent alcohol prevention trial, involving 12 schools in California • Compared with controls, participants in a normative education programme reduced their alcohol and marijuana use • Without normative education, resistance training was not effective in reducing drug use • Resistance training enhanced knowledge, skills and intentions for resisting peer pressure • Normative training improved students' perceptions of conservative norms for drugs use and increased their self-efficacy beliefs for refusing alcohol if offered • The more accurately programme guidelines were followed, the greater the gains in acquisition of knowledge, skills and self-efficacy beliefs for resisting peer pressure

Table 13.4 continued

Study no.	Study type	Authors	Year	N per group	No. of sessions	Group differences	Key findings
4	LST	Botvin et al.	1990a	1. LST-B-P = 200 2. LST-P = 200 3. LST-B = 200 4. LST = 200 5. C = 200	30 sessions	1 > 2 > 3 > 5 > 4	• This study evaluated a smoking, alcohol and drug use prevention life skills programme, the adolescent alcohol prevention trial, involving students from 10 suburban New York schools • Participants in a peer-led life skills training programme to prevent drug abuse showed greater gains than those in teacher-led programmes • When peer-led life skills training programmes were followed by periodic booster sessions, significantly less drug use occurred, an outcome that did not occur in peer-led programmes where booster sessions were not offered • Teacher-led programmes in which booster sessions were offered led to increased rates of alcohol use • For females, teacher-led programmes with booster sessions effectively reduced drug use • Gains were maintained at 1-year follow-up
5	LST	Botvin et al. Botvin et al.	1990b 1995a	1. LST = 762 2. LST + T-V = 848 3. C = 1,142	30 sessions	1 = 2 > 3	• This study evaluated a smoking, alcohol and drug use prevention life skills programme involving students from 56 middle-class schools in New York State • Compared with controls, participants in an adult-led resistance skills training programme reported reductions in tobacco, alcohol and marijuana 1 year after the start of the programme and 6 years later at the end of high school • The greatest gains were made by participants who got all elements of the programme • There was no difference in the outcome of programmes where teachers were trained by research project staff or video
6	LST	Botvin et al.	1995b	1. LST-CF = 252 2. LST = 252 3. C = 252	23 sessions	1 > 2 > 3	• This study evaluated a smoking, alcohol and drug use prevention life skills programme for students from ethnic minorities involving 6 New York city public schools • Compared with controls, participants in both adult-led and peer-assisted resistance skills training programmes reported a reduction in alcohol but not marijuana use 1 and 2 years after the start of the programmes • The greatest gains were made by participants in the culturally focused programme • Both programmes led to reductions in intentions to drink alcohol and stronger anti-alcohol attitudes

7	MSP	Pentz et al. Johnson et al.	1990 1990	1. MSP = 1,536 2. MSP-L = 1,536 3. C = 2,304	10 sessions for children Parent training Community leader training Mass media coverage	1 > 2 = 3	• This study evaluated a smoking, alcohol and drug use prevention programme, the Kansas City arm of the Midwestern Prevention Project involving 42 schools • Compared with controls, youngsters who participated in a multisystemic drug abuse prevention programme implemented with a high degree of adherence showed a reduction in smoking, alcohol use and marijuana use after 1 year • Youngsters in programmes implemented with low levels of adherence did not differ from controls at 1-year follow-up • At 3-years follow-up, high and low risk participants continued to show reduced rates of smoking and marijuana use
8	MSP	Chou et al.	1998	1. MSP = 557 2. C = 516	10 sessions for children Parent training Community leader training Mass media coverage	1 > 2	• This study evaluated a smoking, alcohol and drug use prevention programme, the Marion County, Indianapolis arm of the Midwestern Prevention Project involving 57 schools • Compared with controls, high-risk youngsters with a history of smoking, drinking or marijuana use who participated in a multisystemic drug abuse prevention programme showed a reduction in smoking and alcohol use after 6 months, but these gains were lost at 3.5-year follow-up
9	MSP	Perry et al. Perry et al. Williams & Perry	1996 2000 1998	1. MSP = 1,175 2. C = 1,175	24 sessions for children Parent training Teacher-training Peer-training Community task force training	1 > 2	• The Project Northland intervention programme which targeted 24 school districts in Northeast Minnesota aimed to prevent alcohol use, not minimize alcohol use • Compared with controls, participants in a 3-years multisystemic intervention programme reported less alcohol use, less combined alcohol and cigarette use; more negative attitudes to alcohol use; and better parent–child communication about the negative consequences of alcohol use • Gains were maintained at 5.5-year follow-up • The programme had no effect on rates of cigarette smoking (independent of alcohol use or marijuana use)

Notes
RS = resistance skills training. NE = normative education. LST = life skills training. MSP = multisystemic programme. AF = affective education. -P = peer-led. -B = booster sessions. -CF = culturally focused. -L = programme offered with a low level of integrity. C = control or comparison group. T-V = teachers trained by video.

normative education programme and an affective education programme in eight schools in Los Angeles. They found that compared with controls and participants in the affective education programme, participants in a resistance skills and normative education programme delayed the onset of their smoking, alcohol and marijuana use and these gains were maintained a year after the programme had ended. In contrast, at follow-up participants in the affective education programme were involved in significantly more drug use. The resistance skills and normative education programme focused on teaching youngsters the skills to recognize and deal with external social pressures to use drugs and to establish conservative norms for drug use. The affective education programme taught youngsters skills to manage negative internal states such as anxiety, depression, stress and low self-esteem.

In the adolescent alcohol prevention trial, involving twelve schools in California, Hansen and colleagues compared the efficacy of a resistance skills programme, a normative education programme and a programme that combined both of these components (Hansen & Graham, 1991; Hansen et al., 1991). They found that without normative education, resistance training was not effective in reducing drug use. Resistance training enhanced knowledge, skills and intentions for resisting peer pressure. Normative training improved students' perceptions of conservative norms for drug use and increased their self-efficacy beliefs for refusing alcohol if offered.

The more accurately programme guidelines were followed, the greater the gains in acquisition of knowledge, skills and self-efficacy beliefs for resisting peer pressure. The results of this study highlight the value of establishing conservative norms in drug abuse prevention programmes in addition to teaching resistance skills.

Post-programme effect sizes based on self-reports of cigarette, alcohol and drug use at between one and two years after programme completion across the three studies ranged from 0 to 0.7 with a mean of 0.3, indicating that the average participant fared better afterwards than 62% of controls. Two- to five-year follow-up effect sizes for cigarette, alcohol and drug use ranged from 0 to 0.3 with a mean of 0.1, indicating that the average participant fared better at follow-up than only 54% of controls. In the single study where knowledge and attitudes to drug use were assessed the average two-year post-programme effect size was 0.2 but at five years this had reduced to 0, indicating that the average participant fared better after the programme than 58% of controls and no better than controls after five years.

Life skills

In three studies, life skills training programmes were evaluated (Botvin et al., 1990a, 1990b, 1994, 1995a, 1995b). In all three studies, in addition to being trained in specific drug refusal skills for managing advertising and peer pressure to smoke, drink and use other drugs, participants learned a range of more general decision-making, communication, social problem-solving, and stress management skills to enhance their self-control, social competence and self-esteem.

Compared with controls Botvin et al. (1990b, 1995a) found that participants in an adult-led life skills training programme used less alcohol, tobacco and other drugs at six-year follow-up and that the greatest benefits were reaped by participants who completed the full programme. Programmes in which teachers were trained by video or research staff did not differ in their effectiveness. Participants in this study were students from 56 middle-class schools in New York State.

To determine the impact of peer leadership and booster sessions on the efficacy of their life-skills training programme, Botvin et al. (1990a) compared adult- and peer-led life skills programmes with and without booster sessions. They found that greatest reductions in drug-using behaviour and positive changes in drug-using attitudes and beliefs at one-year follow-up were made by participants in peer-led life-skills training programmes with booster sessions. Overall, teacher-led programmes in which booster sessions were offered led to increased rates of alcohol use, but for females, teacher-led programmes with booster sessions effectively reduced drug use.

To find out if their life-skills training programme was effective with youngsters from ethnic minorities as well as white middle-class adolescents, Botvin et al. (1994, 1995b) compared the effectiveness of their life skills programme with a culturally focused peer-assisted version of the life skills programme for students from black and Latino ethnic minorities in six New York city public schools. They found that compared with controls, participants in both programmes reported a reduction in alcohol but not marijuana use one and two years after the start of the programmes. The greatest gains were made by participants in the culturally focused peer-assisted programme. Both programmes led to reductions in intentions to drink alcohol and stronger anti-alcohol attitudes. In the culturally focused programme in addition to routine life skills training, a peer-assisted story telling and video component was used. Mythic stories from Greek, African and Spanish culture and stories based on inner city culture were used to demonstrate and model different skills. In the stories the hero used skills to gradually overcome obstacles and achieve goals.

Post-programme effect sizes for self-reports of cigarette, alcohol and drug use one to two years after intervention ranged from 0 to 0.9. The mean effect size across the two studies for which data were available was 0.3, indicating that the average life skills programme participant reported less cigarette, alcohol and drug use than 62% of controls one to two years after intervention. Two- to six-year follow-up effect sizes for cigarette, alcohol and drug use ranged from 0 to 0.5 with a mean of 0.1, indicating that the average life skills programme participant reported less cigarette, alcohol and drug use two to six years after intervention than only 54% of controls.

Post-programme effect sizes for knowledge and attitudes towards cigarette, alcohol and drug use after intervention ranged from 0 to 0.4. The mean effect size across the three studies was 0.2. Thus, the average life skills programme participant reported greater knowledge and stronger anti-drug attitudes than 58% of controls after intervention. The average effect size for knowledge and attitudes towards cigarette, alcohol and drug use at two-year follow-up was 0.4, indicating that the average life skills programme participant reported greater knowledge and stronger anti-drug attitudes two years after intervention than 66% of controls.

Multisystemic programmes

The efficacy of multisystemic programmes was determined in the remaining three studies (Pentz et al., 1990; Johnson et al., 1990; Chou et al., 1998; Perry et al., 1996, 2000; Williams & Perry, 1998).

Two of these evaluated different arms of the Midwestern Prevention Programme (Pentz et al., 1990; Johnson et al., 1990; Chou et al., 1998). This programme involved a 10-session classroom-based resistance skills training component; a parent training component focusing on parenting skills, parent–adolescent communication, and school-based drug abuse prevention policy; a community leader training component which aimed to help leaders organize a drug abuse task force; and a mass media campaign involving TV, radio and newspaper coverage with news items, talk show items, commercials and a student video competition in which students produced videos covering the classroom curriculum.

In the Kansas City arm of the Midwestern Prevention Project, Pentz et al. (1990; Johnson et al., 1990) found that compared with controls, youngsters who participated in this multisystemic drug abuse prevention programme implemented with a high degree of adherence showed a reduction in smoking, alcohol use and marijuana use after one year. Youngsters in programmes where the classroom component was implemented with low levels of adherence did not differ from controls at one-year follow-up. At three-year follow-up, high- and low-risk participants continued to show reduced rates of smoking and marijuana use (Johnson et al., 1990).

In the Marion County, Indianapolis, arm of the Midwestern Prevention Project, Chou et al. (1998) found that compared with controls, high-risk youngsters with a history of smoking, drinking or marijuana use who participated in the multisystemic drug abuse prevention programme showed a reduction in smoking and alcohol use after six months, but these gains were lost at three and a half years' follow-up.

In Project Northland, Perry et al. (1996, 2000; Williams & Perry, 1998) found that compared with controls, participants in a three-year multisystemic intervention programme reported less alcohol use, less combined alcohol and cigarette use, more negative attitudes to alcohol use, and better parent–child communication about the negative consequences of alcohol use. The programme had no effect on rates of cigarette smoking (independent of alcohol use) or marijuana use. The Project Northland intervention programme targeted twenty-four school districts in Northeast Minnesota. The aim of the programme was to prevent alcohol use, not harm reduction through minimizing alcohol use. The programme involved a classroom-based component, a family-based component, a peer group-based component, and a community-based component. In each of the three years of the programme, children completed a school-based curriculum of four to eight sessions in which they learned resistance skills, life skills, evolved conservative norms for alcohol use, actively generated leisure activity alternatives to alcohol use, and worked with a theatrical company to develop an educational play about avoiding alcohol use. Peer leaders were involved in the school-based aspect of the programme. The school-based curriculum was linked with home practice. Parents were mailed a newsletter regularly to give information on the prevention of alcohol use, outline details of the programme, and give direct behavioural guidance on prevention of alcohol use. In addition, occasional evening meetings were convened at the school and were attended by children, parents and teachers in which the focus was on aspects of the Project Northlands Curriculum and related activities. In the community-based component, project staff recruited and trained local drug abuse prevention task forces. Members included local government officials, law enforcement officers, health professionals, educational professionals, clergy, adolescents, youth workers and others. The task forces took steps to ensure that the sale of alcohol to minors was reduced, that teen abstinence was rewarded, and that alcohol-free activities and centres for adolescents were developed within the community.

Post-programme effect sizes based on self-reports of cigarette, alcohol and drug use at between one and two years after programme completion across the three multisystemic studies ranged from 0.1 to 0.6 with a mean of 0.3, indicating that the average participant fared better afterwards than 62% of controls. At 3–5½-year follow-up, effect sizes for cigarette, alcohol and drug use ranged from -0.9 to 0.3 with a mean close to 0, indicating that the average participant fared no better at follow-up than controls.

Conclusions

Between 5 and 10% of teenagers under nineteen have drug problems serious enough to require clinical intervention. One strategy for preventing youngsters joining this minority is to provide school-based prevention programmes which aim to prevent or reduce usage of gateway drugs: nicotine, alcohol and marijuana. These gateway drugs are invariably the first step on the road to serious drug problems for those youngsters that eventually develop such difficulties. From this review a number of conclusions may be drawn about the effectiveness of school-based programmes. First, prevention programmes for young teenagers can reduce their use of gateway drugs such as alcohol, nicotine and marijuana over periods of up to two years. These gains are not sustained over longer periods, where programmes and booster sessions cease after two years. Second, effective programmes inform youngsters accurately about the immediate effects of drugs without inducing anxiety about long-term dangers; establish conservative norms for drug use; teach specific drug refusal skills; and also teach general social problem-solving skills. In addition, effective programmes may target members of youngsters' social systems including the peer group, family, school and community. Third, effective programmes are delivered by trained staff or peer leaders who accurately follow manualized curricula and involve active teaching methods which include group discussion and modelling, rehearsal, role-play and giving corrective feedback on skills usage. Fourth, effective programmes begin in early adolescence, include multiple training sessions (10–30) and also include multiple booster sessions in mid-adolescence. Furthermore effective programmes are delivered in such a way that the chances of all pupils getting a full 'dose' of the programme are maximized. Finally, effective programmes are developmental and culturally sensitive, incorporated into the ongoing school curriculum and are rigorously evaluated. A summary of the key elements of effective drug abuse prevention programmes is given in Table 13.5.

Implications for policy and practice

These findings have clear implications for policy and practice. Young teenagers should routinely participate in peer-led programmes of up to 30 sessions in which they receive accurate information about the immediate effects of drugs and conservative normative information about drug use, and learn drug refusal skills and general social problem-solving skills. These programmes should involve active teaching methods and multiple booster sessions in mid-adolescence, and should be integrated into the school curriculum so that most youngsters attend all classes. These school-based programmes should be the nucleus of wider multisystemic programmes which involve members of youngsters' significant social systems.

Implications for research

Effect sizes in Table 13.3 are relatively small compared with those in similar tables in other chapters of this volume. It is clear that school-based drug abuse prevention programmes, while effective, have a less pronounced impact on drug use than prevention programmes described in other chapters have on the target problems they address. Thus, process studies are required which investigate the mechanisms and processes that underpin the effectiveness of such drug abuse prevention programmes and this information may be used to enhance programme effectiveness.

A strong argument may be made for focusing research on harm reduction rather than abstinence-oriented multisystemic adolescent drug abuse prevention programmes. This is because risk-taking in general and substance abuse in particular are normative behaviours for many adolescents. Adolescents

Table 13.5 Key elements of effective drug abuse prevention programmes

Resistance skills and normative education	• Skills to identify social pressure to use drugs and skills to resist such pressure • Accurate knowledge about prevalence of drug use to help develop conservative drug use norms
Life skills	• Assertiveness skills • Skills for improving self-control and self-esteem • Stress management skills • Social communication and problem-solving skills • Decision-making skills • Skills for developing social alternatives to drug use
Multisystemic involvement	• Peer-leader involvement in programme delivery • Peer group projects exploring alternatives to drug use • Home–school liaison about drug use prevention policy • Parent–child homework assignments about drug abuse prevention • Parent training in parent–adolescent communication, limit setting and supervision • Community involvement in drug abuse prevention task force
General design features	• Adequate training, support and supervision of teachers, peer leaders and programme staff • Manualized programme curricula • Monitoring of accurate programme implementation • Active training methods (modelling, rehearsal, corrective feedback, reinforcement and extended practice) • Begin at the transition from primary to secondary school when youngsters are aged 11–13 • Extend over at least a school year and include booster sessions annually throughout high school • Incorporated into existing school curriculum • Developmentally staged • Socially and culturally acceptable to the community, particularly where youngsters are from ethnic minorities • Rigorously evaluated and feedback of evaluation given to implementation team and participants

who experiment with various 'gateway' drugs, but do not progress to drug abuse or addiction, are characterized by a number of protective factors. These include social skills and skills required for emotional self-regulation. They also include membership of non-deviant peer groups and membership of supportive well-organized families in which there is consistent discipline and moderate levels of supervision based in a supportive community. Research on multisystemic school-based drug abuse prevention programmes should examine the degree to which enhancing these protective factors contributes to harm reduction.

Assessment resources

Kaiminer, Y., Wagner, E., Plummer, E. & Seifer, R. (1993). Validation of the Teen Addiction Severity Index (T-ASI). Preliminary Findings. *American Journal of Addictions*, 3, 250–254.

Mayer, J. & Filstead, W. (1979). The adolescent alcohol involvement scale: An instrument for measuring adolescent use and misuse of alcohol. *Journal of Studies in Alcohol*, 40, 291–300.

Oetting, E.R., Beauvais, F., Edwards, R. & Waters, M. (1984). *The Drug and Alcohol Assessment System*. Western Behavioural Studies, Colorado State University, Fort Collins, Colorado.

Pechacek T., Fox B., Murray D. & Leupker, A. (1984) Review of techniques for measurement of smoking behaviour in behavioural health. In J. Matazarro, J. Herd, N. Miller & S. Weiss (Eds.), *A Handbook of Health Enhancement and Disease Prevention* (pp. 729–754). New York: Wiley.

Skinner, H. (1982). The drug abuse screening test. *Addictive Behaviour* 7, 363–371.

Winters, K. (1989). *Personal Experience Screening Questionnaire*. Los Angeles, CA: Western Psychological Services.

Winters, K. & Henly, G. (1989). *Personal Experience Inventory*. Los Angeles, CA: Western Psychological Services.

Programme resources

Botvin, G. (2001). Life skills training manuals. (Available from Dr Gilbert Botvin, New York Hospital, Cornell University Medical Centre, 1300 York Avenue, New York, NY 10021. *http://www.lifeskillstraining.com/*)

Schope, J., Weimer, M., Dielman, L. Smith, A. et al. (1987). *Substance Use Prevention Education and Alcohol Misuse Prevention: Curricula for 5th, 6th and 7th grades and Booster Sessions*. Ann Arbor: University of Michigan. (Contact Dr Jean Schope, Transportation Institute, University of Michigan, 2901, Baxter Road, Ann Arbor, MI 48109–2150.)

Hansen, W. and colleagues (1991). *Project SMART Drug Abuse Prevention Programme*. (Contact Dr William Hansen, Department of Public Health Sciences, Bowman Gray School of Medicine, Winston Salem, North Carolina, 27157.)

Hansen, W. and colleagues (1989). *Project STAR Drug Abuse Prevention Programme*. (Contact Dr William Hansen, Department of Public Health Sciences, Bowman Gray School of Medicine, Winston Salem, North Carolina, 27157.)

Hansen, W. and colleagues (1989). *ALL STARS Drug Abuse Prevention Programme*. (Tanglewood Research Inc. 7–17 Albert Pick Road, Suite D, Greensborough, NC 27409. Tel (336) 662–0090. *www.tanglewood.net*.)

Williams, C. (2000). Project Northland Alcohol Prevention Curriculum for grades 6–8. Minneapolis, MN: Hazelden. (Available from *www.hazelden.org*. Information on programme materials is available from Professor Cheryl Perry Division of Epidemiology, School of Public Health, University of Minnesota, 1300 S Second Street, Suite 300, Minneapolis, MN 55454. Tel (612) 624–1818. Email *perry@epivax.epi.umn.edu*.)

14 Prevention of teenage pregnancy, STDs and HIV infection

Nodlaig Moore, Attracta McGlinchey and Alan Carr

Risky sexual behaviour is a highly significant problem throughout the world. Unintentional teenage pregnancy, sexually transmitted diseases (STDs) and human immunodeficiency virus (HIV) infection are the principal negative outcomes of risky sexual behaviour. Each of these outcomes, in turn, may have negative consequences for health, well-being and development. In recent years there has been a proliferation of programmes to prevent risky sexual behaviour and encourage safe sexual practices. Unfortunately the effectiveness of many of these remains untested (Carr, 2001a). The aim of this chapter is to review methodologically robust research studies on the efficacy of programmes which aim to prevent or minimize risky sexual behaviour, draw reliable conclusions about the effectiveness of these, and outline the implications of these conclusions for policy and practice.

Unintentional teenage pregnancy

From a biological perspective, early pregnancy is not harmful to either the mother or the child. However, complications during teenage pregnancy are common and teenage pregnancy may have many negative consequences in the socioeconomic and psychological domains (Coleman & Roker, 1998; Coley & Chase-Lansdale, 1998). Complications of teenage pregnancy include higher risk of anaemia, toxaemia and hypertension; low birth weight; higher risk of perinatal mortality; and higher risk of spontaneous abortions in other pregnancies. At a socioeconomic level, girls who have children early in their teens tend to drop out of education early, have poorer employment prospects and are more likely to become dependent on welfare subsidies and live in poverty. Children of teenage mothers are more vulnerable to abuse and neglect, to developmental delays, to educational underachievement and to behavioural problems. The majority of fathers of children from teenage pregnancies have little or no contact with their children or partners and provide little or no financial support. Most relationships between teenage mothers and the fathers of their children are short term and teenage mothers are more likely later in life to become separated or divorced.

Sexually transmitted diseases

Sexually transmitted diseases in adolescence include chlamydia, genital warts, gonorrhoea, herpes, syphilis, vaginitis, hepatitis B and HIV infection leading to AIDS. Most of these conditions cause discomforting symptoms, especially genital discomfort. Some STDs – such as chlamydia, gonorrhoea, syphilis and vaginitis – can be cured. Others – such as herpes and genital warts – cannot and so there is increased probability that they will be transmitted to other sexual partners. In females, cervical dysplasia and cervical carcinoma often result from sexually transmitted infection with the human papilloma virus. Genital tract ulceration associated with STD infections increases the likelihood of HIV transmission (King, 1988).

HIV infection

HIV infection has devastating long-term biological and psychological consequences. At a biological level, HIV infection may evolve into acquired immunodeficiency syndrome (AIDS) which even with aggressive treatment is ultimately a fatal condition (Brown et al., 2000). Around 13–23% of HIV-infected children and adolescents develop progressive encephalopathy which is characterized by impaired brain growth, progressive motor dysfunction, and loss or plateauing of developmental milestones with deficits in IQ and language development. The duration between HIV infection and the development of AIDS is variable. Once AIDS develops there is a radical reduction in quality of life associated with an increase in the rate of infections and illness, the requirement for aggressive medical treatment, and the inevitability of a shortened life span.

Epidemiology

In the UK the National Survey of Sexuality and Lifestyles has led to a number of important epidemiological findings about adolescent sexuality (Wellings et al., 1994). The average age of first sexual intercourse has declined over the past twenty to thirty years from age twenty-one to seventeen for women and from twenty to seventeen for men. One in five youngsters under sixteen years are sexually active. Youngsters from working-class families and those of lower educational level have sexual intercourse on average two years earlier than middle-class youngsters with higher educational aspirations. About a quarter of teenagers use no method of contraception. The younger a teenager is, the less likely he or she is to use contraception. Up to 50% of sexually active youngsters under sixteen use no contraception. The condom is the most popular method of contraception with more than half of youngsters using this method and about a fifth using the contraceptive pill. Among teenagers, unintentional teenage pregnancy, sexually transmitted diseases and HIV infection are, unfortunately, surprisingly common problems.

Unintentional teenage pregnancy

Birth rates for fifteen- to nineteen-year-old women in the mid-1990s in the UK were 32 per 1,000 and in the USA they were 57 per 1,000 (Nitz, 1999). Britain has the highest rate of teenage pregnancy in Europe (Coleman & Roker, 1998). About two-thirds of pregnant adolescent girls have abortions. About a third of adolescent mothers go on to have repeat pregnancies within two years (Nitz, 1999).

Sexually transmitted diseases

Rates of STDs among adolescents are difficult to determine. In the USA only the reporting of gonorrhoea and syphilis is mandatory (D'Angelo & Di Clemente, 1996). In the early 1990s for fifteen- to nineteen-year-olds, the rates of gonorrhoea were 882 per 100,000 for males and 1,044 per 100,000 for females. In the early 1990s for fifteen- to nineteen-year-olds the rates of syphilis were 18 per 100,000 for males and 35 per 100,000 for females. Community surveys show that the rates of chlamydia are 5% among college students, and 11% among inner-city adolescents (Rosenthal et al., 1994).

HIV infection

In the late 1990s there were more than seven million cases of AIDS reported worldwide and one million of these were youngsters (Brown et al., 2000). While exact prevalence data are unavailable, it is estimated that for every one reported case of AIDS there are three HIV-positive young people. Thus, there are three million young people worldwide who are HIV positive. Historically, HIV and AIDS initially proliferated among homosexual males and intravenous drug abusers. However, in Europe and America, HIV infection rates are currently increasing most rapidly among heterosexuals and young people in ethnic minorities. In parts of Africa with high HIV prevalence rates, life expectancy has dropped dramatically. For example, in a rural area of Uganda where the prevalence of HIV infection is about 10%, life expectancy has dropped from sixty to forty-three years as a result of AIDS-related deaths.

Aetiology

Numerous psychological theories have been constructed to explain how sexually risky behaviour develops and how it may be modified so that youngsters engage in safer sexual practices. Two of the more comprehensive theories, deserving elaboration, are the behavioural-ecological model of sexual behaviour (Hovell et al., 1994) and the AIDS risk reduction model (Catania et al., 1990).

Behavioural-ecological model of sexual behaviour

The behavioural ecological model argues that risky and safe sexual behaviours are determined by proximal and distal antecedents and consequences within youngsters' social-ecological systems and also by a range of background predisposing factors (Hovell et al., 1994). The model is based on a large body of empirical research evidence reviewed by Hovell and colleagues which supports the assertions made throughout this section. The model incorporates both systemic and cognitive behavioural models of the development and modification of risk-related sexual behaviour, which either implicitly or explicitly underpin the programmes evaluated in the latter half of this chapter.

Background predisposing factors include biologically determined characteristics such as gender or stage of physical development; socioeconomic status; cultural norms concerning sexual behaviour; and personal history of reinforcement for safe and risky sexual behaviours. Late adolescent and young adult males are more likely to engage in sexually risky behaviour, whereas younger adolescents and females are not. Youngsters from low socioeconomic status groups, from cultures that endorse promiscuity, and those with a personal history where risky behaviours such as not using condoms or having multiple sexual partners were reinforced are more likely to engage in sexually risky behaviour. Youngsters from higher socioeconomic groups, with higher educational aspirations, from cultures that endorse traditional or religious values with a personal history where safe behaviours such as abstinence or using condoms or having few sexual partners were reinforced are more likely to engage in safe sexual behaviour.

Distal antecedents of safe and risky sexual behaviour may be identified within the family, school and peer group. Chronic parent–child conflict, lack of parental supervision and poor parent–child communication are among the important family-based distal antecedents of sexually risky behaviour. In contrast, family-based distal antecedents of safe sexual behaviour include co-operative parent–child relationships, age-appropriate parental supervision and good parent–child communication.

Within schools, distal antecedents of sexually risky behaviour include low achievement orientation and the absence of sex education, or sex education that focuses on information giving rather than skills training for safe sex. In contrast, school-based distal antecedents of safe sexual behaviour include high achievement orientation and sex education which focuses on skills training for safe sex.

Within the peer group, distal antecedents of sexually risky behaviour include a group norm or peer pressure which supports sexually risky behaviour or other risky problem behaviours including drug and alcohol abuse and rule breaking. Distal antecedents within the peer group for safe sexual behaviour include a group norm or peer pressure which supports safe sexual behaviour and opposes other risky problem behaviours. The media – TV, radio, films, magazines and newspapers – present models for sexual behaviour that are commonly fantasy-based and rarely involve detailed attention to the practices essential for safe sex. In this sense, the media may present individuals with distal antecedents for risky sexual behaviour. On occasion, the media, through documentaries and responsible reporting, present information on practices essential for safe sex and in such instances offer distal antecedents for safe sexual behaviour.

Proximal antecedents of risky and safe sexual behaviour include personality traits, attitudes, beliefs, knowledge, skills, and behaviour patterns along with those of sexual partners. High levels of sensation-seeking and unconventionality and low levels of self-esteem are the main personality traits that predispose to sexually risky behaviour. In contrast, safe sexual practices are more likely where individuals show low levels of sensation seeking and unconventionality and high self-esteem. Sexually risky behaviour is associated with positive attitudes to such behaviour based on beliefs that the costs of safe sex are far higher than the benefits of risky sex, and also on low self-efficacy beliefs concerning the use of safe sex skills. In contrast, safe sexual behaviour is associated with positive attitudes to safe sex based on beliefs that the benefits of safe sex are far higher than the costs of risky sex, and also on high self-efficacy beliefs concerning the use of safe sex skills. Inaccurate knowledge about safe sex, lack of skills for safe sex (such as condom use skills and sexual assertiveness skills), and involvement in broader patterns of risky behaviour (such as drug and alcohol abuse and delinquency) are other proximal antecedents of risky sexual behaviour. In contrast, other proximal antecedents of safe sexual behaviour include accurate knowledge about safe sex, well-developed skills for safe sex and the absence of other risky behaviour patterns. A further proximal antecedent of risky sexual behaviour is coercion to engage in risky sexual practices (particularly by males). In contrast, partner support for safe sexual behaviour is a further proximal antecedent of safe sex.

Risky or safe sexual behaviour may be maintained by the overall net reinforcing or punishing effect of proximal and distal consequences of such behaviours. Possible positive reinforcing proximal consequences for risky sexual behaviour include heightened sexual pleasure, particularly for the male, and increased opportunities for interspersing episodes of foreplay between episodes of sexual intercourse when condoms are not used. Possible negative or punishing consequences of safe sexual practices including sexual assertiveness and condom use include interpersonal conflict, decreased sexual sensitivity for the male and decreased sexual pleasure for the male. Deviant peer group approval for unsafe sexual practices is a particularly important possible reinforcing distal consequence of risky sexual behaviour.

Possible positive reinforcing proximal consequences for safe sexual behaviour include the knowledge that infection and unwanted pregnancy will be avoided. Possible negative or punishing distal consequences of risky sexual practices include infection, unwanted pregnancy and disapproval from the family, the community and members of non-deviant peer groups.

The behavioural-ecological model of sexual behaviour offers a framework for a range of preventative measures to reduce the incidence of risky sexual practices within communities. Strategies based on the behavioural-ecological model include targeting groups with high-risk profiles on background, distal and proximal antecedent variables; family interventions and parent training to improve parent–child cooperation and communication and parental supervision; school-based programmes which include safe sex skills training and the enhancement of a school's overall achievement orientation; peer-group-based safe sex skills training led or facilitated by respected and popular peers; and media campaigns that advocate safe sex and give information on safe sex skills. In this chapter the focus will be on reviewing evidence for the effectiveness of school-based programmes, although it is recognized that such programmes represent only a single element of the comprehensive community-wide multisystemic preventative approach suggested by the behavioural-ecological model of sexual behaviour.

AIDS risk reduction model

The AIDS risk reduction model (ARRM) reflects an integration of the health beliefs model, the theory of reasoned action, the theory of planned behaviour, protection motivation theory, the social influence model and social learning theory as applied to the development and modification of sexual risk taking. All of these theories which are integrated within the ARRM have implicitly or explicitly influenced the development of inter-vention programmes evaluated in the studies reviewed in the latter half of this chapter. The ARRM pinpoints three stages through which people pass in changing their behaviour with respect to using condoms (Catania et al., 1990; Sheeran et al., 1999). These are labelling, commitment and enactment.

In the labelling stage people become aware that unprotected sex may lead to AIDS. The labelling stage is associated with a number of psychological processes. There is an increase in knowledge about AIDS transmission and prevention. There is an increase in knowledge about personal susceptibility to AIDS infection and people realize 'It could happen to me'. There is an increased awareness of the severity of the consequences of AIDS by for example realizing 'It could be fatal'. There is also an increase in fear about becoming infected with AIDS. During the labelling phase people may review their past lives and evaluate the degree to which their past behaviour has placed them at risk for AIDS. In particular they may review the period of their lives for which they have been sexually active, the number of previous sexual partners, and the frequency with which they have had sex. A variety of cues to action may trigger the process of labelling one's sexual behaviour as problematic. These include exposure to information about AIDS through school- or media-based programmes, contact with people who are HIV positive, or having tests for HIV or other STDs.

In the second stage of the ARRM, a firm commitment is made to use condoms in the future during sex and this commitment is crystallized as an expressed intention to use condoms when having sex. A key factor in this decision-making process is developing the belief that a condom is effective in preventing HIV infection. However, people may be deterred from developing this belief by a variety of factors. They may decide not to use condoms because they are embarrassed about buying them; embarrassed about using them; or because they believe condoms will reduce sexual pleasure. They may also decide not to use condoms because they use other contraceptive methods, such as the pill, and be reluctant to combine this with condom use. A variety of social pressures may influence a person's decision to use condoms. If a person's partner and friends have positive attitudes to condom use, this may help a person make a firm commitment to use condoms in future. Developing commitment to use condoms in the future is influenced by a person's confidence that he or she can effectively use condoms, that is, a sense of self-efficacy for condom use. This confidence or self-efficacy concerning condom use is influenced by personal experiences of successfully using condoms in the past.

In the third stage of the ARRM – the enactment stage – people take active steps to prepare to use condoms. They learn how to use them, carry them and communicate with their partners about using them as a way of avoiding HIV or other STDs. They also plan to use condoms with partners where the risk of HIV infection is high, particularly casual sexual partners or those with a history of intravenous drug use. They also make plans to deal with barriers to condom use such as drug or alcohol intoxication or high levels of sexual arousal.

Empirical studies of condom use show that variables at all three stages of the ARRM are associated with eventual condom use, but the strongest associations are between those processes important for commitment and enactment and condom use (Sheeran et al., 1999). Thus, knowledge about HIV and AIDS that promotes labelling of risky sex as a problem is not as important for eventual condom use as the processes of making a commitment and planning to use condoms. Strategies which facilitate commitment and motivation enhancement include encouraging positive attitudes to condoms and promoting the view that peers and partners also accept condoms as a method of preventing HIV infection. Strategies which facilitate enactment include preparatory skills training which focuses on encouraging youngsters to carry condoms, coaching them in appropriate condom-use skills, and the skills required to communicate effectively with sexual partners about their use. In view of the preventative strategies entailed by the ARRM, it is not surprising that many school-based programmes which aim to reduce sexually risky behaviour include psychoeducation, and/or communications skills training, and/or behavioural skills training as their main components. An outline of these components is given in Table 14.1.

Table 14.1 Main components of prevention programmes for reducing sexually risky behaviours

Area	Topic
Psychoeducation	• Nature, presentation and transmission of AIDS and sexually transmitted diseases (STDs) • Facts about pregnancy and contraception • Risk factors for teenage pregnancy, and STD infection, and HIV infection • Condom use • Mutual monogamy • Partner reduction • STD treatment
Communication skills training	• Speaking and listening skills for enhancing interpersonal communication • Negotiation training for co-operating with partners about sexual risk reduction • Assertiveness training and refusal skills training to manage peer pressure for sexual risk taking
Behavioural skills training	• Anticipating peer pressure for sexual risk taking • Anticipating impact of drug and alcohol use on sexual risk taking • Problem-solving plans for sexually risky situations • Buying, carrying and using condoms effectively

Previous reviews

Reviews of empirical studies that have evaluated programmes which aim to reduce risky sexual behaviour conclude that effective programmes cover certain specific content areas and are delivered using certain specific training processes (Choi & Coates, 1994; Di Clemente & Peterson, 1994; Franklin et al., 1997; Kim et al., 1997; Miller et al., 1992; Kirby, 1992, 1997; Kirby et al., 1994; Nitz, 1999).

The most effective programmes for preventing risky sexual behaviour involve general psychoeducation about contraception, teenage pregnancy, STDs and HIV infection. They also cover specific psychoeducation about safe sex, condom use, mutual monogamy, reducing the number of sexual partners and treatment of STDs. Effective programmes cover communication and sexual assertiveness skills training to equip adolescents to deal with partners' requests for unsafe sex. In addition effective programmes include behavioural skills training. This training covers skills for risk reduction which involves anticipating the impact of peer pressure and drug and alcohol use on risky sexual behaviour and developing problem-solving strategies for dealing with these anticipated high-risk situations and also condom-use skills training.

Effective programmes use a variety of active training techniques including instruction, modelling, rehearsal, role-play, corrective feedback, homework assignments and discussion. They are sufficiently long to allow participants to gain the skills required to practise safe sex. Effective programmes provide opportunities to weigh up the costs and benefits of risky and safe sexual behaviour. Effective programmes may include peer leaders who model safe sex skills and facilitate youngsters participating in the programme to rehearse the skills that have been modelled and to learn from corrective feedback. Effective programmes include activities to address the power of the media and other social influences on sexual behaviour and incorporate activities to strengthen individual and group norms against risky sexual behaviour. Effective programmes are culturally sensitive and age appropriate. Thus, for younger adolescents the aim of programmes may be to help youngsters delay the onset of sexual activity whereas with older adolescents the aim may be to increase condom use. Effective programmes are offered by staff and peer leaders who believe in the value and effectiveness of their programmes. One common argument against sexuality programmes for adolescents and children has been that exposing youngsters to information about sex will encourage them to engage in sexual activity. Previous reviews of the literature in this area do not support this hypothesis.

The confidence that may be placed in the conclusions of these reviews is tempered by the fact that they are based on studies that vary widely in methodological robustness. All of the reviews cited above included both well and poorly designed studies.

Method

The goal of this chapter was to review a selection of well-designed studies of the effectiveness of school-based programmes the aim of which was to prevent sexually risky behaviour associated with teenage pregnancy, sexually transmitted disease and HIV infection. A computer-based literature search of the PsychLit database was conducted. The search was confined to English language journals and covered the period 1977–2000. The main search terms were *AIDS, HIV, STD, teenage pregnancy* and *adolescent pregnancy*. These were combined with the terms *prevention, evaluation, review, education* and *effectiveness*. In addition, a manual search of the bibliographies of all recent review papers on adolescent STD/HIV/pregnancy prevention programmes was conducted. Studies were selected for inclusion in this review if they were group designs (as opposed to single case designs); included a fairly homogeneous group of cases; contained a control or comparison group; and included pre- and post-intervention measures. Of forty-four studies identified which met these criteria, twenty were selected for review. These were selected for their methodological sophistication and also for the design features of the prevention programmes which they evaluated. The group of twenty studies included three subgroups with different programme design features. The first of these contained studies of psychoeducational programmes; the second included studies of programmes that contained psychoeducational and communications skills training components; and the third included studies of programmes which involved behavioural skills training along with psychoeducational and communications skills training components.

Characteristics of the studies

The characteristics of the twenty selected studies in which the efficacy of primary prevention programmes for teenage pregnancy, STD infection, and HIV infection was evaluated are outlined in Table 14.2. Two studies evaluated exclusively psychoeducational programmes (Huszti et al., 1989; Schinke et al., 1990). Seven studies evaluated programmes which contained psychoeducation and communication skills training components (Aplasca et al., 1995; Di Clemente et al., 1989; Levy et al., 1995; Boyer et al., 1997; Howard & McCabe, 1990; Schinke et al., 1981; Bayne Smith, 1994). Eleven studies evaluated programmes which contained psychoeducation, communication and behavioural skills training components (Kipke et al., 1993; Caceres et al., 1994; Walter & Vaughan, 1993; Kirby et al., 1991; Hubbard et al., 1998; Barth et al., 1992; St Lawrence et al., 1995a, 1995b; Fawole et al., 1999; Schaalma et al., 1996; Jemmott et al., 1992). In five of these eleven studies video modelling was used to teach communication and behavioural skills. All twenty studies were published between 1981 and 1999. In all, 12,613 youngsters participated in these studies; 6,930 participated in intervention programmes and 5,683 were assigned to control or comparison groups. Participants ranged from eleven to twenty years of age; 49% of cases were male and 51% were female. The ethnicity of participants was reported in twelve studies. Ethnic groups represented in these studies included whites, Latinos, Filipinos, Chinese, African Americans, Native Americans, Caribbean blacks, Asians and West Indians. The programme sites for nineteen studies were high schools. In two of these studies programmes were conducted after school hours (Kipke et al., 1993, Jemmott et al., 1992). One programme was conducted in a drug treatment facility (St Lawrence et al., 1995a). Programme duration was variable and ranged from one hour to eighteen sessions plus a six-week career mentorship.

Methodological features

The methodological features of the twenty studies included in this review are presented in Table 14.3. All studies selected contained a control or comparison group and participants were randomly assigned to these groups or an intervention group in 65% of the studies. In 90% of the studies intervention and control/comparison groups were demographically similar and all groups were assessed before and after the intervention. Data for three- to six-month follow-up was reported in four studies (Jemmott et al., 1992; Walter & Vaughan, 1993; Schinke et al., 1981; Barth et al., 1992), one study provided

Table 14.2 Characteristics of studies of prevention programmes for reducing sexually risky behaviours

Study no.	Study type	Authors	Year	N per group	Mean age and range	Gender	Family characteristics	Programme setting	Programme duration
1	PE	Huszti et al.	1989	1. PE-HE = 153 2. PE-HE + VT = 131 3. C = 164	16 y 14–17 y	M 44% F 56%	NR	Secondary school	1 h
2	PE	Schinke et al.	1990	1. PE-HE = 18 2. PE-SD = 19 3. C = 23	16 y	M 43% F 56%	AA 37% H 27% CB 15% O 22%	Job training programme	3 × 1 h
3	PE + CST	Aplasca et al.	1995	1. PE-HE + CST = 420 2. C = 384	15 y	M 45% F 55%	RC 87% HSMEd. 53%	Secondary school	12 × 40 min over 6 w
4	PE + CST	Di Clemente et al.	1989	1. PE-HE + CST + VT = 366 2. C =273	13.8 y	M 54% F 46%	W 17% AA 11% L 3% A 58% O 11%	Secondary school	3 × 1 h
5	PE + CST	Levy et al.	1995	1. PE-HE + CST + VT = 1,001 2. C = 668	13 y	M 52% F 48%	AA 60% W 24% H 12% O 4%	Secondary school	10 × 1 h 5 booster sess
6	PE + CST	Boyer et al.	1997	1. PE-HE + CST + VT = 210 2. PE-HE = 303	14 y 13–17 y	M 41% F 59%	C 30% L 20% AA 16% O 18% W 10% F 6%	Secondary school	3 × 1 h
7	PE + CST	Howard & McCabe	1990	1. PE-S + CST + VT = 395 2. C = 141	13–14 y	NR	AA 99% LIC 51%	Secondary school	10 sess
8	PE + CST	Schinke et al.	1981	1. PE-HE + CST + VT = 18 2. C = 18	16 y	M 47% F 53%	—	Secondary school	14 × 1 h

Table 14.2 continued

Study no.	Study type	Authors	Year	N per group	Mean age and range	Gender	Family characteristics	Programme setting	Programme duration
9	PE + CST	Bayne Smith	1994	1. PE + CST + VT = 60 2. C = 60	15 y	M 26% F 74%	AA 43% WI 31% H 23% O 3%	Secondary school	18 × 1 h over 8 w 6 w career mentorship
10	PE + CST + BST	Kipke et al.	1993	1. PE-HE + CST + BST = 41 2. C = 46	14 y	M 45% F 55%	L 59% AA 41%	Secondary school	3 × 90 min
11	PE + CST + BST	Caceres et al.	1994	1. PE-HE + CST + BST = 604 3. C = 609	16 y 11–21 y	M 49.8% F 50.2%	RC 75%	Secondary school	7 × 2 h over 7 w
12	PE + CST + BST	Walter & Vaughan	1993	1. PE-HE + CST + BST = 667 2. C = 534	16 y 12–20 y	M 42% F 58%	AA 37% H 35% W 13% A 11% O 4%	Secondary school	6 × 1 h
13	PE + CST + BST	Kirby et al.	1991	1. PE-HE + CST + BST = 429 2. PE-HE = 329	15 y	M 47% F 53%	W 62% L 20% A 9% AA 2% NA 2% O 5%	Secondary school	15 × 1 h
14	PE + CST + BST	Hubbard et al.	1998	1. PE-HE + CST + BST = 106 2. PE-HE = 106	15–16 y	M 48% F 52%	W 85% AA 14%	Secondary school	16 × 1 h
15	PE + CST + BST	Barth et al.	1992	1. PE-HE + CST + BST = 586 2. PE-HE = 447	15 y	M 51% F 49%	W 61% AA 2% L 21% A 9% O 6% HSMEd 72%	Secondary school	15 × 1 h
16	PE + CST + BST	St Lawrence et al.	1995a	1. PE-HE + CST + BST + VT = 17 2. PE-HE = 17	16 y 13–17 y	M 73% F 26%	W 84% AA 16%	Residential drug treatment facility	6 × 1.5h over 6 w

17	PE + CST + BST	St Lawrence et al.	1995b	1. PE-HE + CST + BST + VT = 123 2. PE-HE = 123	15.3 y	M 28% F 72%	LIC 82%	Secondary school	8 × 2 h over 8 w
18	PE + CST + BST	Fawole et al.	1999	1. PE-HE + CST + BST + VT = 223 2. C = 217	17 y	M 45% F 55%	Y 98% MS 53%	Secondary school	6 × 4 h over 6 w
19	PE + CST + BST	Schaalma et al.	1996	1. PE-HE + CST + BST + VT = 1258 2. PE-HE = 1149	15–16 y	—	NR	Secondary school	4 × 1 h
20	PE + CST + BST	Jemmott et al.	1992	1. PE-HE + CST + BST + VT = 85 2. P = 72	15 y	M 100%	MYMEd 13	Secondary school	5 × 1 h

Notes
PE-HE = psychoeducation, health educator led. PE-S = psychoeducation, student led. PE-SD = psychoeducation self-directed. VT = video training. BST = behavioural skills training. CST = communication skills training. C = control. P = attention placebo control group. W = White. AA = African American. L = Latino. A = Asian. NA = Native American. O = other. CB = Caribbean Black. WI = West Indian. H = Hispanic. C = Chinese. F = Filipino. RC = Roman Catholic. Yorubas. Ms = Moslems. MYMEd = mean years of maternal education. HSMEd = secondary school maternal education. LIC = lowest income category. sess = session. min = minute. w = week. y = year. h = hour. m = month. NR = not recorded.

Table 14.3 Methodological features of studies of prevention programmes for reducing sexually risky behaviours

Feature	Study number S1	S2	S3	S4	S5	S6	S7	S8	S9	S10	S11	S12	S13	S14	S15	S16	S17	S18	S19	S20
Control or comparison group	1	1	1	1	1	1	1	1	1	1	1	1	1	1	1	1	1	1	1	1
Random assignment	1	1	1	0	1	0	0	0	1	1	1	1	0	0	0	1	1	1	1	0
Diagnostic homogeneity	0	0	0	0	0	0	0	0	0	0	0	0	0	0	0	0	0	0	0	0
Demographic similarity	1	1	0	0	0	0	0	0	1	0	0	0	1	1	1	0	1	0	0	1
Pre-treatment assessment	1	1	1	1	1	1	1	1	1	1	1	1	1	1	1	1	1	1	1	1
Post-treatment assessment	1	1	1	1	1	1	1	1	1	1	1	1	1	1	1	1	1	1	1	1
3-month follow-up assessment	0†	0	1	0	0	0	1‡	1‡	0	0	1	1	1‡*	1*	1‡	0	1‡§	0	0	1
Children's self-report	1	1	1	1	1	1	1	1	1	1	1	1	1	1	1	1	1	1	1	1
Parents' ratings	0	0	0	0	0	0	0	0	0	0	0	0	0	0	0	0	0	0	0	0
Teachers' ratings	0	0	0	0	0	0	0	0	0	0	0	0	0	0	0	0	0	0	0	0
Trainer ratings	0	0	0	0	0	0	0	0	0	0	0	0	0	0	0	0	0	0	0	1
Researcher ratings	0	0	0	0	0	0	0	0	0	0	0	0	0	0	0	0	0	0	0	0
Deterioration assessed	0	0	0	0	0	0	0	0	0	0	0	0	0	0	0	0	0	0	0	0
Drop-out assessed	0	0	1	1	1	1	1	0	1	1	1	1	1	1	1	1	1	1	1	1
Clinical significance of change assessed	0	0	0	0	0	0	0	0	0	0	0	0	0	0	0	0	0	0	0	0
Experienced therapists or trainers used	1	1	1	1	1	1	1	1	1	1	1	1	1	1	1	1	1	1	1	1
Programmes were equally valued	0	0	0	0	0	0	0	0	0	0	0	0	0	0	0	0	0	0	0	0
Programmes were manualized	1	1	1	1	1	1	1	1	1	1	1	1	1	1	1	1	1	1	1	1
Supervision was provided	0	0	0	0	0	0	0	0	1	1	0	1	0	1	1	0	1	0	0	0
Programme integrity checked	0	1	1	0	0	0	0	0	0	0	0	0	0	0	0	1	0	0	0	1
Data on concurrent treatment given	0	0	0	0	0	0	0	0	0	0	0	0	0	0	0	0	0	0	0	0
Data on subsequent treatment given	0	0	0	0	0	0	0	0	0	0	0	0	0	0	0	0	0	0	0	0
Total	8	9	10	7	8	7	8	7	10	9	9	10	9	10	10	9	11	8	8	11

Notes

S = study. 1 = design feature was present. 0 = design feature was absent. † = 1-month follow-up. ‡ = 6-month follow-up. § = 12-month follow-up. * = 18-month follow-up.

follow-up data eighteen months after the intervention (Hubbard et al., 1998), and two studies included follow-up data for two time periods, i.e. six and twelve months (St Lawrence et al., 1995b) and six and eighteen months (Kirby et al., 1991). Participants' self-report ratings were obtained in all studies and in two studies researchers' ratings were reported (Kipke et al., 1993; Schinke et al., 1981). Domains in which self-reported assessments were conducted across the twenty studies include knowledge, attitudes, behavioural intentions, self-efficacy, communication skills, sexual behaviour and contraception use. To assess communication skills in two studies participants' responses to vignettes were evaluated (Boyer et al., 1997; Schinke et al., 1981) and in two studies videotaped role-plays were rated (Kipke et al., 1993, Schinke et al., 1981). To assess sexually risky behaviour in three studies, risk behaviour surveys were used (St Lawrence et al., 1995b; Bayne Smith,1994; Di Clemente et al., 1989). Sixty per cent of studies assessed drop-out rates and 50% checked programme integrity. All programmes were conducted by experienced trainers and 70% of the programmes were manualized. In only two studies, the fact that trainers received supervision was reported (Howard & McCabe, 1990; Caceres et al., 1994). From a methodological perspective this was a methodologically robust group of studies and so reasonably reliable conclusions may be drawn from them.

Substantive findings

Treatment effect sizes and outcome rates for the twenty studies are presented in Table 14.4. A narrative summary of key findings from each study is given in Table 14.5.

Psychoeducation

Two studies evaluated the impact of psychoeducational programmes involving didactic instruction led by a health educator or peer (Huszti et al., 1989; Schinke et al., 1990). Huszti et al. (1989) evaluated the effects of an hour-long oral presentation about AIDS and a second programme which included an oral presentation and an information video *AIDS: Acquired Immune Deficiency Syndrome* (Walt Disney, 1986). Compared with controls, participants in both psychoeducational programmes showed significant gains in knowledge of AIDS, attitudes to people with AIDS, and attitudes to the practice of safe sex. Greatest gains were made by female participants, and greater gains were made in knowledge rather than attitudes. Effect sizes across the two programmes based on post-programme assessments of knowledge and attitudes ranged from 0.5 to 1.9 with a mean of 1.1. Effect sizes based on assessments conducted a month after the programme ranged from 0.1 to 1.6 with a mean of 0.7. Thus, the average participant in these two psychoeducational programmes showed greater gains in sexual-risk-related knowledge and attitudes after the programmes

Table 14.4 Summary of results of treatment effect sizes of studies of prevention programmes for reducing sexually risky behaviours

	Study number and condition										
	Psychoeducation				Psychoeducation and communication skills training						
Variable	Study 1	Study 2			Study 3	Study 4	Study 5	Study 6	Study 7	Study 8	Study 9
	PE-HE v C	PE-HE+ VT v C	PE-HE v C	PE-SD v C	PE-HE+ CST v C	PE-HE+ VT v C	PE-HE+ VT+CST v C	PE-HE+ VT+CST v C	PE-SE+ VT+CST v C	PE-HE+ VT+CST v C	PE-HE+ VT+CST v C
Improvement after programme											
Knowledge	1.9	1.9	—	—	0.2	0.8	—	0.1	—	1.0	—
Attitudes towards those with AIDS/HIV	0.7	0.8	—	—	0.2	0.2	—	—	—	—	—
Attitudes towards practising safe sex	0.5	0.6	—	—	—	—	—	—	—	—	—
Self-efficacy beliefs about practising safe sexual behaviour	—	—	—	—	—	—	—	0.1	—	0.8	—
Communication (refusal and negotiation) skills	—	—	—	—	—	—	—	—	—	—	—
Intentions to practise safe sex	—	—	—	—	—	—	0.4	—	—	1.0	—
Reduced frequency of sexual intercourse	—	—	0.5	0.3	—	—	0.2	—	—	—	0.4
Reduced frequency of unprotected sexual intercourse	—	—	—	—	—	—	—	—	—	—	—
Delay initiation of sexual intercourse	—	—	—	—	—	—	0.3	0.3	—	—	—
Use of condom	—	—	—	—	—	—	—	—	0.3‡	—	—
Improvement at follow-up											
Knowledge	1.6	1.2	—	—	—	—	—	—	—	—	—
Attitudes towards those with AIDS/HIV	0.3	0.4	—	—	—	—	—	—	—	—	—
Attitudes towards practising safe sex	0.3	0.3	—	—	—	—	—	—	—	—	—
Self-efficacy beliefs about practising safe sexual behaviour	—	—	—	—	—	—	—	—	—	0.7	—
Communication (refusal and negotiation) skills	—	—	—	—	—	—	—	—	—	—	—
Intentions to practise safe sex	—	—	—	—	—	—	—	—	—	—	—
Reduced frequency of sexual intercourse	—	—	—	—	—	—	—	—	—	—	—
Reduced frequency of unprotected sexual intercourse	—	—	—	—	—	—	—	—	—	—	—
Delay initiation of sexual intercourse	—	—	—	—	—	—	—	—	—	—	—
Use of condom	—	—	—	—	—	—	—	—	—	1.0	—

Notes

PE-HE = psychoeducation, health educator led. PE-S = Psychoeducation, student led. PE-SD = psychoeducation, self-directed. VT = video training. BST = behavioural skills training. CST = communication skill training. C = control. P = attention placebo control group. ‡ Sexually inexperienced at pre-test.

Table 14.4 (continued) Summary of results of treatment effect sizes of studies of prevention programmes for reducing sexually risky behaviours

	Study number and condition										
	Psychoeducation, communication skills training and behavioural skills training										
	Study 10	Study 11	Study 12	Study 13	Study 14	Study 15	Study 16	Study 17	Study 18	Study 19	Study 20
Variable	PE-HE+ CST+ BST	PE-HE+ CST+ BST	PE-HE+ CST+ BST	PE-HE+ CST+ BST	PE-HE+ CST+ BST	PE-HE+ CST+ BST	PE-HE+ CST+ BST	PE-HE+ CST+ BST+VT	PE-HE+ CST+ BST+VT	PE-HE+ CST+ BST+VT	PE-HE+ CST+ BST+VT
	v C	v C	v C	v PE-HE	v PE-HE	v PE-HE	v PE-HE	v PE-HE	v PE-HE	v PE-HE	v P
Improvement after programme											
Knowledge	0.8	0.6	—	0.2	—	0.9	0.5	0.4	1.4	0.4	0.5
Attitudes towards those with AIDS/HIV	0.3	0.4	—	—	—	—	—	—	0.9	—	—
Attitudes towards practising safe sex	—	0.4	—	—	—	—	0.2	0.2	—	—	0.2
Self-efficacy beliefs about practising safe sexual behaviour	0.2	0.6	—	—	—	—	0.5	0.3	—	0.1	—
Communication (refusal and negotiation) skills	0.7	0.6	—	—	—	—	—	0.5	—	—	—
Intentions to practise safe sex	—	0.3	—	—	—	—	—	—	0.2	0.2	0.4
Reduced frequency of sexual intercourse	—	—	—	—	—	—	—	0.5	—	—	—
Reduced frequency of unprotected sexual intercourse	—	—	—	—	—	—	—	—	—	—	—
Delay initiation of sexual intercourse	—	—	—	—	0.3‡	—	—	—	0.2	—	—
Use of condom	—	—	—	—	0.6‡	—	—	0.1	—	—	—
Improvement at follow-up											
Knowledge	—	—	0.5	—	—	—	—	0.5		—	0.2
Attitudes towards those with AIDS/HIV	—	—	—	—	—	—	—	0.0	—	—	—
Attitudes towards practising safe sex	—	—	—	—	—	—	—	0.0	—	—	—
Self-efficacy beliefs about practising safe sexual behaviour	—	—	0.1	—	—	—	—	—	—	—	—
Communication (refusal and negotiation) skills	—	—	—	—	—	—	—	0.2	—	—	—
Intentions to practise safe sex	—	—	—	—	—	0.2	—	—	—	—	0.2
Reduced frequency of sexual intercourse	—	—	—	—	—	0.3‡	—	—	—	—	0.2
Reduced frequency of unprotected sexual intercourse	—	—	—	0.2‡	—	—	—	0.2	—	—	—
Delay initiation of sexual intercourse	—	—	—	0.2‡	—	—	—	—	—	—	—
Use of condom	—	—	—	—	—	0.2	—	0.2	—	—	—

Notes

PE-HE = psychoeducation, health educator led. PE-S = psychoeducation, student led. VT = video training. BST = behavioural skills training. CST = communication skill training. C = control. P = attention placebo control group. ‡ Sexually inexperienced at pre-test.

Table 14.5 Summary of key findings of studies of prevention programmes for reducing sexually risky behaviours

Study no.	Authors	Year	N per group	No. of sessions	Group differences	Key findings
1	Huszti et al.	1989	1. PE-HE = 153 2. PE-HE + VT = 131 3. C = 164	1 h	1 = 2 > 3	• Compared with controls, participants in the regular and video training psychoeducational programmes showed significantly greater knowledge after the programme and at 1-month follow-up • Compared with controls, both programmes led to increased positive attitudes towards people with AIDS but this declined between the end of the programme and follow-up • Participants in both programmes reported favourable attitudes to practising safe sex after the programmes but these gains were lost at follow-up
2	Schinke et al.	1990	1. PE-HE = 18 2. PE-SD = 19 3. C = 23	3 × 1 h	1 > 2	• Compared with controls and participants in the self-directed psychoeducation group, participants in the health educator led psychoeducational programme reported an increase in their intentions to use condoms • Compared with controls and participants in a health educator led programme, participants in the self-directed psychoeducational programme reported a greater valuing of AIDS education
3	Aplasca et al.	1995	1. PE-HE + CST = 420 2. C = 384	12 × 40 min over 6 w	1 > 2	• Compared with controls, participants in the psychoeducational programme combined with communication skills training showed greater knowledge and more positive attitudes towards those with AIDS, but no improvement in intentions to practise safe sex
4	Di Clemente et al.	1989	1. PE-HE + CST + VT = 366 2. C = 273	3 × 1 h	1 > 2	• Compared with controls, after the intervention participants in the psychoeducational programme combined with communication skills training showed increased knowledge about safe and risky sexual behaviour and more positive attitudes (e.g. showing greater tolerance for those with AIDS)
5	Levy et al.	1995	1. PE-HE + CST + VT = 1,001 2. C = 668	10 × 1 h 5 booster sessions	1 > 2	• Compared with controls, participants in the psychoeducational programme combined with communication skills training were significantly more likely to consider using condoms with foam if they intended on being sexually active in the year following the programme • After the programme, compared with controls, participants were significantly more likely to report ever using condoms with foam and they also reported being marginally less sexually active in the past month
6	Boyer et al.	1997	1. PE-HE + CST + VT = 210 2. PE-HE = 303	3 × 1 h	1 > 2	• Compared with those who received psychoeducation only, participants in the psychoeducational programme combined with communication skills training showed increased condom use, knowledge of sexually risky behaviour, and self-efficacy for safe sexual behaviour
7	Howard & McCabe	1990	1. PE-S + CST + VT = 395 2. C = 141	10 sess	1 > 2	• Compared with controls, participants in the psychoeducational programme combined with communication skills training who were not sexually active before the programme were significantly more likely to continue to postpone sexual activity through to the end of 9th grade

#	Study	Year	Groups	Duration	Result	Outcomes
8	Schinke et al.	1981	1. PE-HE + CST + VT = 18 2. C = 18	14 × 1 h	1 > 2	• Compared with controls, participants in the psychoeducational programme combined with communication skills training showed improvements in knowledge about sexually risky behaviour, negotiation skills, and refusal skills • At 6-month follow-up, compared with controls, programme participants had more favourable attitudes towards practising preventive behaviours and were using more effective contraception methods
9	Bayne Smith	1994	1. PE-HE + CST + VT = 60 2. C = 60	18 × 1 h over 8 w 6 w career mentorship	1 > 2	• Compared with controls, participants in the psychoeducational programme combined with communication skills training who were sexually active showed a significant decrease in the frequency of sexual intercourse and an increase in contraception use
10	Kipke et al.	1993	1. PE-HE + CST + BST = 41 2. C = 46	3 × 90 min	1 > 2	• Compared with controls, participants in the psychoeducational programme combined with communication and behavioural skills training showed positive changes in knowledge and attitudes regarding AIDS; increased self-efficacy for safe sexual behaviours; and improved negotiation and refusal skills
11	Caceres et al.	1994	1. PE-HE + CST + BST = 604 3. C = 609	7 × 2 h over 7 w	1 > 2	• Compared with controls, participants in the psychoeducational programme combined with communication and behavioural skills training showed positive changes in knowledge and attitudes regarding AIDS and safe sex; increased self-efficacy for safe sexual behaviours; and stronger intentions to practise safe sex
12	Walter & Vaughan	1993	1. PE-HE + CST + BST = 667 2. C = 534	6 × 1 h	1 > 2	• Compared with controls, participants in the psychoeducational programme combined with communication and behavioural skills training showed greater knowledge about safe sex; increased self-efficacy for safe sexual behaviours; and reduced involvement in sexually risky behaviour
13	Kirby et al.	1991	1. PE-HE + CST + BST = 429 2. PE-HE = 329	15 × 1 h	1 > 2	• Compared with those that received psychoeducation only, participants in the psychoeducational programme combined with communication and behavioural skills training showed positive changes in knowledge about safe sex • Compared with controls participants who had not initiated sexual intercourse before the programme reported lower rates of sexual intercourse 18 months after the programme
14	Hubbard et al.	1998	1. PE-HE + CST + BST = 106 2. PE-HE = 106	16 × 1 h	1 > 2	• Compared with those that received psychoeducation only, participants in the psychoeducational programme combined with communication and behavioural skills training who had not initiated sexual intercourse before the programme significantly delayed the initiation of sexual intercourse • Compared with controls, more participants in the psychoeducational programme combined with communication and behavioural skills training who were sexually active before the programme engaged in safe sexual behaviour after the programme
15	Barth et al.	1992	1. PE-HE + CST + BST = 586 2. PE-HE = 447	15 × 1 h	1 > 2	• Compared with those that received psychoeducation only, participants in the psychoeducational programme combined with communication and behavioural skills training showed stronger intentions to practice safe sex and better communication with parents after the programme and at 6-month follow-up • Compared with those that received psychoeducation only, more participants in the psychoeducational programme combined with communication and behavioural skills training who were sexually active before the programme used contraceptives after the programme • The multimodal programme had no effect on frequency of sexual intercourse or pregnancy scares

Table 14.5 continued

Study no.	Authors	Year	N per group	No. of sessions	Group differ-ences	Key findings
16	Lawrence et al.	1995a	1. PE-HE + CST + BST + VT = 17 2. PE-HE = 17	6 × 1.5 h over 6 w	1 > 2	• Compared with those that received psychoeducation only, participants in the psychoeducational programme combined with communication and behavioural skills training showed a more internal locus of control; greater knowledge about sexually risky behaviour; better attitudes regarding safe sex; increased self-efficacy for safe sexual behaviours; and decreases in sexually risky behaviour
17	Lawrence et al.	1995b	1. PE-HE + CST + BST + VT = 123 2. PE-HE = 123	8 × 2 h over 8 w	1 > 2	• Compared with those that received psychoeducation only, participants in the psychoeducational programme combined with communication and behavioural skills training showed greater knowledge about sexually risky behaviour; more positive attitudes regarding safe sex; increased self-efficacy for safe sexual behaviours; and decreased rates of sexually risky behaviour
18	Fawole et al.	1999	1. PE-HE + CST + BST + VT = 223 2. C = 217	6 × 4 h over 6 w	1 > 2	• Compared with controls, participants in the psychoeducational programme combined with communication and behavioural skills training showed greater knowledge about sexually risky behaviour; more favourable attitudes towards safe sex; and decreases in sexually risky behaviour (reduced number of sexual partners and increased condom use)
19	Schaalma et al.	1996	1. PE-HE + CST + BST + VT = 1258 2. PE-HE = 1149	4 × 1 h	1 > 2	• Compared with those that received psychoeducation only, participants in the psychoeducational programme combined with communication and behavioural skills training showed greater knowledge and more favourable attitudes concerning sexually risky behaviour; stronger intentions to practise safe sex; and decreases in sexually risky behaviour
20	Jemmott et al.	1992	1. PE-HE + CST + BST + VT = 85 2. P = 72	5 × 1 h	1 > 2	• Compared with controls, participants in the video training psychoeducational programme combined with communication and behavioural skills training showed positive changes in knowledge and attitudes concerning sexually risky behaviour; stronger intentions to practise safe sex; and at 3-month follow-up decreases in sexually risky behaviour (lower frequency of sexual intercourse, fewer sexual partners, and more frequent use of condoms)

Notes
PE-HE = psychoeducation, health educator led. PE-S = psychoeducation, student led. PE-SD = psychoeducation self-directed. VT = video training. BST = behavioural skills training. CST = communication skills training. C = control. P = attention placebo control group. sess = session. min = minute. w = week. y = year. h = hour. m = month.

than 86% of controls, and at one-month follow-up fared better than 76% of controls.

Schinke et al. (1990) evaluated the effects of a health-educator-led and a self-instructional psychoeducational programme. In both programmes participants received a comic-format, self-instructional guide on AIDS and safe and risky sex. Those in the health-educator-led programme also completed three instructional sessions in which they received AIDS information and were taught a four-step approach to cognitive problem-solving (i.e. SODA – Stop, Options, Decision, Action). Compared with controls both programmes led to stronger intentions to use condoms in future, but greatest gains in this domain were made by participants in the health-educator-led programme. Participants in the self-directed programme rated the value of AIDS education more highly than participants in the other programme and controls. Effect sizes based on intentions to use condoms after the programme ranged from 0.3 to 0.5 with a mean of 0.4, indicating that after these programmes the average participant fared better than 66% of controls.

From these two studies it may be concluded that psychoeducational programmes can increase knowledge about safe and risky sexual behaviour, promote favourable attitudes towards people with AIDS and the practice of safe sex, and strengthen intentions to use condoms.

Psychoeducation and communication skills training

In seven studies the effects of prevention programmes which contained both psychoeducational and communication skills training components were evaluated (Aplasca et al., 1995; Di Clemente et al., 1989; Levy et al., 1995; Boyer et al., 1997: Howard et al., 1990: Schinke et al., 1981: Bayne Smith, 1994). In these studies, didactic methods and group discussion were used for psychoeducation which focused on information about STDs, AIDS and safe and risky sexual behaviour. Live modelling and/or video modelling, rehearsal, role-playing and corrective feedback were used to train participants in using communication skills. These skills included speaking and listening skills, negotiation skills for solving interpersonal problems, and sexual assertiveness training. This type of assertiveness training typically focused on refusal skills.

Across all six studies and all domains (knowledge, attitudes, beliefs, intentions and behaviour) effect sizes ranged from 0.1 to 1.0 with a mean of 0.4 for improvement after the programme and from 0.3 to 1.0 with a mean of 0.7 for improvements at follow-up. Thus, overall the average participant in these programmes for preventing risky sexual behaviour which included psychoeducational and communications skills training made greater gains in the domains of knowledge, attitudes, beliefs, intentions and behaviour than 66% of controls after the programme and 76% of controls at three- to six-month follow-up.

With respect to increased knowledge about safe and risky sex, effect sizes ranged from 0.1 to 1.0 with a mean of 0.5 for improvement after the programme. Thus, overall the average participant in these prevention programmes had gained more knowledge than 69% of controls.

With respect to improvement in attitudes towards those with HIV and AIDS, the mean effect size was 0.2 after the programme. Thus, overall the average participant in these prevention programmes showed more favourable attitudes than 58% of controls. The effect size for attitudes towards practising safe sexual behaviour at follow-up was 0.7 in the only study where this variable was evaluated. Thus the average participant in this programme had a more favourable attitude toward safe sexual practices than 76% of controls.

With respect to self-efficacy beliefs about safe sexual practices, effect sizes ranged from 0.1 to 0.8 with a mean of 0.5 for improvement after the programme. Thus, overall the average participant in these prevention programmes reported greater self-efficacy beliefs than 69% of controls.

Intentions to practise safe sex were assessed in only one study and here the effect size was 0.4 after the programme, indicating that the average programme participant had stronger intentions to practise safe sex after the programme than 66% of controls.

Average effect sizes for the frequency of sexual intercourse and for the use of condoms after the programme were 0.3 in both instances. Thus, the average programme participant had sex less frequently and used a condom more often after the programme than 62% of controls. At 3–6-month follow-up in the only study where condom use was assessed the effect size was 0.1, indicating that the average programme participant reported using a condom more often at follow-up than 54% of controls.

For sexually inactive youngsters, the effect size for delaying the onset of sexual intercourse was 0.3 in the only study in which this variable was assessed. Thus, the average sexually inexperienced programme participant reported delaying the onset of sexual activity at follow-up longer than 62% of controls.

From these seven studies it may be concluded that prevention programmes which contain both psychoeducational and communication skills training components can favourably influence knowledge, attitudes, beliefs and intentions relevant to sexually risky behaviour and increase the practice of safe sexual behaviour.

Psychoeducation communication and behavioural skills training

Eleven studies evaluated the effectiveness of prevention programmes with psychoeducation, communication and behavioural skills training as the main components (Kipke et al., 1993; Caceres et al., 1994; Walter & Vaughan, 1993; Kirby et al., 1991; Hubbard et al., 1998; Barth et al., 1992; St Lawrence et al., 1995a, 1995b; Fawole et al., 1999; Schaalma et al., 1996; Jemmott et al., 1992). In all of these studies, didactic methods and group discussion were used for psychoeducational training. Live modelling and/or video modelling, rehearsal, role-playing and corrective feedback were used to train participants in using both communication skills and behavioural skills for practising safe sex. Behavioural skills training focused on anticipating and avoiding or escaping from sexually risky situations, and buying, carrying and using condoms.

Across all eleven studies and all domains (knowledge, attitudes, beliefs, intentions and behaviour) effect sizes ranged from 0.1 to 1.4 with a mean of 0.4 for improvement after the programme and from 0 to 0.5 with a mean of 0.2 for improvements at follow-up. When separate effect sizes were calculated for the subgroup of studies in which control groups received no intervention, and for the subgroup of studies in which the comparison group received psychoeducation only, the mean effect sizes were similar to those for the total group of eleven studies. Thus, overall the average participant in these programmes for preventing risky sexual behaviour which included psychoeducation, communication and behavioural skills training made greater gains in the domains of knowledge, attitudes, beliefs, intentions and behaviour than 66% of cases in control and comparison groups after the programme and 58% of cases in control and comparison groups at follow-up.

With respect to increased knowledge about safe and risky sex, effect sizes ranged from 0.2 to 1.4 with a mean of 0.7 for improvement after the programme and a mean of 0.4 at follow-up. Thus, overall the average participant in these prevention programmes had gained more knowledge than 76% of cases in control and comparison groups after intervention and 66% at follow-up.

With respect to improvement in attitudes towards those with HIV and AIDS, effect sizes ranged from 0.3 to 0.9 with a mean effect size of 0.5 after the programme. Thus, overall the average participant in these prevention programmes showed more favourable attitudes than 69% of cases in control and comparison groups. Effect sizes for attitudes towards practising safe sexual behaviour ranged from 0.2 to 0.4 with a mean of 0.3 after intervention and at follow-up the effect size was 0 in the only study where this variable was evaluated. Thus, the average participant in these programmes had a more favourable attitude toward safe sexual practices than 62% of cases in control and comparison groups after intervention, but these gains were lost at follow-up.

With respect to self-efficacy beliefs about safe sexual practices, effect sizes ranged from 0.1 to 0.6 with a mean of 0.3 for improvement after the programme and 0.1 at follow-up. Thus, overall the average participant in these prevention programmes reported greater self-efficacy beliefs than 62% of cases in control and comparison groups after intervention, but these gains were lost at follow-up.

With respect to intentions to practise safe sex, effect sizes ranged from 0.2 to 0.4 with a mean of 0.3 for improvement after the programme and 0.2 at follow-up. Thus, overall the average participant in these prevention programmes reported stronger intentions to practise safe sex than 62% of cases in control and comparison groups after intervention and 58% at follow-up.

With respect to communication skills, effect sizes ranged from 0.2 to 0.7 with a mean of 0.6 for improvement after the programme and 0.2 at follow-up. Thus, overall the average participant in these prevention programmes was rated as having better communication skills than 73% of cases in control and comparison groups after intervention and 58% at follow-up.

In the only study in which reports of reduced frequency of sexual intercourse were evaluated after intervention, the effect size was 0.2 and the mean effect size at follow-up based on results from two studies was 0.3. Thus, the average programme participant had sex less frequently after the programme than 58% of cases in control and comparison groups after intervention and 62% at follow-up.

In the only study in which reports of reduced frequency of unprotected sexual intercourse were evaluated after intervention, the effect size was 0.5 and the mean effect size at follow-up based on results from two studies was 0.2. Thus, the average programme participant had unprotected sex less frequently after the programme than 69% of cases in control and comparison groups after intervention and 58% at follow-up.

For sexually inactive youngsters, the effect size for delaying the onset of sexual intercourse was 0.2 after intervention in the only study in which this variable was assessed at that time and 0.3 at follow-up in the only study in which this variable was assessed at that time Thus, the average sexually inexperienced programme participant reported delaying the onset of sexual activity after intervention longer than 58% of controls and 62% at follow-up.

With respect to condom use, effect sizes ranged from 0.1 to 0.6 with a mean of 0.3 for improvement after the programme and 0.2 at follow-up. Thus, overall the average participant in these prevention programmes reported more frequent condom use than 62% of cases in control and comparison groups after intervention and 58% at follow-up.

From these eleven studies it may be concluded that prevention programmes which contain psychoeducational and communication and behavioural skills training components can favourably influence knowledge, attitudes, beliefs and intentions relevant to sexually risky behaviour and increase the practice of safe sexual behaviour.

Conclusions

From this review the following conclusions may be drawn. First, relatively brief classroom-based prevention programmes can favourably influence knowledge, attitudes, beliefs and intentions relevant to sexually risky behaviour. They can increase knowledge about safe and risky sexual behaviour. They can improve attitudes towards people with HIV and AIDS and improve attitudes towards practising safe sex and reducing sexual risk taking. They can increase self-efficacy beliefs about practising safe sex, and in particular reducing the number of partners, decreasing the frequency of unprotected sex, and increasing the frequency of condom use. These programmes can also strengthen intentions to practise safe sex and reduce the frequency of sexual risk taking.

Second, classroom-based prevention programmes can modify sexually risky behaviour. Specifically these programmes can delay the onset of sexual activity in sexually inexperienced young adolescents, and decrease the frequency of unprotected sex in sexually active adolescents mainly by increasing the frequency of condom use.

Third, prevention programmes that include both psychoeducation and skills training are more effective than those that involve psychoeducation only. All effective programmes include communications training which covers speaking and listening skills, negotiation skills and sexual assertiveness training. Some effective programmes include training in the behavioural skills required for avoiding or escaping from sexually risky situations and also the skills required for acquiring, carrying and using condoms.

Fourth, the positive impact of prevention programmes to reduce sexual risk taking diminishes over time, so follow-up sessions should probably be routinely included in clinical or educational practice.

Fifth, effective programmes do not contaminate adolescents and lead to promiscuous attitudes and behaviour.

Sixth, effective programmes are firmly grounded in robust psychological theories of which the behavioural-ecological model of sexual behaviour (Hovell et al., 1994) and the AIDS risk reduction model (Catania et al., 1990) mentioned earlier in this chapter are good exemplars.

Seventh, while there was no definitive evidence concerning the optimum duration of programmes, it is probably best practice to opt for longer rather than shorter programmes.

Eighth, training is probably important for effective programme delivery and a range of personnel including health educators and teachers may be effective instructors.

Implications for policy and practice

The implications of these conclusions for policy and practice are clear. Classroom-based programmes for preventing sexual risk taking should be routinely included in secondary school curricula. Such programmes should include psychoeducation communication and behavioural skills training as the main components. Didactic methods and group discussion may be used for psychoeducational training. However, live modelling and/or video modelling, rehearsal, role-playing and corrective feedback should be used to train participants in using both communication skills and behavioural skills for practising safe sex. These skills include anticipating and avoiding or escaping from sexually risky situations, and buying, carrying and using condoms. Programmes for younger adolescents should focus particularly on delaying the onset of sexual intercourse and those for older teenagers should focus on the avoidance of unprotected sexual intercourse.

Implications for research

Studies that evaluate the impact of prevention programmes on safe and risky sexual behaviour, pregnancy, HIV and STD infection over follow-up periods that span years rather than months should be a research priority since these are more valid indicators of programme effectiveness than measures of knowledge, attitudes, beliefs and intentions concerning sexual risk taking.

Future evaluation studies should include assessments of programme integrity. In such studies, training sessions are recorded and blind raters use programme integrity checklists to evaluate the degree to which sessions approximate manualized training curricula. Such integrity checks allow researchers to say with confidence the degree to which a pure and potent version of their programme has been evaluated.

Studies that examine the impact of design features that may make programmes more effective are required. For example, the impact of using curricula that are developmentally staged with different versions for younger and older adolescents and the impact of including peer assistants in programme delivery deserve evaluation.

Studies are required which investigate the mechanisms and processes which underpin programme effectiveness. It is clear that there is wide variability in teenagers' responses to sexual risk-taking prevention programmes. Following training, some youngsters practise safe sex while others do not. The determinants of these different outcomes requires careful investigation.

There is a need to design and evaluate programmes for adolescents who have been shown to be particularly vulnerable to teenage pregnancy, STD infection and HIV infection, such as those involved in drug abuse. These programmes must involve methods of engaging these hard-to-reach youngsters in intervention.

Assessment resources

Breener, N., Collins, J., Kann, L. & Warren, C. (1995). Reliability of the Youth Risk Behaviour Survey Questionnaire. *Journal of School Health*, 141(6), 575–580.

Carey, M., Morrison-Beedy, D. & Johnson, B. (1997). The HIV Knowledge Questionnaire: Development and evaluation of a reliable, valid and practical self-administered questionnaire. *AIDS and Behaviour*, 1, 61–74.

Kelly, J.A., St Lawrence, J.S., Hood, H.V. & Brasfield, T.L. (1989). An objective test of AIDS risk behaviour knowledge: Scale development, validation, and norms. *Journal of Behaviour Therapy and Experimental Psychiatry*, 20, 227–234.

Miller, W.R. & Lief, H.L. (1979). The Sex Knowledge and Attitude Test (SKAT). *Journal of Sex and Marital Therapy*, 5, 282–287.

Sacco, W.P., Levine, B., Reed, D.L. & Thompson, K. (1991). Attitudes about condom use as an AIDS-relevant behaviour: Their factor structure and relation to condom use. *Psychological Assessment: A Journal of Consulting and Clinical Psychology*, 3, 276–272.

Torabi, M.R. & Yarber, W. (1992). Alternate forms of HIV prevention attitude scale for teenagers. *AIDS Education and Prevention*, 4, 172–182.

Programme resources

Carr, A. (2001). *Preventing Sexually Risky Behaviour in Adolescence*. Leicester: British Psychological Society.
Di Clemente, R. & Peterson, J. (1994). *Preventing Aids: Theories, Methods and Behavioural Interventions*. New York: Plenum.
ETR Associates (1998). *Safer Choices: Preventing HIV, Other STD and Pregnancy*. Santa Cruz, CA: ETR Associates.
Kelly, J. (1995). *Changing HIV Risk Behaviour: Practical Strategies*. New York: Guilford.

Films

Hoffman, J. (Producer) & Life, R. (Director) (1989). *Seriously Fresh*. (Available from SELECT Media, 225, Lafayette St., Suite 1102, New York, NY 10012.)
Hoffman, J. (Producer) & Barrett, N. (Director) (1991). *Are you with me?*. (Available from AIDSFILMS (SELECT Media) New York.)
Walt Disney Educational Media (producer) (1986). *AIDS; acquired immunodeficiency syndrome*. Burbank, CA: Walt Disney Educational Media.

Resources for clients

Coleman, J. (1995). *Teenagers and Sexuality*. London: Hodder and Stoughton.
Madaras, L. (1989). *What's Happening to My Body? A Growing up Guide for Parents and Sons*. London: Penguin.
Stoppard, M. (1992). *Everygirl's Life-guide*. London: Dorling Kindersley.

15 Prevention of post-traumatic adjustment problems in children and adolescents

Siofradh Enright and Alan Carr

The aim of this chapter is to review methodologically robust research studies on the effectiveness of programmes for preventing adjustment problems in children who have been exposed to trauma, draw reliable conclusions about the effectiveness of these, and outline the implications of these conclusions for policy and practice.

Trauma which may give rise to debilitating psychological reactions includes violence and abuse, natural disasters such as earthquakes and hurricanes, major transportation accidents, and life-threatening illnesses or life-endangering medical procedures (Perrin et al., 2000).

Acute stress reactions and post-traumatic stress disorder (PTSD) are the principal psychological disorders that occur following traumatic events (APA, 1994; WHO, 1992). Acute stress reactions are short-lived and subside within a month, whereas PTSD persists beyond a month's duration. Both conditions are characterized by hyperarousal, intrusive anxiety-provoking memories of the stressful event, and attempts to suppress these distressing memories or avoid situations which lead to recollection of the trauma.

Following traumatic events, it is often youngsters' attempts to avoid both internal and external anxiety-provoking stimuli that lead to adjustment problems. Attempts to avoid external stimuli, such as people, places, objects and events that remind the child of the trauma, may lead to the development of a constricted lifestyle. Attempts to avoid repetitive intrusive memories, thoughts, images and emotions during wakefulness and trauma-related nightmares during sleep may lead to extreme clinginess and a refusal to separate from parents, particularly at bed time, sleep avoidance and exhaustion, drug and alcohol abuse, and emotional blunting. Not surprisingly, PTSD has a profound effect on academic performance, since youngsters find it difficult to attend school, interact with peers and concentrate on academic work.

Epidemiology

The lifetime prevalence rate for PTSD is 1–14% (APA, 1994). Given that between 50% and 70% of people experience traumatic events in their lives, it may be assumed that exposure to trauma is a necessary but insufficient condition for the occurrence of this disorder (Perrin et al., 2000).

Aetiology

Intrusions that typify acute stress reactions and PTSD probably reflect a difficulty in processing traumatic memories and encoding them appropriately (Van Der Kolk et al., 1999). Children with PTSD engage in an ongoing approach–avoidance struggle with respect to stimuli that remind them of the trauma. This approach–avoidance conflict probably reflects competing drives to avoid further danger but also the need to process intense emotional information through exposure and rehearsal and integration into the overall worldview. The strategies adopted by individuals suffering from acute stress reactions and PTSD to avoid or suppress intrusions may inhibit rather than facilitate the processing of traumatic memories.

Characteristics of traumatic events, the child's attibutional and coping styles, the availability of social support, the child's gender, and the child's history of psychological disorder all determine whether or not PTSD occurs and the severity and chronicity of symptomatology (Wolfe, 1998, Perrin et al., 2000). The frequency, suddenness and degree of life-threateningness of the trauma are the main trauma variables associated with the severity of symptomatology. Terr (1991) distinguishes between type I PTSD, which develops in response to a single traumatic event, and type II PTSD, which develops in response to repeated traumatization and is associated with long-term adjustment problems. With type I PTSD the more sudden and life-threatening the trauma, the more severe the PTSD symptoms. A depressive or pessimistic attributional style and the absence of social support both render youngsters more vulnerable to PTSD. Previous psychological difficulties and female gender are important predisposing vulnerability factors. High ability, an optimistic attributional style, good problem-solving skills and the availability of social support on the other hand are significant protective factors. Where parents have been exposed to the same trauma as their children, the children's symptoms persist longer in cases where parents show protracted PTSD symptomatology. But where parents are skilled at processing their own emotions and managing their PTSD symptoms, they are better at helping their children do so. PTSD may persist for up to four years and recur at anniversaries or at times of stress.

Intervention

From reviews of the literature in PTSD in children and adults a number of conclusions may be drawn (Foa & Meadows, 1997; Keane, 1998; Perry & Azad, 1999; Perrin et al., 2000; Pfefferbaume, 1997; Yule, 1994; Yehuda et al., 1998). Psychological and pharmacological intervention can reduce adjustment problems in adults and children who have had traumatic experiences.

Effective psychological treatments for PTSD and acute stress reactions in adults and children all involve exposure to distressing memories of traumatic events until anxiety subsides while concurrently offering support and preventing the use of avoidance strategies during the exposure to, and processing of, traumatic memories. Coping skills training may be offered to help individuals manage anxiety during exposure to trauma-related cues and memories. Safety skills training may be offered to abused children to reduce anxiety associated with the possibility of further abuse in the future. Their parents may be offered behavioural parent training to help manage trauma-related behavioural problems and also to foster a home environment which encourages children not to avoid trauma-related cues and memories. In addition to these interventions, individuals may need to engage in grief work so as to restructure their world view in such a way that it incorporates the reality of the trauma they have suffered and the major losses that this has entailed. Finally, where youngsters have developed constricted lifestyles or drug-related problems, these secondary problems may also need to be addressed. Key elements of programmes shown in previous reviews to be effective are summarized in Table 15.1.

Table 15.1 Elements of PTSD prevention programmes

Graded exposure	• Psychoeducation about the occurrence of traumatic intrusive thoughts and images; and the negative effects of avoidant coping strategies
	• Exposure to increasingly anxiety-provoking situations
	• Exposure to external stimuli and cues that bring traumatic memories into consciousness
	• Imaginal exposure to traumatic events
	• Provision of support and encouragement to use coping skills during graded exposure
Coping skills training	• Relaxation skills training
	• Cognitive coping skills training
Safety skills training for CSA survivors	• Recognizing potentially abusive situations
	• Avoiding potentially abusive situations
	• Escaping from potentially abusive situations
Behavioural parent training for CSA survivors	• Managing children's anxiety and avoidant behaviour
	• Dealing with children's anger and aggressive or oppositional behaviour
	• Reducing children's oversexualized behaviour
	• Training in using reward systems, time out and response cost procedures
Grief work	• Integrating information about trauma-related losses into the overall worldview and self-image (without denial or exaggeration)
	• Developing a lifestyle that is not wholly determined by denial or exaggeration of the significance of the trauma and the losses it has entailed

Graded exposure

Exposure procedures all involve recalling as vividly as possible visual, auditory, somatic and verbal memories of the trauma and holding these in consciousness. Recounting recollections in words or through a variety of artistic media including writing, painting, drawing, drama and so forth may be used here as well as visualization. Exposure to cues or external stimuli that bring traumatic memories into consciousness may also be used. The site of the trauma may be visited and video or audio recordings of trauma-related stimuli may be used. Commonly exposure is facilitated in a gradual way with children being exposed to a graded hierarchy of increasingly challenging situations. Progression to situations which evoke high levels of anxiety occurs after situations which evoke lower levels of anxiety have been mastered.

Typically graded exposure is combined with support and psychoeducation. Support procedures all involve the proximity of a trusted person during the exposure procedure and receiving encouragement and reinforcement for undergoing exposure procedures. With children, support may be provided by therapists along with parents, siblings, peers and teachers. Psychoeducation for children and their families is typically required to help them manage the exposure and support procedures and to help the child feel safe and secure between intervention sessions. Psychoeducation focuses on explaining the nature of anxiety and PTSD; the inevitability of intrusive anxiety-provoking thoughts and images; the natural tendency to try to avoid these; the exacerbating effect of using avoidant coping strategies; the graded exposure process as a healthy alternative to avoidant coping; and the need for parents, peers and teachers to be supportive of children during graded exposure and recovery.

Eye movement desensitization and reprocessing (EMDR; Shapiro, 1989) is a treatment protocol in which traumatized individuals are helped to engage in saccadic eye movements during imaginal exposure to traumatic events. The procedure deserves mention because currently there is considerable controversy about whether it is more effective than other exposure techniques and whether it involves different mechanisms from those that underpin other exposure techniques (Herbert et al., 2000). There are a few uncontrolled case studies suggesting that EMDR may be effective for childhood PTSD (Coco & Sharpe, 1993; Greenwald, 1994; Muris & deJongh, 1996).

Coping skills training

To help youngsters manage anxiety evoked during exposure to trauma-related cues and memories, intervention programmes may include coping skills training. The aim of this training is equip the child with relaxation and cognitive coping skills to reduce anxiety. With relaxation skills training, youngsters learn a sequence of exercises that reduce muscle tension. With cognitive coping skills training children learn to challenge fearful or threatening cognitions and to appraise anxiety-evoking situations in less threatening ways.

Safety skills training

Where the trauma to which children have been exposed involves sexual abuse or violence, safety skills training may be included as an integral part of the treatment programme. Safety skills training involves helping children identify those situations where abuse might potentially occur and helping them develop assertiveness and help-seeking skills to avoid or escape from these potentially traumatic situations.

Behavioural parent training

Parents of traumatized children may be offered behavioural parent training. This aims to help parents manage trauma-related behavioural problems including aggression, defiance and oversexualized behaviour (in the case of child sexual abuse (CSA)). It also helps parents to foster a home environment which encourages children not to avoid trauma-related cues and memories. Parents learn the skills necessary to help their children avoid developing a restricted lifestyle. Behavioural parenting training involves coaching parents to pinpoint adaptive behaviours (such as approaching feared situations or dealing with interpersonal situations in non-aggressive or non-sexualized ways) and systematically reinforcing these adaptive behaviours. It also involves coaching parents in using time-out and response-cost systems to reduce the frequency of avoidant, aggressive or oversexualized behaviour.

Grief work

Traumatic events, particularly natural disasters such as earthquakes, or major transportation accidents such as the sinking of a ship, may involve major losses including bereavement and homelessness. For traumatized children, difficulties may arise in adequately integrating traumatic experiences and information about trauma-related losses into their overall worldview and self-image. Grief work may facilitate this process of integration. The goal of such grief work is to achieve a view of the world in which the losses associated with the trauma are accepted rather than denied or exaggerated and to develop a lifestyle that is not wholly determined by denial or exaggeration of the significance of the trauma and the losses it has entailed.

  Where youngsters deny the significance of traumatic events, the losses entailed by them, and their effects on them, they may use an avoidant coping style. In the short term, they may benefit by avoiding psychological distress, but in the long term this coping style may lead to costly adjustment problems. Avoidance of anxiety-provoking memories and feelings may lead to difficulties experiencing tender emotions, since these too become excluded from consciousness. Avoidant coping can lead to difficulty with anger control and emotional regulation since, periodically, material excluded from consciousness may re-enter unbidden. Finally, drug abuse and alcohol abuse may offer a way for youngsters to pharmacologically exclude unwanted material from consciousness.

An alternative and equally problematic adaptation is to incorporate the experience of the trauma, and the losses entailed by it, without processing it sufficiently, into the cognitive representation of the world so that the youngster's view of the world and the self is permeated by danger, threat, powerlessness and guilt. Beliefs in a foreshortened future and consequent difficulties in career planning in adolescence and making long-term relationships are common recurring themes for youngsters who have experienced PTSD. Survivor guilt is another theme commonly associated with this adaptation.

Critical incident stress debriefing

Critical incident stress debriefing (CISD) is a preventative intervention which aims to facilitate the processing of traumatic memories immediately after a major trauma and so prevent the development of acute stress reactions and PTSD (Wessely et al., 1998). CISD is part of an overall management strategy for dealing with trauma which is offered within 24–72 hours of a critical incident to groups of up to fifteen participants. CISD involves a series of distinct stages which incorporate some of the elements mentioned above. In the *Introduction Stage* the leader establishes an authoritative bond with the group, states the objectives of the meeting, and invites participants to become involved in the confidential debriefing process. During the *Fact Stage* participants are invited to outline the facts of the critical incident. A chronology of events is clarified and the roles of participants during the critical incident are established. Within the *Thought Stage* of CISD participants are invited to describe their 'first thought' during the incident and the differing personal appraisals of all participants of the critical incident are clarified. During the *Reaction Stage* participants describe their emotional reactions and sensory experiences, images and impressions during the critical incident. This process commonly involves emotional ventilation and this promotes group cohesion and support. During the *Symptom Stage* participants are invited to describe cognitive, emotional, physical or behavioural symptoms that they have experienced since the critical incident. Coping skills, including relaxation exercises, managing intrusive memories and mobilizing social support are considered during the *Teaching Stage*. In the final *Re-Entry Stage* outstanding questions are addressed, lessons learned from the debriefing process are summarized and transition to the normal environment is facilitated often through informal rituals such as sharing light refreshments. Reviews of studies of the effectiveness of CISD with adults conclude that the evidence is equivocal (Wessely et al., 1998) and few studies evaluating the efficacy of CISD with children have been conducted.

Intervention formats

A variety of formats have been developed for PTSD treatment and prevention programmes. Such programmes may be offered on an individual, group or family basis. In multimodal intervention programmes some combination of all three formats may be used. In CISD a group format is commonly used.

Method

The aim of the present review was to identify effective programmes for preventing adjustment problems in youngsters exposed to trauma. PsychLit, CINALH and Medline database searches of English language journals for the years 1977 to 2000 were conducted to identify studies in which such prevention programmes were evaluated. The terms *trauma*, *PTSD*, *abuse*, *sexual abuse*, *violence*, *stress*, and *disaster* limited to the term *child*, were combined with terms such as *programme*, *study*, *evaluation*, *effect*, *treatment-outcome*, *intervention*, *therapy*, *CBT*, *EMDR* and *critical incident debriefing*. A manual search through the bibliographies of all recent reviews, and relevant journals was also conducted. Studies were selected for review if they had a group design which included a treatment and control or comparison group; if at least ten cases were included in each group; and if reliable pre- and post-treatment measures were included. Using these criteria seven studies were initially selected. One study in which there was no control group but which involved seventeen cases using single case design methodology was also included, yielding a total of eight studies.

Characteristics of the studies

The characteristics of the eight studies reviewed in this chapter are set out in Table 15.2. All of the studies were published between 1986 and 1998, with six published between 1996 and 1998. Participants in four of the studies were child sexual abuse (CSA) survivors, the majority of whom has been subjected to repeated abuse (Berliner & Saunders, 1996; Deblinger et al., 1996; Cohen & Mannarino, 1996, 1998). Participants in the other studies were earthquakes survivors in Armenia and Italy (Goenjian et al., 1997; Galante & Foa, 1986); survivors of the sinking of the ship *Jupiter* in Greece (Yule, 1992); and survivors of single incident stressors in the USA such as road traffic accidents, gunshot injury, fires, severe storms, severe illness or traumatic bereavement (March et al., 1998). Seven hundred and five youngsters participated in these eight studies and 323 received treatment with the remainder being in control groups. Participants' ages ranged from three to eighteen years. Three-quarters of the participants were female and one quarter were male. From the five studies where data were available, it may be concluded that 61% of participants were Caucasian, 30% were African-American and the remainder were from Hispanic and other ethnic minority groups. Half of the studies

Table 15.2 Characteristics of PTSD prevention studies

Study no.	Trauma	Authors	Year	N per group	Mean age and range	Gender	Ethnicity and class	Trauma details	Level of prevention	Programme setting	Programme duration
1	Abuse	Berliner & Saunders	1996	1. GE + CST + ST-G = 48 2. ST-G = 32	8 y 4–13 y	M 10% F 90%	Caucasian 73% African-American 8% Other 18%	Sexual abuse Multiple episodes 75% Physical abuse 20%	Tertiary	Outpatient clinic	10 × 90 min sess over 3 m
2	Abuse	Deblinger et al.	1996	1. GE + CST + SST + BPT = 22 2. GE + CST + SST = 24 3. BPT = 22 4. C = 21	9 y 7–13 y	M 17% F 83%	Caucasian 72% African-American 20% Other 8% PTSD 71% Major depression 29% Oppositional 30%	Sexual abuse 1 episode 18% 2–10 episodes 47% 11–50 episodes 22% >50 episodes 13%	Tertiary	Outpatient clinic	1. 24 × 45 min sess over 3 m 2. 12 × 45 min sess over 3 m 3. 12 × 45 min sess over 3 m
3	Abuse	Cohen & Mannarino	1996 1997	1. GE + CST + SST + BPT = 39 2. ST = 28	5 y 3–7 y	M 42% F 58%	Caucasian 54% African-American 42% Other 4% Middle SES	Sexual abuse 1 episode 25% 2–5 episodes 26% 6–10 episodes 15% >10 episodes 29%	Tertiary	Outpatient clinic	12 × 90 min sess over 3 m
4	Abuse	Cohen & Mannarino	1998	1. GE + CST + SST + BPT = 30 2. ST = 19	11 y 7–15 y	M 31% F 69%	Caucasian 59% African-American 37% Other 4% Middle SES	Sexual abuse 1 episode 36% 2–5 episodes 21% 6–10 episodes 8% >10 episodes 33% Physical abuse 43%	Tertiary	Outpatient clinic	12 × 90 min sess over 3 m
5	Disaster	Yule	1992	1. GE + CST-G = 24 2. C = 15	11–18 y	F 100%	—	Ship sinking	Secondary	School	1 debriefing sess. + 2 open group sess
6	Disaster	March et al.	1998	1. GE + CST-G = 17	12 y 10–15 y	M 33% F 66%	Caucasian 47% African-American 41% Other 12% Symptoms duration 2 y	Single incident stressors RTA Accidental injury Severe illness Criminal gunshot injury Traumatic bereavement House fire Severe storms	Tertiary	School	18 × 90 m group sess over 5 m

Table 15.2 continued

Study no.	Trauma	Authors	Year	N per group	Mean age and range	Gender	Ethnicity and class	Trauma details	Level of prevention	Programme setting	Programme duration
7	Disaster	Goenjian et al.	1997	1. CST + GW-G + I = 35 2. C = 29	11.5 y	M 35% F 65%	—	Earthquake	Secondary	School	4×30 min group sess + 2×60 m individual sess over 3 w
8	Disaster	Galante & Foa	1986	1. CISD-G = 62 2. C = 238	7 y	—	—	Earthquake	Secondary	School	7×60 min group sess. over 7 m

Notes
GE + CST + SST + BPT = graded exposure with coping skills training and safety skills training offered conjointly to children with their non-offending parents plus behavioural parent training. GE + CST + SST = Graded exposure with coping skills training and safety skills training offered to children only. BPT = behavioural parent training for non-offending parents. GE + CST + ST-G = graded exposure with coping skills training and supportive therapy offered in a group format to children only. ST-G = supportive group therapy for children. GE + CST-G = graded exposure with coping skills training offered to children in a group therapy format. CST + GW-G + I = coping skills training and grief work offered in group and individual therapy formats. CISD-G = critical incident stress debriefing offered in a group format. min = minute. sess = sessions. w = week. m = month. y = year.

evaluated school-based programmes and half evaluated programmes conducted in outpatient settings. In three studies, programmes were at a secondary prevention level, aiming to prevent the onset of PTSD symptoms. In five studies, the interventions were at a tertiary level of prevention, aiming to prevent PTSD symptoms from persisting. In six of the eight studies, graded exposure and coping skills training were included in the treatment protocol and in three of these safety skills training for CSA survivors and behavioural parent training were also part of the treatment package. One study evaluated a psychotherapeutic approach that included grief work and coping skills training as the main elements and in one study the effectiveness of critical incident stress debriefing was assessed. Programmes ranged in duration from three to twenty-four sessions over periods ranging from three weeks to seven months.

Methodological features

Methodological features of the eight studies are given in Table 15.3. Seven of the investigations were comparative group outcome studies with a control group, and in four of these studies, cases were randomly assigned to groups. A multiple baseline across setting and time design was used in the eighth study. In three studies cases were diagnostically homogeneous, with participants meeting criteria for PTSD. In six studies participants in treatment and control groups were shown to be demographically similar. In seven studies pre-treatment assessments were conducted. In five studies post-treatment assessments were conducted and in six studies follow-up assessments were completed at least five months after treatment. Follow-up data at six months were reported by March et al. (1998); at five to nine months by Yule (1992); at one year by Cohen and Mannarino (1997) and Galante and Foa (1986); at two years by Berliner and Saunders (1996); and at three years by Goenjian et al. (1997). In five studies multiple measures of participants' symptomatology provided by a combination of child, parent, teacher, therapist and researcher ratings were reported. Six studies assessed participant deterioration during therapy and all eight studies analysed drop-out rates. Data on the clinical significance of change were provided in seven studies. In all studies experienced therapists or trainers with formal training or therapy qualifications delivered treatments. In three studies a methodologically robust crossover design was used, where therapists trained in the delivery of both comparison and experimental conditions swapped conditions halfway through therapy, thus controlling for specific therapist effects. Five of the eight studies evaluated treatments that had been formally documented in a manual or explicit treatment protocol, and in all of these studies programme integrity was also assessed. Formal supervision of therapists delivering treatments was a feature of five studies. Information on whether or not children or other family members were receiving concurrent psychological or pharmacological treatment was given in three studies, while in only one study were data given regarding

Table 15.3 Methodological features of PTSD prevention studies

| | Study Number | | | | | | | |
Feature	S1	S2	S3	S4	S5	S6	S7	S8
Control or comparison group	1	1	1	1	1	0	1	1
Random assignment	1	1	1	1	0	0	0	0
Diagnostic homogeneity	0	1	0	0	0	1	0	0
Demographic similarity	1	0	1	1	1	0	1	1
Pre-treatment assessment	1	1	1	1	0	1	1	1
Post-treatment assessment	1	1	1	1	0	1	0	0
5-month follow-up assessment	1	0	1	0	1	1	1	1
Children's self-report	1	1	1	1	1	1	1	0
Parents' ratings	1	1	1	1	0	0	0	0
Teachers' ratings	0	0	0	0	0	1	0	1
Therapist or trainer ratings	0	0	0	0	0	1	0	0
Researcher ratings	0	1	0	0	0	0	0	0
Deterioration assessed	1	1	1	1	0	1	1	1
Drop-out assessed	1	1	1	1	1	1	1	1
Clinical significance of change assessed	1	1	1	1	0	1	1	1
Experienced therapists or trainers used	1	1	1	1	1	1	1	1
Programmes were equally valued	1	0	1	1	0	0	0	0
Programmes were manualized	1	1	1	1	0	1	0	0
Supervision was provided	1	1	1	1	0	0	1	0
Programme integrity checked	1	1	1	1	0	1	0	0
Data on concurrent treatment given	0	1	0	0	0	1	1	0
Data on subsequent treatment given	0	0	1	0	0	0	0	0
Total	16	16	17	15	6	14	11	9

Notes
S = study. 1 = design feature was present. 0 = design feature was absent.

whether participants, or their family members, engaged in further treatment following the intervention evaluated in the study. Overall, the eight studies included in this review were methodologically fairly robust, with those involving CSA survivors being slightly more methodologically robust than studies involving survivors of disasters and accidents.

Assessment instruments

In the studies selected for review, PTSD symptomatology was evaluated using rating scales and DSM diagnostic criteria or self-report instruments such as the Impact of Events Scale (Horowitz et al., 1979). General adjustment was commonly evaluated using the Child Behaviour Checklist (Achenbach, 1991) which yields scores on scales which assess internalizing behaviour problems (emotional problems) and externalizing behaviour problems (conduct problems). In studies of CSA survivors, the Child Sexual Behaviour Inventory was commonly used (Friedrich et al., 1992). The revised fear survey schedule was commonly used to evaluate sources of anxiety (Ollendick, 1983). The State-Trait Anxiety Inventory (Spielberger, 1973) or similar instruments were used to evaluate generalized anxiety. The Children's Depression Inventory (Kovacs, 1992) or similar scales were used to evaluate self-reported depressive symptoms.

Substantive findings

Effect sizes and improvement rates for the eight studies are given in Table 15.4 and a narrative summary of key findings is given on Table 15.5.

CSA survivors

Treatment programmes for survivors of repeated CSA were evaluated in four studies (Berliner & Saunders 1996; Deblinger et al., 1996; Cohen & Mannarino 1996, 1998). In all of these studies therapy involved graded exposure and coping skills training along with other treatment components such as supportive group therapy, safety skills training or behavioural parent training.

Berliner and Saunders (1996) found that CSA survivors who participated in a programme involving graded exposure, coping skills training and supportive group therapy fared no better after treatment and at one- and two-year follow-up than those who received routine supportive group therapy. The equivalence of the two treatments may have been due to the fact that the majority of children in the study did not show clinically significant levels of anxiety or PTSD symptomatology before treatment. It may be that programmes involving graded exposure and coping skills training are more effective than supportive therapy only in cases where clinically significant PTSD symptomatology is present at the beginning of treatment.

Deblinger et al. (1996) found that compared with a control group referred to social services, seven- to thirteen-year-old CSA survivors with clinically significant PTSD symptomatology who participated in a programme involving graded exposure, coping skills training, safety skills training and behavioural parent training showed fewer PTSD symptoms after therapy. The programme is described in Deblinger and Hefin (1996) *Treating Sexually Abused Children and their Non-Offending Parents: A Cognitive Behavioural Approach*. Only 16% of children who met the criteria for PTSD before treatment continued to meet these criteria after treatment. The study also included a group who received behavioural parent training for the non-offending parent only and a group who received a graded exposure programme without behavioural parent training. Where non-offending mothers participated in behavioural parent training only, 36% of children who had significant behaviour problems before treatment continued to do so after treatment, but

Table 15.4 Summary of results of treatment effects and outcome rates from PTSD prevention studies

	Study type, number and condition							
	CSA survivors				Disasters and accident survivors			
Variable	Study 1	Study 2	Study 3	Study 4	Study 5	Study 6	Study 7	Study 8
	GE + CST + ST-G v ST-G	GE + CST + SST + BPT v C	GE + CST + SST + BPT v ST	GE + CST + SST + BPT v ST	GE + CST-G v C	GE + CST-G v BL	CST + GW-G + I v C	CISD-G v C
Improvement after programme								
Children's self-report								
PTSD	—	—	—	—	—	—	—	—
Fears (FSS)	0.3	—	—	—	—	—	—	—
Anxiety	0.0	0.4	—	0.2	—	1.0	—	—
Depression	-0.1	0.6	—	0.5	—	0.6	—	—
Parents' ratings								
CBCL–Internalizing	-0.4	0.3	0.7	0.3	—	—	—	—
CBCL–Externalizing	-0.6	0.5	0.3	0.1	—	—	—	—
CSBI–Oversexualized behaviour	-0.4	—	0.5	0.2	—	—	—	—
Teachers' ratings	—	—	—	—	—	—	—	—
Therapists' PTSD ratings	—	—	—	—	—	2.0	—	—
Researchers' PTSD ratings	—	0.9	—	—	—	1.8	—	—
Improvement at 6m–1year follow-up								
Children's self-report								
PTSD	—	—	—	—	1.0	—	—	—
Fears (FSS)	0.3	—	—	—	0.6	—	1.4	—
Anxiety	0.4	—	—	—	0.1	1.4	—	—
Depression	0.2	—	—	—	0.2	0.9	0.8	—
Parents' rating								
CBCL–Internalizing	-0.3	—	0.4	—	—	—	—	—
CBCL–Externalising	-0.2	—	0.5	—	—	—	—	—
CSBI–oversexualized behaviour	-0.1	—	0.4	—	—	—	—	—
Teachers' ratings	—	—	—	—	—	—	—	—
Therapists' PTSD ratings	—	—	—	—	—	3.0	—	1.4
Researchers' PTSD ratings	—	—	—	—	—	2.3	—	—

Positive clinical outcomes							
% improved after treatment	19% v 15%	84% v 70%	78% v 53%	29% v 11%	57%	—	—
% improved at 6 m–3 y follow-up	31% v 26%	—	89% v 63%	—	86%	72% v 31%	28% v 0%
Negative clinical outcomes							
% Deterioration	5%	7%	9%	3%	0%	0%	—
% Drop-out	31%	10%	15%	37%	17%	0%	0%

Notes

GE + CST + SST + BPT = graded exposure with coping skills training and safety skills training offered conjointly to children with their non-offending parents plus behavioural parent training. GE + C-ST + SST = graded exposure with coping skills training and safety skills training offered to children only. BPT = behavioural parent training for non-offending parents. GE + CST + ST-G = graded exposure with coping skills training and supportive therapy offered in a group format to children only. ST-G = supportive group therapy for children. GE + CST-G = graded exposure with coping skills training offered to children in a group therapy format. CST + GW-G + I = coping skills training and grief work offered in group and individual therapy formats. CISD-G = critical incident stress debriefing offered in a group format. CBCL = Child Behaviour Checklist. CSBI = Child Sexual Behaviour Inventory. FSS = Fear Survey Schedule.

Table 15.5 Summary of key findings from PTSD prevention studies

Study no.	Authors	Year	N per group	Programme duration	Group differences	Key findings
1	Berliner & Saunders	1996	1. GE + CST + ST-G = 48 2. ST-G = 32	10 × 90min sess over 3 m	1 = 2	• CSA survivors who participated in a programme involving graded exposure, coping skills training and supportive group therapy fared no better after treatment and at 2-year follow-up than those that received routine supportive group therapy
2	Deblinger et al.	1996	1. GE + CST + SST + BPT = 22 2. GE + CST + SST = 24 3. BPT = 22 4. C = 21	1. 24 × 45 min sess over 3 m 2. 12 × 45 min sess over 3 m 3. 12 × 45 min sess over 3 m	1 = 2 > 3 = 4	• Compared with cases where behavioural parent training only occurred and cases in the control group referred to social services, CSA survivors who participated in programmes involving graded exposure, coping skills training and safety skills training (with our without behavioural parent training) showed fewer PTSD symptoms after therapy • Only 16% of children who met these criteria for PTSD before treatment continued to meet these criteria after treatment in a programme involving graded exposure, coping skills training and safety skills training • Where mothers participated in behavioural parent training only 36% of children who had significant behaviour problems before treatment continued to do so after treatment but where mothers did not receive behavioural parent training 80% of children continued to have behaviour problems after treatment • Where mothers participated in behavioural parent training only 36% of children who had major depression symptoms before treatment continued to do so after treatment but where mothers did not receive behavioural parent training 62% of children continued to have major depression symptoms after treatment
3	Cohen & Mannarino	1996 1997	1. GE + CST + SST + BPT = 39 2. ST = 28	12 × 90 min sess over 3 m	1 > 2	• Compared with the control group who received supportive therapy only, after treatment and at 1-year follow-up, CSA survivors who participated in a programme involving graded exposure, coping skills training and safety skills training and behavioural parent training showed marked improvements on the Child Behaviour Checklist and the Child Sexual Behaviour Inventory • One year after treatment, only 7% of treated cases scored in the clinical range on the total behaviour problem scale of the CBCL compared with 30% of controls • One year after treatment, only 4% of treated cases scored in the clinical range on the Child Sexual behaviour Inventory compared with 40% of Controls
4	Cohen & Mannarino	1998	1. GE + CST + SST + BPT = 30 2. ST = 19	12 × 90 min sess over 3 m	1 > 2	• Compared with the control group who received supportive therapy only, after treatment CSA survivors who participated in a programme involving graded exposure, coping skills training and behavioural parent training showed improvements on the Children's Depression Inventory and the Child Behaviour Checklist

	Author	Year	Groups (N)	Sessions	Outcome	Findings
5	Yule	1992	1. GE + CST-G = 24 2. C = 15	1 debriefing sess + 2 open group sess	1 > 2	• Compared with untreated controls, 5–9 months after attending 1 debriefing session and 2 open group sessions, child survivors of the sinking of the ship *Jupiter* showed fewer PTSD symptoms on the Impact of Events Scale and fewer fears on a modified version of the Fear Survey Schedule
6	March et al.	1998	1. GE + CST-G =17	18 × 90 m group sess over 5 m	Post > baseline	• After group-based treatment and at 6-month follow-up, children who had been exposed to a range of single incident traumas (such as RTA, serious illness or bereavement) and who participated in group based graded exposure and coping skills training showed reduced PTSD symptomatology, anxiety and depression compared with baseline measures • 57% of cases no longer met the criteria for PTSD immediately after treatment, and 86% of participants were free of PTSD symptoms at 6-month follow-up
7	Goenjian et al.	1997	1. CST + GW-G + I = 35 2. C = 29	4 × 30 min group sess + 2 × 60 m individual sess over 3 w	1 > 2	• Compared with controls, child earthquake survivors who participated in the therapeutic programme involving group and individual sessions focusing on coping skills training and grief work showed greater improvement in post-traumatic stress symptoms and depressive symptomatology • 18 months after treatment, rates of PTSD amongst the treated group were 28%, (down from 60%), compared with 69% of untreated cases (which were up from 52%)
8	Galante & Foa	1986	1. CISD-G = 62 2. C = 238	7 × 60 min group sess. over 7 m	1 = 2	• Compared with controls, children who attended seven monthly 1-hour debriefing sessions following a devastating earthquake were found to show fewer PTSD symptoms and behaviour problems

Notes

GE + CST + SST + BPT = graded exposure with coping skills training and safety skills training offered conjointly to children with their non-offending parents plus behavioural parent training. GE + C-ST + SST = graded exposure with coping skills training and safety skills training offered to children only. BPT = behavioural parent training for non-offending parents. GE + CST + ST-G = graded exposure with coping skills training and supportive therapy offered in a group format to children only. ST-G = Supportive group therapy for children. GE + CST-G = graded exposure with coping skills training offered to children in a group therapy format. CST + GW-G + I = coping skills training and grief work offered in group and individual therapy formats. CISD-G = critical incident stress debriefing offered in a group format. RTA = road traffic accident.

where mothers did not receive behavioural parent training, 80% of children continued to have behaviour problems after treatment. Behaviour problems were assessed with the Child Behaviour Checklist (Achenbach, 1991). Where mothers participated in behavioural parent training only, 36% of children who had major depression symptoms before treatment continued to do so after treatment, but where mothers did not receive behavioural parent training, 62% of children continued to have major depression symptoms after treatment. Depression was assessed with the Children's Depression Inventory (Kovacs, 1992).

Cohen and Mannarino (1996, 1997) found that compared with the control group who received supportive therapy only, after treatment and at one-year follow-up, three- to seven-year-old CSA survivors who participated in a programme involving graded exposure, coping skills training, safety skills training and behavioural parent training showed marked improvements on the Child Behaviour Checklist (Achenbach, 1991) and the Child Sexual Behaviour Inventory (Friedrich et al., 1992). The treatment protocol is described in Cohen and Mannarino (1993). One year after treatment, only 7% of treated cases scored in the clinical range on the total behaviour problem scale of the Child Behaviour Checklist compared with 30% of controls. One year after treatment, only 4% of treated cases scored in the clinical range on the Child Sexual Behaviour Inventory compared with 40% of controls.

In a second study with adolescents Cohen and Mannarino (1998) found that compared with the control group who received supportive therapy only, teenage CSA survivors who participated in a programme involving graded exposure, coping skills training and behavioural parent training showed improvements on the Children's Depression Inventory (Kovacs, 1992) and the Child Behaviour Checklist (Achenbach, 1991) after treatment.

From the results of these four studies, summarized in Tables 15.4 and 15.5, the following conclusions may be drawn. First, the findings of the first study differ from those of the other three, insofar as the graded exposure programme and the control group who received supportive group therapy had similar outcomes. This probably reflected the initial low intensity of participants' PTSD symptomatology in this study, and the relatively severe symptoms of cases in the other three studies. Second, the graded exposure programmes evaluated in the other three studies were significantly more effective in preventing the persistence of post-traumatic symptoms and adjustment problems than supportive therapy of referral to social services. These highly effective graded exposure programmes included coping skills training, safety skills training and behavioural parent training.

Third, in the short term these programmes reduced self-reported anxiety and depression. Averaging across the two studies for which self-report data were available, the effect size after programme completion was 0.4, indicating that the average youngster who participated in these programmes reported lower levels of anxiety and depression immediately afterwards than 66% of controls.

Fourth, in the short term these programmes led to reductions in parent-reported internalizing, externalizing and sexual behaviour problems. Averaging across the three studies for which parent-report data were available, the effect size after programme completion was 0.4, indicating that the average youngster who participated in these programmes showed lower levels of behaviour problems immediately afterwards than 66% of controls. One-year follow-up parent-report data were available for only one study. Averaging across internalizing, externalizing and sexual behaviour problems, in this study, the effect size was 0.4, indicating that the average treated youngster showed lower levels of behaviour problems a year after the programme than 66% of controls.

Fifth, in all three studies rates of clinically significant improvement after treatment for youngsters who participated in graded exposure programmes were higher than those for youngsters who participated in support groups or were referred to social services. The average improvement rate was 64% for youngsters who completed graded exposure programmes and 45% for youngsters in control conditions. Pre-adolescents had better improvement rates than adolescents. In the single study where one-year follow-up data on clinically significant improvement were available, 89% of youngsters who completed graded exposure programmes were clinically improved compared with 63% of youngsters in control conditions.

Sixth, deterioration rates averaged 6% and drop-out rates averaged 21% across the three studies.

Disaster and accident survivors

Treatment programmes for survivors of disasters and accidents were evaluated in four studies (Yule, 1992; March et al., 1998; Goenjian et al., 1997; Galante & Foa, 1986).

Yule (1992) found that compared with untreated controls, 5–9 months after attending one debriefing session and two open group sessions, child survivors of the sinking of the ship *Jupiter* showed fewer PTSD symptoms on the Impact of Events Scale (Horowitz et al., 1979) and fewer fears on a modified version of the Fear Survey Schedule (Ollendick, 1983).

March et al. (1998) found that after treatment and at six-month follow-up, children who had been exposed to a range of single incident traumas and who participated in group-based graded exposure and coping skills training showed reduced PTSD symptomatology, anxiety and depression compared with baseline measures. Fifty-seven per cent of cases no longer met the criteria for PTSD immediately after treatment, and 86% of participants were free of PTSD symptoms at six-month follow-up. Participants in this study were survivors of traumas in the USA such as road traffic accidents, gunshot injury, fires, severe storms, severe illness or traumatic bereavement.

Goenjian et al. (1997) found that compared with controls, child earthquake survivors in Armenia who participated in a therapeutic programme involving group and individual sessions focusing on coping skills training and grief work showed greater improvement in post-traumatic stress symptoms and depressive symptomatology.

Galante and Foa (1986) found that compared with controls, children who attended seven monthly one-hour debriefing sessions following a devastating earthquake in Italy showed fewer PTSD symptoms and behaviour problems.

From the results of these four studies summarized in Tables 15.4 and 15.5, the following conclusions may be drawn. First, programmes evaluated in these studies were effective in preventing the persistence of post-traumatic symptoms and adjustment problems. These highly effective programmes included the following elements: graded exposure, coping skills training, and grief work. A combination of group therapy and individual therapy formats were used.

Second, for the single study in which short-term data were available, averaging across self-report anxiety and depression data and therapist and researcher PTSD ratings an effect size of 1.3 was obtained, using baseline and post-treatment data to calculate effect sizes. Thus the average treated cases fared better than 90% of cases prior to treatment.

Third, in the long term these programmes reduced self-reported PTSD symptomatology, fears, anxiety and depression. Averaging across the three studies for which self-report data were available, the effect size six months to a year after programme completion was 0.8. This indicates that the average youngster who participated in these programmes reported lower levels of PTSD symptomatology, fears, anxiety and depression than 79% of controls six months to a year after programme completion.

Fourth, in the long term these programmes led to reductions in behaviour problems and symptoms as rated by teachers, therapists and researchers. Averaging across the two studies for which such data were available, the effect size six months to a year after programme completion was 2.2, indicating that the average youngster who participated in these programmes showed fewer problems and symptoms six months to a year after programme completion than 99% of controls.

Fifth, in all three studies where data were provided, rates of clinically significant improvement six months to a year after treatment for youngsters who participated in programmes were higher than those for youngsters in control groups. The average improvement rate was 62% for youngsters who completed treatment and 16% for youngsters in control conditions.

Conclusions

Survivors of traumas such as child abuse, natural disasters and accidents may develop serious psychological problems including acute stress reactions and PTSD. However, from this review it is clear that psychological intervention programmes can prevent the development of such reactions or prevent such reactions from persisting. Such programmes contain the elements listed in Table 15.1.

For pre-adolescent and adolescent CSA survivors, effective tertiary prevention programmes span twelve to twenty-four sessions and involve graded exposure, coping skills training, safety skills training and behavioural parent training. The graded exposure and coping skills training elements reduce PTSD symptomatology while behavioural parent training reduces conduct problems and depression. Safety skills training reduces the probability of further child abuse occurring.

For survivors of natural disasters (such as earthquakes) involving major losses (such as homelessness or bereavement) secondary prevention programmes which include grief work and coping skills training are effective. Critical incident stress debriefing includes both of these elements. Offering at least a portion of the intervention programme in a group format may be important for successful treatment. Effective programmes span three to seven sessions.

For single incident traumas such as accidents and assaults, graded exposure and coping skills training offered in a group format over eighteen sessions is an effective tertiary prevention approach.

Implications for policy and practice

This review has clear implications for policy and practice. Tertiary PTSD prevention programmes should be routinely available to pre-adolescent and adolescent CSA survivors. These programmes should include graded exposure, coping skills training, safety skills training and behavioural parent training. Secondary PTSD prevention programmes should be routinely available for children and adolescents following natural disasters and major accidents or illnesses. Such programmes should involve grief work and coping skills training and may take the form of critical incident stress debriefing (CISD; Wessely et al., 1998).

Implications for research

Studies that examine the impact of design features which may make programmes more effective are required. For example, eye movement desensitization and reprocessing (EMDR; Shapiro, 1989) is enjoying considerable popularity as a treatment for adults with PTSD. Research on children and adolescents evaluating the comparative effectiveness of EMDR combined with behavioural parent training and safety skills training, on the one hand, and graded exposure, coping skills training, safety skills training and behavioural parent training, on the other, would be particularly valuable.

Studies are required which investigate the mechanisms and processes which underpin programme effectiveness. Previous psychological difficulties, a depressive or pessimistic attributional style, the absence of social support, the presence of protracted PTSD in parents exposed to the same trauma, and female gender all render youngsters more vulnerable to protracted PTSD (Perrin et al., 2000). There is a need to design and evaluate programmes for children with such characteristics who are particularly vulnerable to protracted PTSD.

Assessment resources

Classen, C., Kooperman, C., Hales, R. & Spiegel, D. (1998). Acute stress disorder as a predictor of posttraumatic stress symptoms. *American Journal of Psychiatry*, 155, 620–624. (Contains the revised version of the Stanford Acute Stress Reaction Questionnaire, (SARSQ).)

Fletcher, K. (1997). The Childhood PTSD Interview-Child Form. In E. Carlson (Ed.), *Trauma Assessments: A Clinician's Guide* (pp. 248–250). New York: Guilford Press.

Ford, J.D. & Rogers, K. (1997). Empirically based assessment of trauma and PTSD with children and adolescents. In: *Proceedings From the International Society of Traumatic Stress Studies Annual Meeting*, Montreal, November, 1997. (Contains the Traumatic Events Screening Inventory for Children (TESI-C).)

Friedrich, W.N., Grambsch, P., Damon, L., Hewitt, S.K., Koverola, C., Lang, R.A., Wolfe, V. & Broughton, D. (1992) The Child Sexual Behaviour Inventory: Normative and clinical comparisons. *Psychological Assessment*, 4, 303–311.

Horowitz, M.J., Wilner, N. & Alvarez,W. (1979). Impact of Events Scale: a measure of subjective stress. *Psychosomatic Medicine*, 41, 209–218.

Kaufman, J., Birmaher, B., Brent, D., Rao, U., Flynn, C., Moreci, P., Williamson, D. & Ryan, N. (1997). Schedule for Affective Disorders and Schizophrenia for School-Age Children-Present and Lifetime Versions, (K-SADS-PL), PTSD Scale. Initial reliability and validity data. *Journal of the American Academy of Child and Adolescent Psychiatry*, 36, 980–988.

Kovacs, M. (1992). *Children's Depression Inventory (CDI) Manual*. North Tonawanda, NY: Multi-Health Systems.

March, J., Parker, J., Sullivan, K., Stallings, P. & Connors, C. (1997b). The Multidimensional Anxiety Scale for Children (MASC): factor structure, reliability and validity. *Journal of the American Academy of Child and Adolescent Psychiatry*, 36, 554–565.

Nader, K.O., Blake, D., Kriegler, J. & Pynoos, R. (1994). *Clinician Administered PTSD Scale for Children (CAPS-C), Current and Lifetime Diagnosis Version*. Los Angeles: UCLA Neuropsychiatric Institute and National Centre for PTSD.

Nader, K.O., Kriegler, J.A., Blake, D.D., Pynoos, R.S., Newman, E. & Weather, F.W. (1996). *Clinically Administered PTSD Scale, Child and Adolescent Version*. White River Junction, VT: National Centre for PTSD.

Ollendick, T.H. (1983). Reliability and validity of the revised Fear Survey Schedule for Children (FSSC-R). *Behaviour Research and Therapy*, 21, 77–84.

Pynoos, R. & Eth, S. (1986). Witness to violence: The child interview. *Journal of the American Academy of Child and Adolescent Psychiatry*, 25, 306–319.

Pynoos, R.S., Frederick, C., Nader, K., Arroyo, W., Steinberg, A., Eth, S., Nunez, F. & Fairbanks, L. (1992). Life threat and posttraumatic stress in school-age children. *Archives of General Psychiatry*, 44, 1057–1063. (Contains the Child Posttraumatic Stress Reaction Index.)

Reynolds, C.R. & Richmond, B.O. (1985). *Revised Children's Manifest Anxiety Scale Manual, (RCMAS)*. Los Angeles: Western Psychological Services.

Saigh, P.A. (1989). The validity of DSM-III post traumatic stress disorder classification as applied to children. *Journal of Abnormal Psychology*, 198, 189–192.

Spielberger, C.D. (1973). *Preliminary Manual for the State-Trait Anxiety Inventory for Children*. Palo Alto, CA: Consulting Psychologists Press.

Treatment resources

Clark, S.L. (2000). *Group Facilitator Manual for Taming Worry Dragons: A Manual for Children, Parents, and other Coaches*. Vancouver, British Columbia: British Columbia Children's Hospital.

Cohen, J.A. & Mannarino, A.P. (1993). A treatment model for sexually abused preschoolers. *Journal of Interpersonal Violence*, 8, 115–131.

Dadds, M.R., Spence, S.H., Holland, D.E., Barrett, P.M. & Laurens, K.R. (1997). Prevention and early intervention for anxiety disorders: A controlled trial. *Journal of Consulting and Clinical Psychology*, 65, 627–635.

Deblinger, E. & Hefin, A.H. (1996). *Treating Sexually Abused Children And Their Non-Offending Parents: A Cognitive Behavioural Approach*. Thousand Oaks, CA. Sage.

Dwivedi, K. (2000). *Post Traumatic Stress Disorder in Children and Adolescents*. London: Whurr.

Garland, E.J. & Clark, S.L. (1996). *Taming Worry Dragons: A Manual for Children, Parents and other Coaches*. Vancouver, British Columbia: British Columbia Children's Hospital.

Smith, P., Dyregrov, A., Yule, W., Gupta, L., Perrin, S. & Gjestad, R. (1999). *Children and Disaster: Teaching Recovery Techniques*. Bergen, Norway: Children and War Foundation.

Tinker, R. & Wilson, S. (1999). *Through the Eyes of a Child: EMDR with Children*. London: Norton.

16 Prevention of suicide in adolescence

Deirdre Hickey and Alan Carr

Suicide refers to any death that is the result of an act accomplished by the victim, knowing or believing the act will lead to death (Jacobs, 1999). Suicidal thoughts generally precede suicidal acts and many completed suicides are preceded by attempts or parasuicidal gestures. Suicide is not a single event but a process which may follow a number of different paths. For some, the process of suicide begins with passive suicidal ideation and proceeds through stages of active planning and preparation which finally culminate in an act of fatal self-harm. For others, a suicide attempt can be the result of long-lasting suicidal ideation with the intent to die. In some instances suicide is an impulsive act carried out with a readily available method at a time of intense emotional distress, or an indirect way of communicating distress. A variety of psychological, social and biological factors may predispose adolescents to suicide and trigger suicide attempts, some of which will be discussed below. Suicide consistently ranks as one of the leading causes of death for adolescents between fifteen and nineteen years of age (Kalafat, 1997). The dramatic rise of adolescent suicide has led to a proliferation of preventative programmes. The effectiveness of many of these remains untested. The aim of this chapter is to review methodologically robust research studies on the effectiveness of school-based suicide prevention programmes, draw reliable conclusions about the effectiveness of these, and outline the implications of these conclusions for policy and practice.

Epidemiology

In the USA and the UK childhood suicide (for children under fourteen years) is rare. The rate is about 0.8 per 100,000. On the other hand, teenage suicide is not a rare event and is on the increase, particularly among male teenagers. For fifteen- to nineteen-year-old males in the USA and the UK the rates are currently about 13 per 100,000 and 7.6 per 100,000 respectively (Shaffer & Piacentini, 1994). Suicide is more common among males. In Ireland the male–female suicide ratio for the years 1988–1992 was 7:1, the highest of any English speaking country for which WHO statistics are available (Kelleher, 1998). Parasuicide or attempted suicide is a common event. A mean parasuicide event rate of 195/100,000 per year was found in a WHO twelve-centre study covering much of Europe and parasuicide repetition was found to be common (Platt, 1992). Parasuicide is more common among females than males. Over the past two decades there has been an increase in overall suicide rates, with the highest increase (fourfold) occurring among older teenage and young adult males between the ages of fifteen and twenty-four years (Kienhorst et al., 1995). Currently, suicide accounts for 30% of deaths in the 15–24-year age group, and has now surpassed road traffic accidents as the leading cause of death among young men (Birchard, 1999).

Aetiology

Risk and protective factors for adolescent suicide and parasuicide are summarized in Table 16.1, and are based on thorough literature reviews (Berman & Jobes, 1993; Brent, 1997; Cohen et al., 1996; Group for the Advancement of Psychiatry, 1996; Jacobs, 1999; O'Connor & Sheehy, 2000; Rudd & Joiner, 1998; Shaffer & Piacentini, 1994; Traskman-Bendz et al., 1993; Zimmerman & Asnis, 1995). These risk and protective factors fall into the following ten categories:

- suicidal ideation and intention
- method lethality
- precipitating factors
- motivation
- personality-based factors
- disorder-related factors
- historical factors
- family factors
- demographic factors
- biological factors

Suicidal intention and ideation

Suicidal intention may be distinguished from suicidal ideation. Suicidal intention is characterized by

- advanced planning
- precautions against discovery
- lethal method
- absence of help-seeking
- a final act

Thus, when adolescents' attempted suicides are characterized by suicidal intention, there is evidence that they have engaged in advanced planning about taking their own lives and have taken precautions against discovery.

Table 16.1 Risk and protective factors for suicide in adolescence

Risk factors	Domain	Protective factors
• Suicidal intention • Advanced planning • Precautions against discovery • Lethal method • Absence of help-seeking • A final act	Suicidal intention and ideation	• Suicidal ideation (not intention) • Acceptance by adolescent of no-suicide contract • Acceptance by parents and carers of suicide monitoring contract
• Availability of lethal method (guns and drugs)	Method lethality	• Absence of lethal methods
• Loss of parents or partner by death, separation or illness • Conflict with parents or partner • Involvement in judicial system • Severe personal illness • Major exam failure • Unwanted pregnancy • Imitation of other suicides	Precipitating factors	• Resolution of interpersonal conflict with parents or partner that precipitated suicide • Acceptance and mourning of losses that precipitated suicide • Physical and psychological distancing from peers or others who precipitated imitative suicide.
Suicide attempted to serve the function of • Escaping an unbearable psychological state or situation • Gaining revenge by inducing guilt • Inflicting self-punishment • Gaining care and attention • Sacrificing the self for a greater good	Motivation	Capacity to develop non-destructive coping styles or engage in treatment to be better able to • Regulate difficult psychological states • Modify painful situations • Express anger assertively • Resolve conflicts productively • Mourn losses • Manage perfectionistic expectations • Solicit care and attention from others • Cope with family disorganization

Factor type	Risk factors	Protective factors
Personality-based factors	• High level of hopelessness • High level of perfectionism • High level of impulsivity • High levels of hostility and aggression • Inflexible coping style	• Low level of hopelessness • Low level of perfectionism • Low level of impulsivity • Low levels of hostility and aggression • Flexible coping style
Disorder-related factors	• Depression • Alcohol and drug abuse • Conduct disorder • Antisocial personality disorder • Borderline personality disorder • Epilepsy • Chronic painful illness • Multiple co-morbid chronic disorders	• Absence of psychological disorders • Absence of physical disorders • Absence of multiple co-morbid chronic disorders • Capacity to form therapeutic alliance and engage in treatment for psychological and physical disorders
Historical factors	• Previous suicide attempts • Loss of a parent in early life • Previous psychiatric treatment • Involvement in the juvenile justice system	• No history of previous suicide attempts • No history of loss of a parent in early life • No history of previous psychiatric treatment • No history of involvement in the juvenile justice system
Family factors	• Family history of suicide attempts • Family history of depression • Family history of drug and alcohol abuse • Family history of assaultive behaviour • Disorganized unsupportive family • Family deny seriousness of suicide attempts • Family has high stress and crowding • Family has low social support and is socially isolated	• No family history of suicide attempts • No family history of depression • No family history of drug and alcohol abuse • No family history of assaultive behaviour • Well-organized supportive family • Family has low stress • Family has high social support
Demographic factors	• Male • Social class 5 • White (not black) in USA • Weak religious commitment • Early summer	• Female • Social classes 2, 3 or 4 • Black (not white) in USA • Strong religious commitment
Biological factors	• Low levels of serotonin (5-HIAA)	• Normal levels of serotonin (5-HIAA)

There is also evidence that they have used a potentially lethal method such as hanging, self-poisoning, using a gun or jumping from a very dangerous height and have not sought help after making the suicide attempt. Youngsters with suicidal intentions typically have also completed a final act such as writing a suicide note. Where youngsters show all of these features of suicidal intention, there is a high risk of suicide.

With suicidal ideation, in contrast, adolescents report thinking about self-harm and possibly engaging in non-lethal self-harm such as superficial wrist-cutting but have no clear-cut plans about killing themselves. Suicidal intention and ideation probably reflect two ends of a continuum, with states that approximate suicidal intention reflecting a higher level of risk and those approximating suicidal ideation reflecting a lower level of risk.

The absence of suicidal intentions may be considered a protective factor. The acceptance by the adolescent of a verbal or written contract during a suicide risk assessment not to attempt suicide is also a protective factor. The commitment on the part of the parents or carers to monitor the adolescent constantly until all suicidal intention and ideation have abated is a further important protective factor to consider in this domain. This commitment may take the form of an oral or written contract between the clinician and the parents or carers.

Method lethality

The lethality of the method used or threatened is an important factor to consider in assessing risk, with more lethal methods being associated with greater risk. Using a firearm, hanging, jumping from a great height and self-poisoning with highly toxic drugs are considered to be more lethal than cutting or overdosing on non-prescription drugs. Within this domain, the availability of a lethal method such as access to a firearm or highly toxic drugs constitutes an important risk factor for suicide. Self-harm, particularly superficial cutting of the wrists and arms, should be distinguished from potentially lethal incomplete suicide attempts. Non-lethal self-harm of this sort is commonly associated with an attempt to relieve tension or gain attention following an interpersonal crisis. This type of self-harming is often preceded by a sense of emptiness or depersonalization (a sense of not being oneself). It is common among adolescents with a history of abuse or neglect and among adolescents with a history of repeated parasuicidal episodes.

The unavailability of lethal methods such as firearms and toxic drugs is an important protective factor. This protective factor can be put in place by inviting parents to remove guns, drugs and other lethal methods from the household or placing the adolescent in a place where there is no access to lethal methods.

Precipitating events

Suicide attempts are commonly precipitated by interpersonal conflict or loss involving a parent or romantic attachment. Ongoing conflict with parents, particularly if this entails child abuse, is strongly associated with completed suicide. More severe abuse, combined physical and sexual abuse, and chronic abuse are all associated with higher risk. Conflict over disciplinary matters and rule-breaking, particularly if this involves court appearance and imprisonment, are also associated with suicide attempts. For imprisoned adolescents, the risk of suicide attempts is greater during the early part of detention. Loss of parents or a romantic partner through death, long-term separation or severe chronic illness may precipitate attempted suicide. Other loss experiences such as diagnosis of severe personal illness (e.g. being HIV positive) or exam failure may precipitate self-harm. Adolescent pregnancy may also precipitate attempted suicide and may reflect a loss of innocence and a potential focus for intense parent–adolescent conflict.

Suicide, arising from imitation of others, may be precipitated by suicides within the peer group, school or locality or media coverage of suicides.

Repeated attempted suicide (as distinct from completed suicide) is associated with impulsive separation following romantic relationship difficulties or recent court appearance associated with impulsive or aggressive antisocial behaviour.

Protective factors in this domain include the resolution of interpersonal conflict with parents or romantic partner that precipitated suicide; acceptance and mourning of losses that precipitated suicide; and physical and psychological distancing from peers or others who precipitated imitative suicide.

Motivation

Youngsters may be motivated to attempt suicide for a wide variety of reasons. Suicide is usually perceived by youngsters as the only feasible solution to a difficult problem involving interpersonal loss or conflict. In this respect, the act of suicide may be construed as fulfilling one or more functions including

- escaping an unbearable psychological state or situation
- gaining revenge by inducing guilt
- inflicting self-punishment
- gaining care and attention
- sacrificing the self for a greater good

The potential for finding alternative ways of fulfilling the functions of attempted suicide is a protective factor. Thus flexibility about developing new coping styles for solving the problem for which the suicide attempt was a destructive solution places adolescents at lower risk for suicide.

Personality-based risk factors

Personality traits which place adolescents at risk for suicide include hopelessness, perfectionism, impulsivity, aggression and an inflexible coping style. Youngsters who attempt suicide view themselves as incapable of changing their situation and so the future, to them, looks hopeless. Perfectionism is a risk factor for suicide probably because it leads to heightened self-expectations which may be difficult to meet. Suicidal adolescents tend to be inflexible in their coping styles and have difficulties drawing on memories of successfully solving problems in the past and so have a limited repertoire of coping strategies to draw upon. Thus, they resort to strategies which may be ineffective. Their aggression and impulsivity may lead them to engage in self-directed aggression with little reflection on other possible alternatives for solving their difficulties.

Low levels of personality traits which place adolescents at risk for suicide are protective factors in this domain, i.e. low levels of hopelessness, perfectionism, impulsivity, hostility and aggression. It has already been noted in the previous section that the potential for flexibility in finding alternatives to suicide as a way of coping is a protective factor also.

Disorder-related risk factors

The presence of depression is the single strongest health-related risk factor for future suicide. Depression is strongly associated with hopelessness, which paves the way for suicide. Major depression (a recurrent episodic mood disorder) is strongly associated with completed suicide whereas dysthymia (a chronic milder non-episodic mood disorder) is associated with repeated suicide attempts. Other disorders which are risk factors for suicide include alcohol and drug abuse, conduct disorder, antisocial or borderline personality disorders. All of these are more common among impulsive individuals and impulsivity has already been mentioned as a personality-based risk factor for suicide. Epilepsy and chronic painful illness are the two physical conditions which place adolescents at increased risk of suicide. Increased suicide risk is strongly associated with multiple co-morbid chronic psychological and physical disorders.

The absence of psychological or physical disorders and the absence of multiple co-morbid chronic psychological and physical disorders are important protective factors in this domain. So, too, is the capacity to form a good therapeutic alliance and engage in a contract for treatment of disorders including depression, alcohol and drug abuse, conduct disorder, antisocial or borderline personality disorders, epilepsy and chronic painful illness.

Historical risk factors

A history of previous suicide attempts is the single strongest historical risk factor for future suicide. Other historical risk factors include loss of a parent in early life, previous psychiatric treatment and a history of involvement in the juvenile justice system. These three factors are particularly strongly associated with repeated suicidal attempts or parasuicide.

The absence of these historical events is a protective factor, as is a history of good premorbid adjustment.

Family risk factors

A family history of a range of problems notably suicide attempts, depression, drug and alcohol abuse, and assaultive behaviour places youngsters at risk for suicide. In addition youngsters are placed at increased risk of suicide if their families are socially isolated, live in stressful overcrowded conditions and if they deny the seriousness of the youngster's suicidal intentions or are unsupportive of the youngster.

A family history that does not entail suicide attempts, depression, drug and alcohol abuse, and assaultive behaviour is a protective factor. Where the family is well organized and supportive of the youngster and where there are low levels of stress and high level of social support for the family as a whole, these may be considered as protective factors.

Demographic risk factors

Male adolescents are at greater risk for completed suicide while female adolescents are at greatest risk of parasuicide. Males tend to use more lethal methods (guns and hanging) whereas females use less lethal methods (cutting or self-poisoning). Membership of social class five (unskilled workers with low incomes and educational levels) is a risk factor for completed suicide and repeated parasuicide, while membership of social class one (professional and higher managerial employees) is a risk factor for completed suicide only. With respect to ethnicity, in the USA suicide rates are higher for white than black adolescents. With respect to religion, adolescents from communities with lower levels of religious practice are at greater risk for suicide. With respect to seasonality, completed suicide is most common in early summer.

Protective demographic factors include being female; membership of social classes two, three and four; being black (not white) in the USA; and having a strong commitment to religious values and practices.

Biological factors

Serotonin (5-HIAA), a neurotransmitter, has been consistently related to suicidal behaviour. Lower than average levels of serotonin are associated with suicide attempts, poor impulse control, and aggression in both depressed and non-depressed people.

Prevention strategies

Integrative theories of suicide argue that the risk of suicide increases as the number of risk factors increases and the number of protective factors decrease (Carr, 1999, 2001b). However, currently precisely how risk and protective factors interact to determine the occurrence or avoidance of suicide is unclear. A range of adolescent suicide prevention strategies have been developed, in light of the potential risk and protective factors listed above. These include school-based psychoeducational programmes; screening programmes for students at risk; crisis services and hotlines for students at risk; postvention programmes for survivors in social networks where suicide has occurred; and programmes which aim to restrict access to potentially lethal self-harming methods. There is some evidence for the effectiveness of all of these strategies. In this chapter, the focus is exclusively on the effectiveness of school-based psychoeducational programmes.

Previous reviews

From recent reviews of the literature on the effectiveness of school-based suicide prevention programmes, a number of conclusions may be drawn (Berman & Jobes, 1993; Garland et al., 1989; Garland & Zigler, 1993; Kalafat, 1997; Miller & DuPaul, 1996; Shaffer et al., 1988). First, comprehensive psychoeducational programmes for secondary school students hold considerable promise as an effective strategy for preventing adolescent suicide. Second, these programmes, which are usually facilitated by mental health professionals or specially trained teachers, increase awareness about the problem of adolescent suicide, train students to identify adolescents at risk for suicide, educate participants about community mental health services for at-risk adolescents, coach youngsters in the communication, problem-solving and decision-making skills necessary for referring a peer to an appropriate community mental health service, and offer stress management and coping skills training to help youngsters deal with stresses and negative mood states (such as depression and anger) which could contribute to suicide. Programmes that include a narrow curriculum which does not cover this broad spectrum of topics may not be as effective as broadly based programmes.

Third, a range of teaching techniques are used in school-based suicide prevention programmes. These include traditional didactic instruction and group discussion methods and active learning techniques such as video modelling, role-play, and rehearsal. Programmes which rely exclusively on traditional didactic techniques alone and do not use skills training techniques may not be optimally effective.

Fourth, many suicidal youngsters confide their concerns more often to peers than adults, so school-based programmes should offer explicit training in referral skills. They should empower peers to be a link in the referral chain that puts suicidal youngsters in contact with appropriate mental health services.

Fifth, a stress model of suicide is the conceptual cornerstone of most adolescent suicide prevention programmes, because it destigmatizes suicide by distinguishing it from the symptoms of 'mental illness'. That is, in most programmes, suicide is presented as an understandable reaction to extreme psychosocial stress rather than a sign of insanity or the expression of an organically based 'mental illness'. Critics of this approach argue that by destigmatizing suicide and highlighting the increasing prevalence of suicidal behaviour, there is a danger of normalizing suicide. This, they argue, may contribute to possible contagion effects, or unnecessarily increase anxiety about the possibility of suicide within students' peer groups. However, there is little evidence that this is the case.

Sixth, school-based suicide prevention programmes should include early screening, identification and evaluation of suspected suicidal students. Seventh, school-based programmes should be multisystemic and include education programmes for teachers and parents as well as students. Multisystemic programmes also involve networking with community mental health services and monitoring and follow-up procedures.

Method

The aim of the present review was to identify effective classroom-based suicide prevention programmes. A PsychLit database search of English language journals for the years 1977 to 2000 was conducted to identify studies in which suicide prevention programmes were evaluated. The term *suicide*, limited to the term adolescent, was combined with terms such as *prevention*, *programme*, *study*, *evaluation*, *school-based* and *effect*. A manual search through the bibliographies of recent reviews, and relevant journals on adolescent suicide prevention was also conducted. Studies were selected for review if they had a group design, which included a classroom-based treatment and control or comparison group, if at least ten cases were included in each group, and if reliable pre- and post-treatment measures were included. Using these criteria ten studies were selected.

Characteristics of the studies

Characteristics of the studies are set out in Table 16.2. In four studies the impact of child-focused suicide prevention programmes was evaluated (Abbey et al., 1989a; Ciffone, 1993; Hennig et al., 1998; Kalafat & Gagliano, 1996). Six of the studies evaluated multisystemic suicide prevention programmes (Klingman & Hochdorf, 1993; Orbach & Bar-Joseph, 1993; Overholser et al., 1989; Spirito et al., 1988a; Kalafat & Elias, 1994; Nelson, 1987a).

Table 16.2 Characteristics of effective classroom-based prevention studies for suicide prevention in adolescence

Study no.	Study type	Authors	Year	N per group	Mean age and range	Gender	Family characteristics	Programme duration
1	CF	Abbey et al.	1989a	1. GT + BIB -A(T) = 48 2. C = 25	21–24 y	—	—	1. Study for 4w 2. Study for 4w + lectures over 2w
2	CF	Hennig et al.	1998	1. GT + BIB-A(T) = 142 2. C = 163	—	M 57% F 43%	White 66% Hispanic 23% Black 10%	1 × 90 min class
3	CF	Kalafat & Gagliano	1996	1. GT + BIB -A(M) = 52 2. C = 57	—	M 58% F 42%	Middle SES	5 × 1 h classes
4	CF	Ciffone	1993	1. GT + BST + VT-A(M) = 203 2. C = 121	—	M 53% F 47%	Middle SES	1 × 1h class
5	MS-A + M	Orbach & Bar-Joseph	1993	1. GT-A(M) + GT-M = 215 2. C = 178	—	M 45% F 55%	Middle SES	7 × 2 h classes
6	MS'-A + M	Klingman & Hochdorf	1993	1. GT + CBT + VT-A(M) + GT-M = 116 2. C = 121	13–14 y	M 47% F 53%	Low to middle SES	12 × 50min classes over 12 w
7	MS-A + T	Spirito et al.	1988a	1. GT + BST-A(T) + GT-T = 291 2. C = 182	—	M 47% F 53%	Suburban and rural	8 × 1 h classes
8	MS-A + T	Overholser et al.	1989	1. GT + BST-A(T) + GT-T = 215 2. C = 256	14 y	M 53% F 47%	Middle SES	5 × 1 h classes
9	MS-A + P + T	Kalafat & Elias	1994	1. GT + BST + VT-A(T) + GT-T + P = 134 2. C = 119	—	M 57% F 43%	Middle SES	3 × 45 min classes
10	MS-A + P + T	Nelson	1987a	1. GT + BST + VT-A(T) + GT + BST + VT-T + P = 189 2. C = 181	15 y	—	White 49% Hispanic 16% Black 16% Asian 10%	1 × 4 h class

Notes

CF = study of child-focused programme. MS = study of multisystemic programme. GT = group training based on didactic methods and discussion. BST = behavioural skills training, involving listening and/or problem-solving skills. VT = video training where appropriate skills are modeled. BIB = bibliotherapy. CBT = cognitive behavioural training. –A = Training was given to adolescents. –T = training was given to teachers. –P = training was given to parents. (T) = training was given by teachers. (M) = training was given by a mental health professional. C = control group. min = minute. h = hour. w = week. y = year. SES = socio-economic status.

These programmes used multimodal training methods or targeted multiple systems, or both. All of the studies were conducted between 1987 and 1998. Eight of the ten studies were conducted in the USA, while two were conducted in Israel. Across the ten studies there were 3,008 participants, with 1,607 in treatment groups and 1,401 in control groups. The majority of participants were adolescent high school students in grades eight to ten. Based on studies where gender data were given, 53% of participants were male, and 47% were female. In all studies, the programmes were group-based and conducted in school settings. The intensity and duration of programmes ranged from a single one-hour session to twelve weekly fifty-minute sessions. Across the ten studies, four of the interventions were delivered by mental health professionals (school counsellors, psychologists, social workers), five were delivered by school teachers, who had received an average of two days' training (Abbey et al., 1989a; Hennig et al., 1998; Kalafat & Elias, 1994; Overholser et al., 1989; Spirito et al., 1988), and in one study no data were given on the facilitator (Nelson, 1987a).

Methodological features

Methodological features of the ten studies included in this review are presented in Table 16.3. All studies included demographically similar participants and controls. Only three of the ten studies randomly assigned participants to treatment or control groups. Pre- and post-intervention measures were used in all studies. No follow-up data were available for any of the studies. Child self-report measures were used in all studies. The studies evaluated the effectiveness of prevention programmes using measures of adolescent knowledge, attitudes, help seeking, adaptive coping and hopelessness. To assess participants before and after participation in suicide prevention programmes, self-report ratings were used in all studies, parent ratings in two studies, and teacher ratings in one study; researcher ratings were not used in any of the ten studies. In three studies deterioration was assessed and in only two studies drop-out rates were reported. Experienced therapists were used in four studies. This possible shortcoming may be offset by the fact that in all but three of the studies, interventions were manualized so that they could be reliably delivered by teachers and school counsellors. In only one of the programmes was supervision of trainers provided. In all studies information on statistical significance of treatment gains was reported. In two studies information on engagement in concurrent or subsequent treatment was given. Overall this was a methodologically robust group of studies.

Outcome assessment

In these studies knowledge about suicide, attitudes toward suicide and help seeking behaviour were the most common domains within which outcome was evaluated. The Knowledge of Suicide Test (KOST; Abbey et al., 1989b);

Table 16.3 Methodological features of effective classroom-based prevention studies for suicide prevention in adolescence

Feature	S1	S2	S3	S4	S5	S6	S7	S8	S9	S10
	Study number									
Control or comparison group	1	1	1	1	1	1	1	1	1	1
Random assignment	1	0	0	0	0	1	0	0	0	0
Diagnostic homogeneity	0	0	0	0	0	0	0	0	0	0
Demographic similarity	1	1	1	1	1	1	1	1	1	1
Pre-treatment assessment	1	1	1	1	1	1	1	1	1	1
Post-treatment assessment	1	1	1	1	1	1	1	1	1	1
3-month follow-up assessment	0	0	0	0	1	0	0	0	0	0
Children's self-report	1	1	1	1	1	1	1	1	1	1
Parents' ratings	0	0	0	0	0	0	0	0	0	1
Teachers' ratings	0	0	0	0	0	0	0	0	0	1
Therapist or trainer ratings	0	0	0	0	0	0	0	0	0	0
Researcher ratings	0	0	0	0	0	0	0	0	0	0
Deterioration assessed	0	0	0	1	0	1	1	1	0	0
Drop-out assessed	0	1	0	0	1	0	0	0	0	0
Clinical significance of change assessed	1	1	1	1	1	1	1	1	1	1
Experienced therapists or trainers used	1	0	1	0	0	1	0	0	0	0
Programmes were equally valued	0	0	0	0	0	0	0	0	0	0
Programmes were manualized	0	1	0	0	1	1	1	1	1	1
Supervision was provided	0	0	0	0	0	1	0	0	0	0
Programme integrity checked	0	0	0	0	0	0	0	0	0	0
Data on concurrent treatment given	0	1	0	0	0	0	0	0	0	0
Data on subsequent treatment given	0	0	0	0	1	0	0	0	0	0
Total	8	9	7	8	11	11	8	10	7	9

Notes
S = study. 1 = design feature was present. 0 = design feature was absent.

Suicide Prevention Questionnaire (SPQ; Abbey et al., 1989b); Suicide Knowledge Test (SKT; Spirito et al., 1988b); and Suicide Prevention Questionnaire (Nelson, 1987a) were used in these studies to measure suicide-related knowledge. Attitudinal measures included the Attitudes toward Suicide Test (Spirito et al., 1988b), items from the Curriculum Assessment Instrument (Nelson, 1987b) and various customized instruments (e.g., Ciffone, 1993; Hennig et al., 1998). Two forms of help-seeking behaviour were commonly measured: willingness to seek help if suicidal, and willingness to encourage others to seek help if suicidal. Help-seeking behaviours were measured by responses to simulations or suicide-related vignettes in three studies (Abbey et al., 1989a; Kalafat & Elias, 1994; Kalafat & Gagliano, 1996) and in the remaining studies authors developed their own instruments.

Substantive findings

Treatment effect sizes and outcome rates for the ten studies are presented in Table 16.4. A narrative summary of key findings from each study is given in Table 16.5.

Child-focused programmes

In four studies the impact of child-focused suicide prevention programmes was evaluated (Abbey et al., 1989a; Hennig et al., 1998; Kalafat & Gagliano, 1996; Ciffone., 1993). In three of these, the programmes included group instruction and discussion, supplemented with bibliotherapy (Abbey et al., 1989a; Hennig et al., 1998; Kalafat & Gagliano, 1996), while the fourth involved both of these components and behavioural skills training (Ciffone, 1993). Abbey et al. (1989a) found that compared with controls, programme participants showed improved knowledge of suicide on the KOST and SPQ, and correctly identified more suicidal warning signs and intervention strategies. In this study, provision of lectures and handouts on suicide awareness was more effective than handouts alone. Hennig et al. (1998) found that compared with controls, participants in a suicide prevention programme were more likely to recognize symptoms of suicide, intervene appropriately and arrange for professional follow-up. The programme was based on Crabtree's (1990) manual *When Friends are Hurting* and included information on myths and facts about suicide, information on suicide warning signs and instructions on how to establish 'no harm agreements'. A 'no harm agreement' is a peer contract where suicidal adolescents make promises not to hurt themselves before talking with professional counsellors. Kalafat and Gagliano (1996) found that compared with controls, participants in a suicide prevention programme provided more help-seeking responses to vignettes about suicidal and distressed adolescents. Ciffone (1993) found that compared to controls, participants in a suicide prevention programme which included behavioural skills training in addition to group instruction, discussion and bibliotherapy showed improved attitudes related to suicide, help seeking and stigmatization. Males benefited more from the programme than females. The programme included viewing the video *Teens Who Choose Life: The Suicidal Crisis*, which tells the story of a girl who attempted suicide and a boy who completed suicide. A structured discussion followed the viewing, which focused on differences between normal and abnormal adolescent feelings and stresses; self-image concerns; finality of death; the relationship between mental illness and suicide; and adaptive coping skills.

Three specific conclusions may be drawn about the effectiveness of these child-focused suicide prevention programmes. First, with respect to the acquisition of suicide-related knowledge, effect sizes ranged from 0.4 to 2.4 with a mean of 1.4. Thus the average participant showed a greater increase in suicide-related knowledge than 92% of controls. Second, with respect to

Table 16.4 Summary of results of treatment effects and outcome rates for suicide prevention studies

	Study number and type									
	Child focused				Multisystemic					
	Study 1	Study 2	Study 3	Study 4	Study 5	Study 6	Study 7	Study 8	Study 9	Study 10
	GT + BIB-A-(T) v C	GT + BIB-A-(M) v C	GT + BIB-A-(T) V C	GT + BST + VT-A-(M) v C	GT-A-(M) + GT-M v C	GT + CBT + VT A(M) + GT-M v C	GT + BST-A-(T) + GT-T v C	GT + BST-A-(T) + GT-T v C	GT + BST + VT-A-(T) + GT-T + P v C	GT + BST + VT-A-(T) + GT + BST + VT-T + P v C
Increased suicide knowledge	2.4	—	—	0.4	—	0.5	0.9	0.0	0.9	0.3
Improved attitudes to suicide	—	—	—	—	—	—	0.1*	0.2*	0.3	0.3
Willing to seek help if suicidal	—	—	—	0.9	—	—	—	0.0	—	—
Willing to ask others to seek help if suicidal	1.1	1.9	0.8	0.4	—	—	0.0		0.2	—
Increased adaptive coping	—	—	—	—	0.0	0.2	0.0	0.2*	—	—
Decreased hopelessness	—	—	—	—	0.3	—	0.2	0.2*	—	—
Reduced risky behaviour	—	—	—	—	0.3	0.2	—	—	—	—
Improved ego identity	—	—	—	—	1.5	—	—	—	—	—
Drop-out	0%	0%	13	0%	0%	0%	0%	0%	0%	0%

Notes
GT = group training based on didactic methods and discussion. BST = behavioural skills training, involving listening and/or problem-solving skills. VT = video training where appropriate skills are modelled. BIB = bibliotherapy. CBT = cognitive behavioural training. –A = training was given to adolescents. –T = training was given to teachers. –P = training was given to parents. (T) = training was given by teachers. (M) = training was given by a mental health professional. C = control group.
* Improvement for girls only.

Table 16.5 Summary of key findings of effective classroom-based prevention studies for suicide prevention in adolescence

Study no.	Study type	Authors	Year	N per group	Programme duration	Group differences	Key findings
1	CF	Abbey et al.	1989a	1 and 2. GT + BIB -A(T) = 48 3. C = 25	1. Study for 4 w 2. Study for 4 w + lectures over	2 > 1 > 3 2 w	• Compared to controls, participants in the suicide prevention programme showed improved suicide-related knowledge, application of suicide-related knowledge, and suicide intervention response • Provision of lectures and handouts on suicide awareness was more effective than handouts alone
2	CF	Hennig et al.	1998	1. GT + BIB -A(T) = 142 2. C = 163	1 × 90 min class	1 > 2	• Compared to controls, participants in the suicide prevention programme were more likely to recognize symptoms of suicide, intervene appropriately and arrange for professional follow-up
3	CF	Kalafat & Gagliano	1996	1. GT + BIB -A(M) = 52 2. C = 57	5 × 1 h classes	1 > 2	• Compared with controls, participants in the suicide prevention programme provided more help-seeking responses
4	CF	Ciffone	1993	1. GT + BST + VT-A(M) = 203 2. C = 121	1 × 1 h class	1 > 2	• Compared to controls, participants in the suicide prevention programme showed improved attitudes related to suicide for most items, including help seeking and associating suicide with mental illness • Males were more likely than females to seek help from mental health professionals
5	MS -A + M	Orbach & Bar-Joseph	1993	1. GT-A(M) + GT-M = 215 2. C = 178	7 × 2 h classes	1 > 2	• Compared to controls, participants in the suicide prevention programme reported reduced suicidal feelings and increased ability to cope • Compared to controls, participants in the suicide prevention programme showed improved ego identity
6	MS -A + M	Klingman & Hochdorf	1993	1. GT + CBT + VT-A(M) + GT-M = 116 2. C = 121	12 × 50 min classes over 12 w	1 > 2	• Compared to controls, participants in the suicide prevention programme showed increased suicide-related knowledge, improved suicide-related attitudes, a greater reduction in suicide risk, and improved coping skills
7	MS-A + T	Spirito et al.	1988a	1. GT + BST-A(T) + GT-T = 291 2. C = 182	8 × 1 h classes	1 > 2	• Compared to controls, participants in the suicide prevention programme showed improved suicide-related knowledge • Female students benefited more from the suicide prevention programme and expressed less prejudicial attitudes to suicidal peers and increased willingness to assist suicidal peers in seeking counselling
8	MS-A + T	Overholser et al.	1989	1. GT + BST-A(T) + GT-T = 215 2. C = 256	5 × 1 h classes	1 > 2	• Compared to controls, female participants in the suicide prevention programme showed reduced hopelessness, more positive attitudes, and less maladaptive coping • Male participants did not benefit from the programme

Table 16.5 continued

Study no.	Study type	Authors	Year	N per group	Programme duration	Group differences	Key findings
9	MS-A + P + T	Kalafat & Elias	1994	1. GT + BST + VT-A(T) + GT-T + P = 134 2. C = 119	3 × 45 min classes	1 > 2	• Compared with controls, students participating in the suicide prevention programme showed increased suicide-related knowledge, more positive attitudes toward help seeking, increased awareness of potential suicide among peers, and an increased willingness to intervene with troubled peers
10	MS-A + P + T	Nelson	1987a	1. GT + BST + VT-A(T) + GT + BST + VT-T + P = 189 2. C = 181	1 × 4 h class	1 > 2	• Compared to controls, participants in the suicide prevention programme showed increased suicide-related knowledge and more positive suicide-related attitudes • Students who completed the course were better able to recognize the signs and symptoms of a potential suicide crisis and maintain a more informed and helpful attitude towards suicidal peers

Notes
CF = study of child-focused programme. MS = study of multisystemic programme. GT = group training based on didactic methods and discussion. BST = behavioural skills training, involving listening and/or problem-solving skills. VT = video training where appropriate skills are modelled. BIB = bibliotherapy. CBT = cognitive behavioural training. –A = training was given to adolescents –T = training was given to teachers. –P = training was given to parents. (T) = training was given by teachers. (M) = training was given by a mental health professional. C = control group. min = minute. h = hour. w = week.

willingness to encourage others to seek help if suicidal, effect sizes ranged from 0.4 to 1.9 with a mean of 1.1. Thus the average participant showed a greater willingness to encourage others to seek help if suicidal than 86% of controls. Third, in the single study where willingness to seek help if suicidal was evaluated, the effect size was 0.9, indicating that the average participant was more willing to seek help if suicidal than 82% of controls. In summary, child-focused multimodal programmes that include some combination of didactic instruction and discussion, bibliotherapy, and behavioural skills training were effective in increasing suicide-related knowledge, willingness to seek help if suicidal, and willingness to encourage potentially suicidal peers to seek professional help.

Multisystemic programmes

Six studies evaluated multisystemic suicide prevention programmes which included didactic instruction and discussion coupled with behavioural coping skills training for adolescents and other members of their social networks. Two of these studies evaluated programmes for adolescents and mental health professionals (Klingman & Hochdorf, 1993; Orbach & Bar-Joseph, 1993); two evaluated studies where programmes targeted both adolescents and teachers (Overholser et al., 1989; Spirito et al., 1988a); and two evaluated comprehensive programmes which targeted adolescents, teachers and parents (Kalafat & Elias, 1994; Nelson, 1987a).

Orbach and Bar-Joseph (1993) found that compared with controls, participants in a suicide prevention programme facilitated by school counsellors and psychologists who had completed an intensive seven-week training programme, reported reduced suicidal feelings and an increased ability to cope. Compared with controls, participants in the suicide prevention programme showed improvement on the Adolescents Ego-Identity Scale (Tzuriel, 1984). The prevention programme involved exploration of personal and situational factors that contribute to negative mood states and coping skills training. Klingman and Hochdorf (1993) found that compared with controls, participants in a cognitive behavioural suicide prevention programme facilitated by counsellors who had received three hours' intensive training showed increased suicide-related knowledge, improved suicide-related attitudes, a greater reduction in suicide risk, and improved coping skills. In this programme didactic instruction about coping skills was followed by active modelling and rehearsal of these skills, and in the third phase of the programme participants used coping skills in stressful situations, as homework assignments, to regulate negative mood states (Meichenbaum, 1985).

Spirito et al. (1988a) found that compared with controls, participants in a suicide prevention programme facilitated by teachers who had completed an intensive two-day training programme and who followed a programme implementation manual showed improved suicide-related knowledge and decreased hopelessness. Female students benefited more from the programme. They acquired more suicide-related knowledge, expressed less prejudicial attitudes to suicidal peers, and reported an increased willingness to assist suicidal peers in seeking counselling. Within the programme, participants learned factual information about suicide and risk factors, as well as behavioural skills such as active listening and referral techniques to help them assist suicidal peers. Overholser et al. (1989) evaluated the same programme as that investigated by Spirito et al. (1988a) and found that compared with controls, female participants in the suicide prevention programme showed reduced hopelessness, more positive attitudes, and less maladaptive coping. However, male participants did not benefit from the programme.

Positive results were found in two studies which evaluated multisystemic, multimodal programmes which targeted adolescents, teachers and parents and involved video-training, behavioural skills training and didactic group instruction. Kalafat and Elias (1994) found that compared with controls, students participating in the *Lifelines* (Kalafat & Underwood,1989) prevention programme showed increased suicide-related knowledge, more positive attitudes toward help-seeking, increased awareness of potential suicide among peers, and an increased willingness to intervene with troubled peers. Nelson (1987a) found that compared with controls, participants in the *Youth Suicide Prevention Program* showed increased suicide-related knowledge and more positive suicide-related attitudes. Students who completed the course were better able to recognize the signs and symptoms of a potential suicide crisis and maintain a more informed and helpful attitude towards suicidal peers.

A number of specific conclusions may be drawn about the effectiveness of multisystemic, multimodal suicide prevention programmes. First, with respect to the acquisition of suicide-related knowledge, effect sizes ranged from 0 to 0.9 with a mean of 0.5. Thus, the average participant showed a greater increase in suicide-related knowledge than 69% of controls. Second, with respect to risky behaviour, effect sizes ranged from 0.2 to 0.3 with a mean of 0.3. Thus the average participant showed a greater decrease in risky or potentially self-harming behaviour than 62% of controls. Third, with respect to the development of positive attitudes to suicidal peers and decreased personal hopelessness, effect sizes ranged from 0.1 to 0.3 with a mean of 0.2 in each domain. Thus the average participant showed a greater improvement in suicide-related attitudes and hopelessness than 58% of controls. Fourth, in the single study where improved ego identity was evaluated, the effect size was 1.5, indicating that the average participant showed greater improvement in ego identity than 93% of controls. Fifth, with respect to willingness to seek help if suicidal, willingness to encourage others to seek help if suicidal, and increased use of adaptive coping styles, effect sizes ranged from 0 to 0.1 with a mean of 0.1, indicating that programme participants made minimal gains in these domains. Sixth, there was no clear pattern linking programme duration or design to outcome. In summary, multisystemic, multimodal suicide prevention programmes which included didactic instruction and discussion coupled with behavioural coping skills training for adolescents and other members of their social networks were moderately effective in increasing suicide-related knowledge and positive attitudes to suicidal peers while decreasing hopelessness and potentially self-harming risky behaviour.

Conclusion

Currently, suicide accounts for about a third of deaths in the 15–24-year age group, and is the leading cause of death among young men. A variety of psychological, social and biological factors may predispose adolescents to suicide and trigger suicide attempts. From the present review it may be concluded that child-focused multimodal programmes which include some combination of didactic instruction and discussion, bibliotherapy, and behavioural skills training may be very effective in increasing suicide-related knowledge, willingness to seek help if suicidal, and willingness to encourage potentially suicidal peers to seek professional help. Multisystemic prevention programmes which include didactic instruction and discussion coupled with behavioural coping skills training for adolescents and other members of their social networks are moderately effective in increasing suicide-related knowledge and positive attitudes to suicidal peers while decreasing hopelessness and potentially self-harming risky behaviour, particularly among females.

Implications for policy and practice

These conclusions have clear implications for policy and practice. First, classroom-based suicide prevention programmes should be included as part of an overall youth suicide prevention strategic plan which also includes screening programmes for students at risk, crisis services and hotlines for students at risk, postvention programmes for survivors in social networks where suicide has occurred, and programmes which aim to restrict access to potentially lethal self-harming methods.

Second, it is cost-effective to provide students with booklets containing information about suicide before engagement in classroom-based programmes. Such booklets should contain information on suicide myths and facts, warning signs for suicide, risk factors for suicide, and strategies for helping distressed peers obtain help from mental health services. Third, classroom-based programmes of three to twelve hours delivered by specially trained teachers or school counsellors or psychologists should cover a similar curriculum and also include communication, problem-solving, decision-making, and stress management training. Referral skills, particularly those for forming 'no harm agreements' where peers ask suicidal adolescents to make promises not to hurt themselves before talking with professional counsellors, should be a key feature of classroom-based suicide-prevention programmes. Fourth, active teaching methods including video modelling, role-play, rehearsal, corrective feedback and home practice should be used for skills training. Fifth, programmes should include training sessions covering a similar curriculum for teachers, parents and mental health professionals from the school and local community. Sixth, programmes should be delivered by trained personnel, have manualized procedures, and be evaluated using reliable and valid outcome measures.

Implications for research

The studies of suicide prevention programmes reviewed here examined changes in knowledge, attitudes and self-reported use of coping strategies rather than changes in behaviour. Prevention programme outcome studies are required in which large cohorts of adolescents are followed up over time periods spanning up to ten years (from fifteen to twenty-five years of age) and in which rates of parasuicidal behaviour and completed suicide are evaluated, particularly among high-risk groups. Such studies should include reliable referral tracking systems and sufficiently large samples to capture measurable incidence of reporting of suicidal behaviours.

A psychometrically robust and standardized set of instruments to assess suicide-related knowledge and attitudes, willingness to seek and give help, hopelessness, helplessness, depression, suicidality and coping strategies is required for use by all researchers within this field, to make reliable and valid cross-study comparisons possible.

The utility of paper and pencil vignettes to assess the impact of programmes on skill development was demonstrated in this review. Future studies should incorporate these measures, but also evaluate skill acquisition using simulated behavioural role-play vignettes which more closely approximate real-life situations.

Future research should evaluate manualized intervention programmes, in which checklists for programme integrity are made. In such studies, training sessions are recorded and blind raters use programme integrity checklists to evaluate the degree to which sessions approximate manualized procedures. Such integrity checks allow researchers to say with confidence the degree to which a pure and potent version of their programme has been evaluated.

Studies are required which investigate the mechanisms and processes which underpin programme effectiveness. It is clear that there is variability in adolescents' responses to suicide prevention programmes of different types. For example, it is not clear what mechanisms underpinned the fact that effect sizes were greater for child-focused rather than multisystemic programmes in the studies reviewed in this chapter. It is also not clear why females responded better to multisystemic programmes than males. The determinants of these different outcomes require careful investigation. Such research is vital for the development of programmes which are acceptable to, and effective for, male adolescents. After all, it is male adolescents who are at greatest risk for suicide and who have provided the impetus for the development of this entire field of research.

Assessment resources

Abbey, K.J., Madsen, C.H. & Polland, R. (1989). *Knowledge of Suicide Test (KOST), Suicide Prevention Questionnaire (SPQ)*. (Available from K. Abbey, Florida State University, Tallahassee, Florida, FL 32306 (Tel. 806–644–2525).)

Beck, A. and Steer, R. (1991) *Beck Scale for Suicide Ideation*. New York: The Psychological Corporation.

Beck, A.T., Weissman, A., Lester, D. & Trexler, L. (1974). The measurement of pessimism: The Helplessness Scale. *Journal of Consulting and Clinical Psychology*, 42, 861–865.

Birleson, P., Hudson, I., Buchanan, D. & Wolff, S. (1987). Clinical evaluation of a self-rating scale for depressive disorder in childhood (Depression Self-Rating Scale). *Journal of Child Psychology and Psychiatry*, 28, 43–60.

Kazdin, A., Rodgas, A. & Colbus, D. (1986). The Hopelessness Scale for Children: psychometric characteristics and concurrent validity. *Journal of Consulting Clinical Psychology*, 54, 241–245.

Kovacs, M. & Beck, A. (1977). An empirical clinical approach towards definition of childhood depression. In J. Schulterbrandt et al. (Eds.), *Depression in Children*. (pp. 1–25). New York: Raven.

Neimeyer, R.A. & MacInnes, W.D. (1981). Assessing paraprofessional competence with the Suicide Intervention Response Inventory. *Journal of Counseling Psychology*, 28, 176–179.

Nelson, F. (1987). *Curriculum Assessment Instrument*. (Available from Dr Franklyn Nelson, Director of clinical training, The Institute for Studies of Destructive Behaviors and the Suicide Prevention Center, 1041 South Menlo Avenue, Los Angeles, California 90006.)

Rosenbaum, A. (1986). A schedule for assessing self-control behavior. *Behavior Therapy*, 17, 132–142.

Spirito, A., Overholser, J., Ashworth, S., Morgan, J. & Benedict-Drew, C. (1988). *Attitudes Toward Suicide Test and Suicide Knowledge Test (SKT)*. (Available from Dr Spirito, Child & Family Psychiatry, Rhode Island Hospital, 593 Eddy St. Providence, RI 02903.)

Tzuriel, D. & Bar-Joseph, H. (1989). *The Israeli Index of Potential Suicide (IIPS)*. Ramat-Gan: Bar-llan University, Department of Psychology. (Available from Dr Bar-Joseph, Department of Psychology, Bar-Ilan University, Ramat-Gan 52900, Israel.)

Zung, W.W.K. (1974). Index of potential suicide (IPS): A rating scale for suicide prevention. In T. Beck, H. Resnick & D. Lettieri (Eds.), *The Prediction of Suicide* (pp. 221–249). Bowie, MD: Charles Press.

Treatment manuals and resources

Berman, A. & Jobes, D. (1993) *Adolescent Suicide: Assessment and Intervention*. Washington, DC: APA.

Carr, A. (2001). *Depression and Attempted Suicide in Adolescence*. Leicester: British Psychological Society.

Centers for Disease Control (1992). *Youth Suicide Prevention Programs*: *A Resource Guide*. Atlanta, GA: Centers for Disease Control.

Clarke, G., Lewinsohn, P. & Hops, H. (2000). *Leader's Manual for Adolescent Groups. Adolescent Coping with Depression Course*. Portland, OR: Center for Health Research. *http://www.kpchr.org/*

Crabtree, C.R. (1990). *When Friends are Hurting*. (Available from C.R. Crabtree, Texas Tech University, Department of Sociology, Anthropology, and Social Work, P.O. Box 41012, Lubbock, TX, 79409–1012, USA.)

Jacobs, D. (1999). (Ed) *The Harvard Medical School Guide to Suicide Assessment and Intervention*. San Francisco, CA: Jossey Bass.

Kalafat, J. & Underwood, M. (1989). *Lifelines: A School-Based Adolescent Suicide Response Program*. Dubuque, IA: Kendall/Hunt.

Mufson, L., Moreau, D., Weissman, M. & Kerman, G. (1993). *Interpersonal Psychotherapy for Depressed Adolescents*. New York: Guilford.

Stark, K. & Kendall, P. (1996). *Treating Depressed Children: Therapists Manual for ACTION*. Ardmore, PA: Workbook Publishing.

Teens who choose life: The suicidal crisis, part II. Gail chooses life [Video filmstrip]. (1986). Pleasantville, NY: Sunburst Communications. (Available from Sunburst Communications, 39 Washington Avenue, Pleasantville, NY 10570–0040.)

Resources for clients

Clarke, G., Lewinsohn, P. & Hops, H. (2000). *Students' Workbook. Adolescent Coping with Depression Course*. Portland, OR: Center for Health Research. *http://www.kpchr.org/*

Copeland, M.E. & Copans, S.M. (1998). *The Adolescent Depression Workbook*. New Harbinger Publications.

Giovacchini, P. (1983). *The Urge to Die: Why Young People Commit Suicide*. New York: Penguin.

Joan, P. (1986). *Preventing Teenage Suicide: The Living Alternative Handbook*. New York: Human Sciences Press.

Lester, D. (1992). *The Cruelest death: The Enigma of Adolescent Suicide*. New York: Charles Press Publishers.

Orbach, I. (1988). *Children Who Don't Want to Live*. San Francisco, CA: Jossey Bass.

Shamoo, T.K., Patros, P.G. & Rinzler, A. (1997). *Helping your Child Cope with Depression and Suicidal Thoughts*. San Francisco, CA: Jossey Bass.

Stark, K., Kendall, P., McCarthy, M., Stafford, M., Barron, R. & Thomeer, M. (1996). *A Workbook for Overcoming Depression*. Ardmore, PA: Workbook Publishing.

Williams, K. (1995). *A Parents Guide For Suicidal And Depressed Teens: Help for Recognizing if a Child is in Crisis and What to Do*. Hazeldon Information Education.

17 Conclusions

Alan Carr

The objective of this book has been to identify intervention programmes which prevent a range of relatively common psychological problems in childhood and adolescence. In order to identify effective prevention programmes we reviewed over 200 studies involving more than 70,000 children. Furthermore, the studies we selected for review were the most methodologically robust that we could find using both computer and manual searches of the English language literature for the past quarter of a century. We can therefore place considerable confidence in our conclusions which are summarized in this chapter. Our conclusions concern the prevention of the following list of problems:

1. developmental delay in low birth weight infants
2. cognitive delays in socially disadvantaged children
3. adjustment problems in children with physical disabilities
4. adjustment problems in children with sensory disabilities
5. adjustment problems in children with autism
6. challenging behaviour in children with intellectual disabilities
7. physical abuse
8. sexual abuse
9. bullying
10. adjustment problems in children with asthma
11. adjustment problems in children with diabetes
12. teenage drug abuse
13. teenage pregnancy, sexually transmitted diseases and HIV infection
14. post-traumatic adjustment problems in children and adolescents
15. suicide in adolescence

To make the text below more readable, all assertions in this chapter are made unreferenced. References on which assertions are based are contained in relevant chapters of this volume. Furthermore, while we are reasonably confident about the reliability and validity of our conclusions, it is important to stress that all of our conclusions are open to revision in light of new evidence. For example, future programme evaluation studies of autistic children may show that low intensity speech and language intervention programmes are as effective as highly intensive behavioural programmes. So our conclusions are not cast in stone. Rather, they are the best we can offer, today, in light of available scientific evidence.

1. Prevention of developmental delay in low birth weight infants

Low birth weight is a problem that places infants at risk for developmental delay. About 7% of all births in industrialized countries have low birth weights and 1% of children at birth meet the criterion for very low birth weight. Social disadvantage and preterm birth are the main risk factors for low birth weight. Families in which low birth weight infants are born should be engaged in programmes which begin in neonatal intensive care units and involve home visiting, community-based outpatient and preschool follow-up sessions. Such programmes should include child stimulation, parent training and support, and conjoint parent–child sessions to promote secure attachment. Such programmes should be continued throughout the preschool and early school going years until a comprehensive multidisciplinary assessment indicates that the child's development falls within normal limits. Children with a high level of biological vulnerability as indexed by very low birth weights and neurological impairment may require more intensive programmes. Special efforts should be made to help parents stay engaged with these programmes. Home visiting and the provision of transport to day centres may facilitate this.

2. Prevention of cognitive delay in socially disadvantaged children

Children from socially disadvantaged backgrounds show delayed development of cognitive abilities. They obtain lower scores on tests of intelligence, cognitive skills, language development and academic attainment, compared with children who are not reared in poverty. Rates of cognitive delay are about 10% in lower socioeconomic groups compared with 2–3% in higher socioeconomic groups. Four broad types of early intervention programmes have been developed for socially disadvantaged children.

- Home-visiting programmes which aim to help socially disadvantaged parents understand and meet their children's needs for intellectual stimulation, secure attachment, and consistent supervision.
- Preschool programmes which aim to directly provide disadvantaged children with a stimulating preschool environment to compensate for their intellectually impoverished home environment.
- Combined home-visiting and preschool programmes which aim both to enhance the quality of disadvantaged children's home environments and to give them access to enriched preschool environments.

- Multisystemic programmes which attempt to extend support services for children and families into middle childhood.

Multisystemic programmes are the most effective. Overall, the average child who participates in a multisystemic early intervention programme fares better than 93% of children whose families do not participate in this type of programme. In rank order of effectiveness after multisystemic programmes are home-visiting programmes, combined home-visiting and preschool programmes, and programmes that involve preschool enrolment only. Overall, longer programmes are more effective than shorter programmes and the most effective programmes extend beyond five years. Disadvantaged children at risk for cognitive delay should be offered effective early intervention programmes to prevent such delays occurring. Effective programmes involve a comprehensive range of components delivered by a multidisciplinary team who receive continuous training and supervision. Effective programmes are intensive, involving frequent and long-term contact. They involve children's families fully and build upon their cultural beliefs, traditions and practices. Preschools in effective programmes have small child–teacher ratios and modify the curriculum to meet the unique needs of individual children. Effective programmes use manualized curricula to ensure that all staff involved in implementation provide the intervention as intended. Effective programmes also evaluate participants with appropriate assessment instruments before, during and after the intervention and at follow-up to monitor progress and respond to children who are having difficulties benefiting from participation. Effective programmes also include additional supports to maintain initial positive effects.

3. Prevention of adjustment problems in children with cerebral palsy

Cerebral palsy, which affects about 1 in 400 children, is a disorder of movement and posture that results from an insult to, or anomaly of, the immature central nervous system in centres which govern motor activity. Children with cerebral palsy often have other co-morbid disabilities including intellectual disability, seizure disorders, visual and auditory impairments, learning difficulties and behaviour problems. Best practice involves offering comprehensive multidisciplinary rehabilitative programmes of care specifically designed to minimize the impact of the constraints placed by cerebral palsy and co-morbid conditions on the child's physical and psychosocial development. Such programmes may include environmental alterations to manage the musculoskeletal complications of cerebral palsy; the use of carefully designed devices to aid posture and mobility; medication, nerve blocks and motor point blocks and neurosurgery to reduce spasticity; and orthopaedic surgery. In addition to these essentially physical interventions a range of other interventions including neurodevelopmental therapy, infant stimulation, therapeutic electrical stimulation, special education and conductive education should be included in overall multidisciplinary care plans.

To be effective neurodevelopmental therapy must be offered at a high level of intensity with clinic physiotherapy sessions once or twice a week and daily home practice. Such intensive programmes should not be offered until the infant is six months and the effectiveness of this type of treatment for infants is enhanced if it is preceded by an infant stimulation programme during the child's first six months. In toddlers and young children when coupled with inhibitive limb-casting neurodevelopmental therapy is particularly effective in improving the motor functioning of limbs for which inhibitive casts are worn for a set period of time each day. Therapeutic electrical stimulation may be offered as a parent-administered manualized home-based programme to improve gross motor functioning in specific muscles or muscle groups. Special education and conductive education when offered as day programmes are equally effective in promoting cognitive, motor and social development in young children.

4. Prevention of adjustment difficulties in children with sensory impairments

The prevalence of deafness is about 4 per 1,000 and about 1 in every 3,000 children has severe visual impairment. For children with sensory impairments cognitive and social development are invariably more challenging than for children without sensory impairments. In addition, deaf children face particular challenges in developing language and blind children are particularly challenged in developing sensorimotor integration and motor skills. Developmental screening procedures are essential to facilitate early identification of children with sensory impairments. Multisystemic family-based early intervention programmes should be offered to families with children who are detected through screening procedures as having sensory impairments. These multisystemic family-based early intervention programmes should include child-focused and parent-focused components and these components should be offered flexibly on a home-visiting basis and at local health, social or educational centres for families of children with sensory impairments. The SKI*HI curriculum is a good example of this type of intervention. Child-centred interventions should focus on promoting the use of all senses including the impaired sense, especially in the case of visually impaired children. In addition child-centred interventions should focus on training the child in communication skills including oral speech and sign language in the case of deaf children. Child-centred interventions may be taught by an adult with a sensory impairment who acts as an advocate and role model for the child, introducing them to the deaf and blind minority cultures. Parent-centred interventions should provide information on sensory impairment, and coaching in techniques that parents can use to help their children learn communication and social skills. Parent-centred interventions should also provide parents with ongoing personal support and advice on how to access health, social and educational services. For school-aged children, school-based programmes should follow on from home-based child-centred programmes. In school-based programmes, systematic and intensive instruction, tailored to children's unique learning profiles, should be used to promote language development. Social problem-solving skills should also be taught to promote social understanding and behavioural adjustment, as in the PATHS programme. Long-term parent-centred programmes should run in parallel with the child-centred school-based programmes, to provide a forum within which parents can address the various problems that occur as their sensorily impaired children make various life-cycle transitions such as entering puberty and leaving high school.

5. Prevention of adjustment problems in children with autism

A triad of deficits typify most autistic children. These deficits occur in social development, language and behaviour, particularly imaginative or make-believe play. The prevalence rate for autism is 9.6 per 10,000. The outcome for children with autism is poor and up to 60% are unable to lead an independent life. Autistic children with a non-verbal IQ in the normal range and some functional language skills at the age of five have the best prognosis. Under-estimating the potential of children with autism to develop life skills and avoid developing secondary adjustment problems is a major pitfall to be avoided. In order to prevent adjustment problems in children with autism screening and assessment systems which allow for the early detection of autism are vital. Once identified youngsters with autism require intensive intervention. Lovaas's behavioural intervention programme, Schopler's TEACCH programme, and speech- and language-focused programmes all hold promise as secondary preventative interventions for children with autism. Psychological interventions can have marked impact on the cognitive, behavioural and social adjustment of children with autism in the short and long term. Effective interventions are intensive and protracted and occur across multiple contexts including the home and the school or preschool setting, with highly collaborative working relationships between parents, teachers and clinical staff. Effective interventions have an adult to child ratio varying from 1:1 to 1:3, are highly structured and based on theoretically derived procedural treatment manuals. Effective intervention programmes are sufficiently flexible to address the unique profile of needs of each child. They are designed to enhance skills in five key areas: (1) attending to aspects of the environment essential for learning; (2) imitation; (3) language usage; (4) imaginative play; and (5) social interaction. In addition, psychoeducational and relief care support services for parents may be required, although research on this issue is lacking.

6. Prevention of challenging behaviour in children with intellectual disabilities

Challenging behaviour, particularly self-injury, aggression and property destruction, are of central concern to parents and carers of people with intellectual and other developmental disabilities because they are particularly unresponsive to routine care practices and because they place clients, parents and carers at risk of injury. Substantial reductions in challenging behaviour may be achieved using behavioural interventions following rigorous and systematic functional analysis. Through this type of assessment, factors that maintain challenging behaviours may be identified. Individualized behavioural programmes may then be developed based on these assessments and implemented to prevent challenging behaviour from persisting. For children and adolescents with developmental disabilities, both proactive and suppressive interventions can effectively prevent challenging behaviour. Proactive interventions include functional communication training, negative reinforcement, neutralizing routines and instructional manipulation. Suppressive interventions include overcorrection, restraint and punishment. One central practice issue is which category of intervention to consider in any particular case. Interventions that focus on antecedents of challenging behaviour, such as functional communication training, neutralizing routines and instructional manipulation, have been used to good effect with challenging behaviour that is directed at others (such as aggression) and the self (self-injurious behaviour) and in a wide range of community and institutional settings. These interventions, because of their non-coercive and non-aversive nature and their suitability to multiple settings, may be the interventions of first choice when youngsters present with challenging behaviour. In contrast, interventions which focus predominantly on altering the consequences of challenging behaviour such as overcorrection, restraint and punishment have been used exclusively with self-injurious behaviours in predominantly institutional settings in the studies reviewed in this volume. These may therefore be viewed as second line interventions to consider when functional communication training, neutralizing routines and instructional manipulation have not been effective, particularly within institutional settings, and particularly with self-injurious behaviour. Strong ethical justification is required in using these more coercive interventions. For example, where youngsters are engaging in potentially fatal self-injurious behaviour, their use may be ethically justified.

7. Prevention of physical abuse

Because physical child abuse is a violation of children's rights, because it leads to deleterious short- and long-term psychological consequences, and because the prevalence of serious physical abuse is about 10%, the prevention of physical child abuse is imperative. Physical abuse occurs in families characterized by high levels of stress and low levels of support when children place demands on their parents which outstrip parental coping resources, and parents in frustration injure their children. Families at risk for physical child abuse should be identified by screening mothers prenatally. Subsequently they should be engaged in multimodal community-based programmes which begin prenatally and which include home visiting conducted by nurses or paraprofessionals, behavioural parent training, stress management and life skills training until a comprehensive multidisciplinary assessment of risk factors indicates that the risk of physical abuse has been substantially reduced. Participating in home-visiting programmes, particularly those that begin prenatally, can reduce the risk of physical child abuse and child hospitalization by half. Poor, unmarried teenage mothers may derive greatest benefit from home-visiting programmes. Stress management training programmes and behavioural parent training child abuse prevention programmes lead to marked short-term improvements in parental well-being and in parent-reported child welfare and this is sustained at follow-up. Unfortunately the marked short-term improvements in parenting skills which arise from participation in behavioural parent training child abuse prevention programmes are not maintained at follow-up and so ongoing booster sessions are required for gains in parenting skills to be maintained in the long term. Attrition is a problem in all physical child abuse prevention programmes. The lowest drop-out rates occur in home-visiting and inpatient programmes and the highest drop-out rates occur in behavioural parent training programmes conducted on a group basis in community centres rather than parents' homes or inpatient settings. This underlines the importance of ongoing long-term home visiting.

8. Prevention of sexual abuse

Estimates of prevalence rates vary from 2–30% in males and 4–30% in females depending on definitions used and population studied. Sexual abuse has profound short- and long-term effects on psychological functioning. Behaviour problems shown by children who have experienced sexual abuse typically include sexualized behaviour, excessive internalizing or externalizing behaviour problems, school-based attainment problems and relationship difficulties. About a fifth of cases show clinically significant long-term problems which persist into adulthood. Primary prevention programmes which equip pre-adolescent children with the skills necessary for preventing child sexual abuse (CSA) should be routinely included in primary school curricula. These programmes should be developmentally staged with different programme materials for younger and older children, be of relatively long duration spanning a school term, be taught using multimedia materials and active skills training methods, and be multisystemic. That is, programmes should include components which target not only children but also parents, teachers and members of the local health, social and law enforcement services. The curriculum of the parents' and teachers' training components should cover an overview of child abuse and child protection issues, a preview of the children's programme lesson plans, and information on local child protection procedures and the roles of parents and teachers in these procedures. Training is important for effective programme delivery and a range of personnel may be effective instructors. Thus parents, teachers, mental health professionals and law enforcement officers may all take the role of instructors in child abuse prevention programmes provided they are adequately trained. CSA prevention programmes do not lead to increased sexualized behaviour, anxiety or other significant adjustment difficulties.

9. Prevention of bullying

Bullying in schools is a significant problem for a large minority of children. Estimates for the prevalence of being bullied frequently vary from 4 to 13%. Estimates of engaging in frequent bullying range from 1 to 7%. Whole-school bullying prevention programmes effectively reduce both reports of bullying and reports of being bullied in the short term (over periods of an academic year) but also in the longer term over periods of up to three years. To prevent bullying, the whole-school approach to bullying should be routinely introduced into primary and secondary schools. The whole-school approach to bullying incorporates a wide range of strategies at school, class and individual levels within the context of an overall school policy in which the administration of the school, including the board of management, the principal, teachers and other staff along with the pupils, take responsibility for preventing bullying. The anti-bullying school policy must be given the highest priority and be backed up with specific prevention strategies. Particular care should be taken to implement such programmes fully and consistently in accordance with programme guidelines. School staff should be provided with periodic training and consultancy to help them implement programmes effectively. The effectiveness of whole-school bullying prevention programmes is determined by the degree to which the programme integrity is maintained and the degree to which external training, consultancy and support are offered to ensure proper implementation of whole-school bullying prevention programmes.

10. Prevention of adjustment problems in children with asthma

Asthma is one of the most common chronic diseases with a prevalence rate of about 10% among children. Its effects are pervasive and can lead to restrictions in daily activity, absences from school, repeated hospitalization during severe attacks, hypoxia, seizures and brain damage; if left untreated, asthma is potentially fatal. The course of asthma is determined by the interaction between abnormal respiratory system physiological processes to which some youngsters have a predisposition, physical environmental triggers and psychological processes. Psychological interventions for paediatric asthma include:

- Psychoeducation to improve understanding of the condition.
- Relaxation training to help reduce physiological arousal.
- Skills training to increase adherence to asthma management programmes.
- Family therapy to empower family members to work together to manage asthma effectively.

Psychological interventions should be offered in conjunction with routine paediatric management of asthma, particularly where children have severe symptoms, repeated hospitalizations and/or adherence problems. In such cases multisystemic, family-based, psychoeducational programmes which include relaxation and behavioural skills training should be provided. These should typically be clinic based and involve approximately six to eight sessions. Where service demands greatly outweigh available resources, self-administered psychoeducation should be provided as a preliminary measure but this should ideally be followed up with further intervention, particularly where youngsters have severe symptoms or adherence problems. If resources permit and particularly when parents cannot engage in treatment, relaxation training and biofeedback techniques should be made available within the context of child-focused programmes. For children with severe asthma that is not well controlled with conventional treatment methods, family therapy (rather than multiple family group psychoeducation) should be provided. The most effective programmes involve relaxation training (using frontalis biofeedback or self-hypnosis) and family therapy.

11. Prevention of adjustment problems in children with diabetes

Type 1, or insulin-dependent diabetes mellitus (IDDM), is an endocrine disorder typically diagnosed in childhood, characterized by complete pancreatic failure. The prevalence rate is approximately 1.2–1.9 cases per 1,000 children under the age of 20. The long-term outcome of IDDM is associated with devastating complications in some cases, including blindness and leg amputation, particularly those where there has been poor regime adherence. For youngsters with diabetes, blood glucose levels as close as possible to the normal range are achieved through a regime involving a combination of insulin injections, balanced diet, exercise and self-monitoring of blood glucose. For diabetic youngsters five types of psychological intervention programmes can prevent adjustment problems and improve adherence and metabolic control. These are:

- family crisis intervention programmes
- family-based behavioural programmes

- family-based communication and problem-solving skills training programmes
- child-focused coping skills training programmes
- intensive inpatient psychoanalytic psychotherapy.

For newly diagnosed diabetic children family-based multidisciplinary crisis intervention programmes should be routinely offered. Such programmes should include psychoeducation, supportive family counselling, school liaison meetings, home visiting, and peer counselling for newly diagnosed patients from youngsters with experience in managing diabetes. For youngsters who continue to show poor metabolic control during the preadolescent years family-based behavioural programmes may be offered. In these programmes self-care skills are modelled and rehearsed. Initially parents prompt and reinforce skill use, but gradually youngsters take increasing responsibility for self-management of their diabetes regime. In adolescence, where youngsters show poor metabolic control, family-based communication and problem-solving programmes should be offered. Such programmes should include parent simulation exercises in which parents are invited to complete diabetes management tasks while their adolescents act as their 'coaches'. This exercise helps parents to empathize with the challenges faced by their youngsters and facilitates joint problem-solving. Adolescents with poor metabolic control may also be offered coping skills training programmes to develop the skills to cope with peer pressure to violate their diabetic regime. Regular booster sessions should be offered after the completion of such programmes. All of the programmes mentioned so far in this section are relatively brief (ten to thirty sessions). Where brittle diabetes develops, intensive inpatient psychoanalytic psychotherapy three to five times per week over four months should be offered. The cost of such treatment can be justified in terms of the impact such programmes can have in preventing short-term complications and repeated hospitalizations and in the longer term in delaying the onset and progression of serious complications associated with diabetes.

12. Prevention of drug abuse

Between 5 and 10% of teenagers under nineteen have drug problems serious enough to require clinical intervention. One strategy for preventing youngsters joining this minority is to provide school-based prevention programmes which aim to prevent or reduce usage of gateway drugs: nicotine, alcohol and marijuana. These gateway drugs are invariably the first step on the road to serious drug problems for those youngsters that eventually develop such difficulties. Young teenagers should routinely participate in peer-led school-based programmes of up to 30 sessions in which they receive accurate information about the immediate effects of drugs, conservative normative information about drug use, and learn drug refusal skills and general social problem-solving skills. These programmes should involve active teaching methods and multiple booster sessions in mid-adolescence, and should be integrated into the school curriculum so that most youngsters attend all classes. These school-based programmes should be the nucleus of wider multisystemic programmes which involve members of youngsters' significant social systems.

13. Prevention of teenage pregnancy, STDs and HIV infection

Risky sexual behaviour is a highly significant problem throughout the world. Unintentional teenage pregnancy, sexually transmitted diseases, and HIV infection are the principal negative outcomes of risky sexual behaviour. Relatively brief classroom-based prevention programmes can favourably influence knowledge, attitudes, beliefs and intentions relevant to sexually risky behaviour. Specifically these programmes can delay the onset of sexual activity in sexually inexperienced young adolescents and decrease the frequency of unprotected sex in sexually active adolescents mainly by increasing the frequency of condom use.

Classroom-based programmes for preventing sexual risk taking should be routinely included in secondary school curricula. Such programmes should include psychoeducation, communication and behavioural skills training as the main components. Didactic methods and group discussion may be used for psychoeducational training. However, live modelling and/or video modelling, rehearsal, role-playing and corrective feedback should be used to train participants in using both communication skills and behavioural skills for practising safe sex. These skills include anticipating and avoiding or escaping from sexually risky situations, and buying, carrying and using condoms. Programmes for younger adolescents should focus particularly on delaying the onset of sexual intercourse and those for older teenagers should focus on the avoidance of unprotected sexual intercourse. The positive impact of prevention programmes in reducing sexual risk taking diminishes over time, so follow-up sessions should be routinely included in clinical or educational practice. Training is important for effective programme delivery and a range of personnel including health educators and teachers may be effective instructors.

14. Prevention of post-traumatic adjustment problems

Survivors of traumas such as child abuse, natural disasters and accidents may develop serious psychological problems including acute stress reactions and PTSD. However, psychological intervention programmes can prevent the development of such reactions or prevent such reactions from persisting. Tertiary PTSD prevention programmes of twelve to twenty-four sessions should be routinely available to pre-adolescent and adolescent CSA survivors. These programmes should include graded exposure, coping skills training, safety skills training and behavioural parent training. Secondary PTSD prevention programmes should be routinely available for children and adolescents following natural disasters and major accidents or illnesses. Such programmes should include grief work and coping skills training and may take the form of critical incident stress debriefing. Such programmes may span three to seven sessions. Offering at least a portion of the intervention programme in a group format may be important for successful treatment. For single incident traumas such as accidents and assaults, graded exposure and coping skills training offered in a group format over eighteen sessions is an effective tertiary prevention approach.

15. Prevention of suicide in adolescence

Currently, suicide accounts for about a third of deaths in the 15–24-year age group, and is the leading cause of death among young men. A variety of psychological, social and biological factors may predispose adolescents to suicide and trigger suicide attempts. Child-focused multimodal programmes which include some combination of didactic instruction and discussion, bibliotherapy, and behavioural skills training may be very effective in increasing suicide-related knowledge, willingness to seek help if suicidal, and willingness to encourage potentially suicidal peers to seek professional help. Multisystemic prevention programmes which include didactic instruction and discussion coupled with behavioural coping skills training for adolescents and other members of their social networks are moderately effective in increasing suicide-related knowledge and positive attitudes to suicidal peers while decreasing hopelessness and potentially self-harming risky behaviour, particularly among females. Classroom-based suicide prevention programmes should be included as part of an overall youth suicide prevention strategic plan which also includes screening programmes for students at risk, crisis services and hotlines for students at risk, postvention programmes for survivors in social networks where suicide has occurred, and programmes which aim to restrict access to potentially lethal self-harming methods.

It is cost-effective to provide students with booklets containing information about suicide before engagement in classroom-based programmes. Such booklets should contain information on suicide myths and facts, warning signs for suicide, risk factors for suicide, and strategies for helping distressed peers obtain help from mental health services. Classroom-based programmes of three to twelve hours delivered by specially trained teachers or school counsellors or psychologists should cover a similar curriculum and also include communication, problem-solving, decision-making and stress management training. Referral skills, particularly those for forming 'no harm agreements' where peers ask suicidal adolescents to make promises not to hurt themselves before talking with professional counsellors, should be a key feature of classroom-based suicide-prevention programmes. Active teaching methods including video-modelling, role-play, rehearsal, corrective feedback and home practice should be used for skills training. Programmes should include training sessions covering a similar curriculum for teachers, parents and mental health professionals from the school and local community. Finally, programmes should be delivered by trained personnel, have manualized procedures, and be evaluated using reliable and valid outcome measures.

Common themes in effective prevention programmes

Certain common themes emerge from the fifteen sets of conclusions outlined above. These broad themes constitute a set of principles for designing, delivering and evaluating effective psychological prevention programmes.

Prevention programmes based on sound psychological theory, particularly multifactorial systemic theories, can reduce adjustment problems in biologically or psychosocially vulnerable children and adolescents. Multisystemic programmes are particularly effective. These include components that target the individual youngster and members of the significant social systems of which the youngster is a member including the family, school, peer group and community.

Child-focused elements of effective multisystemic programmes equip the child with specific skills or experiences which are important for addressing their biological or psychosocial vulnerability. They do this by reducing personal risk factors and strengthening personal protective factors.

Components of multisystemic programmes that target vulnerable youngsters' families, parents, schools and peer groups aim to enhance the amount of social support these systems can offer vulnerable children or involve members of these systems in providing the child with skills to manage his or her unique vulnerabilities.

Effective multisystemic prevention programmes are delivered by trained staff, parents or peers who are well supervised and who follow manuals which specify the programme curriculum and intervention procedures. Curricula of effective programmes are based on sound psychological theory and are developmentally and culturally matched to participants' age and ethnic status. Effective programmes involve multiple teaching methods such as didactic instruction and discussion on the one hand and modelling, rehearsal, corrective feedback and extended practice on the other. They also use multimedia including verbal presentations, print, video, and drama where appropriate.

Effective programmes are intensive, involving frequent contact, with good child:facilitator ratios, are of longer rather than shorter duration, and involve follow-up booster sessions. They are delivered by credible facilitators. In adolescence this may mean programmes are delivered by peers.

Effective programmes are delivered in a convenient setting. So for mothers with infants, home visiting is an important setting for programme delivery. For adolescents, the school may be the most appropriate setting.

Effective programmes include monitoring procedures, such as frequent staff support and supervision, to ensure that programme integrity is maintained.

Effective programmes also include evaluation procedures to ensure that programme effectiveness is monitored. Evaluation studies should be methodologically robust and score highly on the methodological checklist contained in Chapter 1. The effectiveness of programmes may be enhanced by investigating the relationships between a range of factors and overall outcome, and redesigning programmes in light of findings from such process-based research. Important factors that may have a bearing on outcome and deserve investigation include programme design features (such as curriculum content, programme duration, type of facilitators involved, teaching methods used, programme setting, etc.); characteristics of participants (such as age, gender, level of disability or vulnerability, coping style, etc.); and characteristics of participants' social networks (such as family structure, peer group deviance, type of school, etc.).

These common principles may serve as a template for the development of future psychological prevention programmes.

Bibliography

Abbey, K.J., Madsen, C.H. & Polland, R. (1989a). Short-term suicide awareness curriculum. *Suicide and Life-Threatening Behavior*, 19, 216–222.*

Abbey, K.J., Madsen, C.H. & Polland, R. (1989b). *Knowledge of Suicide Test (KOST), Suicide Prevention Questionnaire (SPQ)*. (Available from K. Abbey, Florida State University, Tallahassee, Florida, FL 32306.)

Abidin, R. (1983). *Parenting Stress Index*. Charlottesville, VA: Pediatric Psychology Press.

Achenbach, T. (1991). *Integrated Guide for the 1991 CBCL/4–18, YSR and TRF profiles*. Burlington: University of Vermont Department of Psychiatry.

Achenbach, T.M. & Edelbroch, C. (1983). *Manual for the Child Behaviour Checklist and Revised Child Behaviour Profile*. Burlington, VT: University Associates in Psychiatry.

Achenbach, T., Phares, V., Howell, C., Rauh, V. & Nurcombe, B. (1990). Seven-year outcome of the Vermont Intervention Programme for low birth weight infants. *Child Development*, 61, 1672–1681.*

Achenbach, T., Howell, C., Aoki, M. & Rauh, V. (1993). Nine-year outcome of the Vermont Intervention Programme for low birth weight infants. *Paediatrics*, 91, 45–55.*

Affleck, G., Tennen, H., Rowe, J., Roscher, B. & Walker, L. (1989). Effects of formal support on mothers' adaptation to the hospital-to-home transition of high-risk infants: The benefits and costs of helping. *Child Development*, 60, 488–501.*

Agosta, J., Close, D., Hops, H. & Rusch, R. (1980). Treatment of self-injurious behaviour through overcorrection procedures. *Journal of the Association for Persons with Severe Handicaps*, 5(1), 5–12.*

Ahmad, Y., Whitney, I. & Smith, P.K. (1991). A survey service for schools on bully/victim problems. In P.K. Smith & D.A. Thomson (Eds.), *Practical Approaches to Bullying*. London: David Fulton.

Airwise National Heart, Lung and Blood Institute (1985). *Living with Asthma: Manual for Teaching Families the Self-Management of Childhood Asthma*. (NIH Institute Publication no. 85–2364). New York: Airwise.

Alpern, G., Ball, T. & Shearer, M. (1986). *Developmental Profile 2*. Los Angeles: Western Psychological Services.

---

* Indicates that the reference is a primary source and contains a description of one of the 200 studies reviewed in Chapters 2–16.

Alsaker, F. (1996). The impact of puberty. *Journal of Child Psychology and Psychiatry*, 37, 249–258.

American Diabetes Association (1990). *Diabetes Support Group for Young Adults: Facilitators Manual*. Alexandria, VA: American Diabetes Association.

American Lung Association Asthma Advisory Group and Edelman, M. (1997). *American Lung Association: Family Guide to Asthma and Allergies*. New York: Little, Brown.

American National Standards Institute (1989). *Specifications for Audiometers (ANSI)*. New York: Acoustical Society of America.

American Psychiatric Association (APA) (1994). *Diagnostic and Statistical Manual of Mental Disorders* (Fourth Edition) (DSM IV). Washington, DC: APA.

Ammerman, R.T. & Hersen, M. (1997). *Handbook of Prevention and Treatment with Children and Adolescents*. New York: Wiley.

Anderson, B.J., Wolf, F.M., Burkhart, M.T., Cornell, R.G. & Bacon, G.E. (1989). Effects of peer-group intervention on metabolic control of adolescents with IDDM – Randomized outpatient study. *Diabetes Care*, 12(3), 179–183.*

Anderson, C. (1986). A history of the Touch Continuum. In M. Nelson & K. Clark (Eds.), *The Educator's Guide To Preventing Child Sexual Abuse* (pp. 15–25). Santa Cruz, CA: Network Publications.

Anderson, C. & Baumann, A. (1988). *A Parents Guide To Sexual Abuse And The Touch Video*. Minneapolis, MN: Illusion Theatre.

Anderson, C., Morris, B. & Robins, M. (1990). *Touch*. Minneapolis, MN: Illusion Theatre.

Anderson, C., Venier, M. & Roderiquez, J. (1992). *Touch Discussion Guide*. Minneapolis, MN: Illusion Theatre.

Anderson, S., Boignon, S. & Davis, K. (1991). *The Oregon Project for Visually Impaired and Blind Preschool Children*. Medford, OR: Jackson Education Service District.

Andrews, S.R., Blumenthal, J.B., Johnson, D.L., Kahn, A.J., Ferguson, C.J., Lasater, T.M., Malone, P.E. & Wallace, D.B. (1982). The skills of mothering: A study of parent child development centers. *Monographs of the Society for Research in Child Development*, 47, 6.*

Aplasca, M.R., Siegel, D., Mandel, J.S., Santana-Arciaga, R.T., Paul, J., Hudes, E.S., Monzon, T. & Hearst, N. (1995). Results of a model AIDS prevention program for high school students in the Philippines. *AIDS*, 9 (suppl 1), 7–13.*

Arthur, G. (1952). *The Arthur Adaptation of the Leiter International Performance Scale*. Beverly Hills, CA: Psychological Service Center Press.

Auerbach, A. (1968). *Parents Learn Through Discussion: Principles and Practice of Parent Group Education*. New York: Wiley.

Auerbach, A. (1971). *Creating a Preschool Center: Parent Development in an Integrated Neighborhood Project*. New York: Wiley.

Aylward, G., Pfeiffer, S., Wright, A. & Verhulst, S. (1989). Outcome studies of low birth weight infants. Published in the last decade: A meta-analysis. *Journal of Pediatrics*, 115, 515–520.

Badger, E. (1968). *Mothers Training Programme in Educational Intervention by Mothers of Disadvantaged Infants*. Washington, DC: National Institute of Education.

Badger, E. (1971). A mothers' training program – the road to a purposeful existence. *Children*, 18, 168–173.

Badger, E. (1973). *Mother's Guide To Early Learning*. Paoli, PA: McGraw-Hill.

Baer, D., (1993). Quasi-random assignment can be as convincing as random assignment. *American Journal on Mental Retardation*, 97(4), 373–379.

Bailey, A., Phillips, W. & Rutter, M. (1996). Autism: Towards an integration of clinical genetic neuropsychological and neurobiological perspectives. *Journal of Child Psychology and Psychiatry*, 37, 89–126.

Bairstow, P., Cochrane, R. & Rusk, I. (1991). Selection of children with cerebral palsy for conductive education and the characteristics of children judged suitable and unsuitable. *Developmental Medicine and Child Neurology*, 33, 984–992.

Bairstow, P., Cochrane, R. & Hur, J. (1993). *Evaluation of Conductive Education for Children with Cerebral Palsy, Final Report*. HMSO Publications: London.*

Baron-Cohen, S. (1995). *Mindblindness: An Essay on Autism and Theory of Mind*. Cambridge, MA: MIT Press.

Barraga, N. (1980). *Program to Develop Efficiency in Visual Functioning*. Louisville, KY: American Printing House for the Blind.

Barrera, M., Rosenbaum, P. & Cunningham, C. (1986). Early home intervention with low birth weight infants and parents. *Child Development*, 57, 20–33.*

Barry, M. (1996). Physical therapy interventions for patients with movement disorders due to cerebral palsy. *Journal of Child Neurology*, 11, Supplement 1, 51–60.

Barth, R. (1991). An experimental evaluation of in-home child abuse prevention services. *Child Abuse and Neglect*, 15, 363–375.*

Barth, R.P., Blythe, B.J., Schinke, S.T. & Schilling, R.F. (1983). Self-control training with maltreating parents. *Child Welfare*, 4, 313–325.*

Barth, R., Hacking, S. & Ash, J.R. (1988). Preventing child abuse: An experimental evaluation of the Child Parent Enrichment Project. *Journal of Primary Prevention*, 8(4), 201–217.*

Barth, R.P., Fetro, J., Leland, N. & Volkan, K. (1992). Preventing adolescent pregnancy with social and cognitive skills. *Journal of Adolescent Research*, 7(2), 208–232.*

Basmajian, J. & Wolf, S. (1990). *Therapeutic Exercise* (Fifth Edition). Baltimore, MD: Williams & Wilkins.

Bayley, N. (1969) *Bayley Scales of Infant Development*. New York: Psychological Corporation.

Bayley, N. (1993). *Bayley Scales of Infant Development* (Second Edition). New York, NY: Psychological Corporation.

Bayne Smith, M.A. (1994). Teen Incentive Program: Evaluation of a health promotion model for adolescent pregnancy prevention. *Journal of Health Education*, 25, 24–29.*

Beck, A. & Steer, R. (1991). *Beck Scale for Suicide Ideation*. New York: The Psychological Corporation.

Beck, A., Ward, C., Mendelson, M., Mock, J. & Erbaugh, J. (1961). An inventory for measuring depression. *Archives of General Psychiatry*, 4, 561–571.

Beck, A.T., Weissman, A., Lester, D. & Trexler, L. (1974). The measurement of pessimism: The Helplessness Scale. *Journal of Consulting and Clinical Psychology*, 42, 861–865.

Beelman, A. & Brambring, M. (1998). Implementation and effectiveness of a home-based early intervention programme for Blind Children and Preschoolers. *Research in Developmental Disabilities*, 19, 225–244.

Bennett, F. (1987). The effectiveness of early intervention for infants at increased biological risk. In M. Gurlanick & F. Bennett (Eds.), *The Effectiveness of Early*

Intervention for At-Risk and Handicapped Children (pp. 79–109). San Diego, CA: Academic Press.

Bereiter, C. & Engleman, S. (1966). *Teaching Disadvantaged Children in the Preschool.* Englewood Cliffs, NJ: Prentice Hall.

Berlin, L., Brooks-Gunn, J., McCarton, C. & McCormick, M. (1998). The effectiveness of early intervention. Examining the risk factors and pathways to enhanced development. *Preventive Medicine*, 27, 238–245. 1988*

Berliner, L. & Elliott, D. (1996). Sexual abuse of children. In J. Briere, L. Berliner, J. Bulkley, C. Jenny & T. Reid (Eds.), *The APSAC Handbook on Child Maltreatment* (pp. 51–71). Thousand Oaks, CA: Sage.

Berliner, L. & Saunders, B.E. (1996). Treating fear and anxiety in sexually abused children: results of a controlled 2-year follow up study. *Child Maltreatment*, 1, 294–309.*

Berman, A. & Jobes, D. (1993). *Adolescent Suicide: Assessment and Intervention.* Washington, DC: APA.

Bernard-Bonnin, A., Stachenko, S., Bonin, D., Charette, C. & Rousseau, E. (1995). Self-management teaching programs and morbidity of pediatric asthma: A meta-analysis. *Journal of Allergy and Clinical Immunology*, 95 (1), 34–41.

Bernbaum, J. & Batshaw, M. (1997). Born too soon, born too small. In M. Batshaw (Ed.), *Children with Disabilities* (Fourth Edition, pp. 115–139). Baltimore, MD: Brookes.

Bernstein, D.A. & Borkovec, T.D. (1973). *Progressive Relaxation Training: A Manual for the Helping Professions.* Champaign: Research Press.

Besag, V. (1992). *We don't have Bullies Here!.* 57 Manor House Road, Jesmond, Newcastle upon Tyne, NE2 2LY.

Bess, F.H. & Humes, L.E. (1995). *Audiology: The Fundamentals.* Baltimore: Williams & Wilkins.

Birchard, K. (1999). Suicide rates in Ireland continue to rise. *Lancet*, February 27, 1.

Birleson, P., Hudson, I., Buchanan, D. & Wolff, S. (1987). Clinical evaluation of a self-rating scale for depressive disorder in childhood (Depression Self-Rating Scale). *Journal of Child Psychology and Psychiatry*, 28, 43–60.

Birnbrauer, J. & Leach, D. (1993). The Murdoch early intervention program after 2 years. *Behaviour Change*, 10(2), 63–74.*

Blair, C. & Ramey, C. (1997). Early intervention for low birth weight infants and the path to second generation research. In M. Gurlanick (Ed.), *The Effectiveness of Early Intervention* (pp. 77–98). Baltimore, MD: Paul Brookes.

Blind Children Centre (1993). *First Steps: A Handbook for Teaching Young Children who are Visually Impaired.* Los Angeles, CA: Blind Children's Centre.

Bloch, J., Gersten, E. & Kornblum, S. (1980). Evaluation of a language programme for young autistic children. *Journal of Speech and Hearing Disorders*, 45, 76–89.*

Boardway, R.H., Delamater, A.M., Tomakowsky, J. & Gutai, J.P. (1993). Stress management training for adolescents with diabetes. *Journal of Paediatric Psychology*, 18(1), 29–45.*

Bobath, B. & Bobath, K. (1972). Cerebral palsy. In P.H. Pearson & C.E. Williams (Eds.), *Physical Therapy Services in The Developmental Disabilities* (pp. 28–185). Springfield, IL: Charles C. Thomas.

Bobath, K. (1980). *A Neurophysiological Basis for the Treatment of Physiotherapy. Clinics in Developmental Medicine No 75* (Second Edition). Philadelphia, PA: Lippincott.

Botvin, G. (1999). Adolescent drug abuse prevention: Current findings and future directions. In C.R. Hartel & M.D. Glantz (Eds.), *Drug Abuse: Origins and Interventions* (pp. 285–308). Washington, DC: APA Books.

Botvin, G. (2001). Life skills training manuals. Available from Dr Gilbert Botvin, New York Hospital, Cornell University Medical Centre, 1300 York Avenue, New York, NY 10021. *http://www.lifeskillstraining.com/*

Botvin, G., Baker, E., Filazzola, A. & Botvin, E. (1990a). A cognitive-behavioural approach to substance abuse prevention: a one year follow-up. *Addictive Behaviours*, 15, 47–63.*

Botvin, G., Baker, E., Dusenbury, L., Tortu, S. & Botvin, E. (1990b). Preventing adolescent drug abuse through a multimodal cognitive behavioural approach: Results of a three year study. *Journal of Consulting and Clinical Psychology*, 58, 437–446.*

Botvin, G., Schinke, S., Epstein, J. & Diaz, T. (1994). Effectiveness of culturally focused and generic skills training approaches to alcohol and drug abuse prevention among minority youths. *Psychology of Addictive Behaviours*, 8, 116–127.*

Botvin, G., Baker, E., Dusenbury, L., Botvin, E. & Diaz, T. (1995a). Long-term follow-up results of a randomized drug abuse prevention trial in a white middle class population. *Journal of the American Medical Association*, 273, 1106–1112.*

Botvin, G., Schinke, S., Epstein, J., Diaz, T. & Botvin, E. (1995b). Effectiveness of culturally focused and generic skills training approaches to alcohol and drug abuse prevention among minority adolescents: Two year follow-up results. *Psychology of Addictive Behaviours*, 9, 193–194.*

Bower, E., McLellan, D.L., Arney, J. & Campbell, M.J. (1996). A randomised controlled trial of different intensities of physiotherapy and different goal-setting procedures in 44 children with cerebral palsy. *Developmental Medicine and Child Neurology*, 38, 226–237.*

Bower, E., Michell, D., Burnett, M., Campbell, M.J. & McLellan, D.L. (2001). Randomized controlled trial of physiotherapy in 56 children with cerebral palsy followed for 18 months. *Developmental Medicine and Child Neurology*, 43, 4–15.*

Boyce, G.C., Smith, T.B. & Casto, G. (1999). Health and educational outcomes of children who experienced severe neonatal medical complications. *Journal of Genetic Psychology*, 160(3), 261–269.

Boyer, C.B., Shafer, M. & Tschann, J.M. (1997). Evaluation of a knowledge- and cognitive–behavioural skills building intervention to prevent STDs and HIV infection in high school students. *Adolescence*, 32(125), 25–42.*

Bradley, C. (1994). *Handbook of Psychology and Diabetes*. Chur, Switzerland: Harwood.

Bradley, R.H. & Caldwell, B.M. (1977). Home Observation for Measurement of the Environment: A validation study of screening efficiency. *American Journal of Mental Deficiency*, 81, 417–420.

Brambring, M. (1989). Methodological and conceptual issues in the construction of a developmental test for blind infants and preschoolers. In M. Brambring, F. Losel & H. Skowronek (Eds.), *Children at risk: Assessment, Longitudinal Research, and Intervention* (pp. 136–154). Berlin, NY: de Gruyter.

Brazelton, T.B., (1973). Neonatal Behavioural Assessment Scale. *Clinics in Developmental Medicine*, 50. Philadelphia: Lippincott Company.

Breener, N., Collins, J., Kann, L. & Warren, C. (1995). Reliability of the Youth Risk Behaviour Survey Questionnaire. *Journal of School Health*, 141(6), 575–580.

Bregman, J. & Gerdtz, J. (1997). Behavioural interventions. In D. Cohen & F. Volk-mar (Eds.), *Handbook of Autism and Pervasive Developmental Disorders* (Second Edition, pp. 606–631). New York: Wiley.

Brent, D. (1997). The aftercare of adolescents with deliberate self-harm. *Journal of Child Psychology and Psychiatry*, 38, 277–286.

Briere, J., Berliner, L., Bulkley, J., Jenny, C. & Reid, T. (1996). *The APSAC Handbook on Child Maltreatment*. Thousand Oaks, CA: Sage.

Bromwich, R. (1983). *Parent Behaviour Progression*. Unpublished manual, California State University, Northridge, CA.

Brooks-Gunn, J., McCarton, C., Casey, P.H., McCormick, M.C., Bauer, C.R., Bern-baum, J.C., Tyson, J., Swanson, H., Bennett, F.C., Scott, D.T., Tonascia, J. & Mein-ert, C.L. (1994). Early intervention in low-birth weight premature infants. Results through age 5 from the Infant Health and Development Program. *Journal of the American Medical Association*, 272, 1257–1262.*

Brown, L., Lourie, K. & Pao, M. (2000). Children and adolescents living with HIV and AIDS. *Journal of Child Psychology and Psychiatry*, 41, 81–96.

Brown, P. (1972). *Parental Information and Attitude Scale For Parents of Hearing-Impaired Children*. Washington, DC: Gallaudet College.

Browne, D. & Peterson, L. (1997). Unintentional injury and child abuse and neglect. In R.T. Ammerman & M. Hersen (Eds.), *Handbook of Prevention and Treatment with Children and Adolescents* (pp. 332–356). New York: Wiley.

Browne, K. & Herbert, M. (1997). *Preventing Family Violence*. Chichester: Wiley.

Bryant, D. & Ramey, C. (1987). An analysis of the effectiveness of early intervention programs for environmentally at-risk children. In M. Guralnick & F. Bennett (Eds.), *The Effectiveness of Early Intervention for At-risk and Handicapped Children* (pp. 33–78). San Diego, CA: Academic Press.

Bryant, D. & Maxwell, K. (1997). The effectiveness of early intervention for disadvan-taged children. In M. Guralnick (Ed.), *The Effectiveness of Early Intervention* (pp. 23–46). Baltimore, MD: Brooks.

Buchanan, N., Cooper, J. & McQuitty, P. (1995). *Childhood Asthma: What it is and what you can do?* Berkeley, C.A: Ten Speed Press.

Burch, G. & Mohr, V. (1980). Evaluating a child abuse intervention program. *Social Casework: The Journal of Contemporary Social Work*, 1980, Feb., 90–99.*

Caceres, C.F., Rosasco, A.M., Mandel, J.S. & Hearst, N. (1994). Evaluating a school-based intervention for STD/AIDS prevention in Peru. *Journal of Adolescent Health*, 15, 582–591.*

Calgary Communities Against Sexual Assault (1995). *Who Do you Tell Programme*. Calgary, Alberta, Canada: Author.

Calderon, R. & Greenberg, M.T. (1997). The effectiveness of early intervention for deaf children and children with hearing loss. In M. Guralnick, *The Effectiveness of Early Intervention*. (pp. 455–482) Baltimore, MD: Brookes.

Caldwell, B. (1970). *Cooperative Preschool Inventory: Revised edition*. Menlo Park, CA: Addison-Wesley.

Caldwell B. & Bradley, R. (1979). *Home Observation for Measurement of the Environ-ment (HOME)*. Little Rock, AK: University of Arkansas.

Caldwell, B. & Bradley, R. (1985). *Home Observation for Measurement of the Environment*. New York: Dorsey Press.

Campbell, F. & Ramey, C. (1994). Effects of early intervention in intellectual and academic achievement: A follow-up study of children from low income families. *Child Development*, 65, 684–698.

Campbell, F. & Ramey, C. (1995). Cognitive and school outcomes for high risk African American students at middle adolescence: Positive effects of early intervention. *American Educational Research Journal*, 32, 743–772.

Campbell, R.V & Lutzker, J.R. (1993). Using functional equivalence training to reduce severe challenging behavior: A case study. *Journal of Developmental and Physical Disabilities*, 5(3), 203–216.*

Campbell, T. & Patterson, J. (1995). The effectiveness of family interventions in the treatment of physical illness. *Journal of Marital and Family Therapy*, 21, 545–583.

Capute, A. & Shapiro, B. (1985). The motor quotient: A method for the early detection of motor delay. *American Journal of Disability in Children*, 139, 940–941.

Carey, M., Morrison-Beedy, D. & Johnson, B. (1997). The HIV Knowledge Questionnaire: Development and evaluation of a reliable, valid and practical self-administered questionnaire. *AIDS and Behaviour*, 1, 61–74.

Carey, W. (1970). A simplified method for measuring infant temperament. *Journal of Pediatrics*, 77, 188–194.

Carney, A.E. & Moeller, M.P. (1998). Treatment efficacy: hearing loss in children. *Journal of Speech, Language and Hearing Research*, 41, 61–84.

Carr, A. (1999). *Handbook of Child and Adolescent Clinical Psychology: A Contextual Approach*. London: Routledge.

Carr, A. (2000). *What Works with Children and Adolescents? A Critical Review of Research on Psychological Interventions with Children, Adolescents and their Families*. London: Routledge.

Carr, A. (2001a). *Preventing Risky Sexual Behaviour in Adolescence*. Leicester, UK: British Psychological Society.

Carr, A. (2001b). *Depression and Attempted Suicide in Adolescence*. Leicester: British Psychological Society.

Carr, A. (2001c). Fathers in family therapy: Lessons from research. In A. Carr (Ed.), *Family Therapy: Readings on Theory, Practice and Research* (pp. 87–106). Wales: Edwin Mellen Press.

Carr, E.G. & Durand, V.M. (1985). Reducing behaviour problems through functional communication training. *Journal of Applied Behavior Analysis*, 28, 111–126.

Carr, E., Robinson, S., Taylor, J. & Carlson, J. (1990). Positive approaches to the treatment of severe behaviour problems in persons with developmental disabilities. A review and analysis of reinforcement based procedures. *Monograph of the Association For Persons with Severe Handicap No. 4* (ERIC Document Reproduction Service No ED 330151).

Carr, E., Levin, L., McConnachie, G., Carlson, J., Kemp, D. & Smith, C. (1994). *Communication Based Intervention for Problem Behaviour. A Users Guide for Producing Postive Change*. Baltimore, MD: Paul H. Brookes.

Carroll, C., Miltenberger, R. & O'Neill, H. (1992). A review and critique of research evaluating child sexual abuse prevention programs. *Education and Treatment of Children*, 15(4), 335–354.

Carter, M. & Ward, J. (1987). Use of overcorrection to suppress self-injurious behaviour. *New Zealand Journal of Developmental Disabilities*, 13(4), 227–242.

Casey, P., Kelleher, K., Bradley, R., Kellogg, K., Kirby, R. & Whiteside, L. (1994). A multifaceted intervention for infants with failure to thrive. A prospective study. *Archives of Pediatric and Adolescent Medicine*, 148(10), 1071–1077.

Castes, M., Hagel, I., Palenque, M., Canelores, P., Carao, A. & Lynch, N.R. (1999). Immunological changes associated with clinical improvement of asthmatic children subjected to psychosocial interventions. *Brain, Behavior and Immunity*, 13, 1–13.*

Catanese, A.A., Coleman, G.J., King, J.A. & Reddihough, D.S. (1995). Evaluation of an early childhood programme based on the principles of conductive education: The Yooralla Project. *Journal of Paediatric Child Health*, 31, 418–422.*

Catania, J., Kegeles, S. & Coates, T. (1990). Towards an understanding of risk behaviour. An AIDS risk reduction model ARRM. *Health Education Quarterly*, 17, 53–72.

Cattell, P. (1960). *The Measurement of Intelligence of Infants and Young Children (Revised Edition)*. New York: Johnson Reprint.

Centers for Disease Control (1992). *Youth Suicide Prevention Programs: A Resource Guide*. Atlanta, GA: Centers for Disease Control.

Central Television (1990). *Sticks and Stones*. Community Unit, Central Television, Broad Street, Birmingham.

Chen, D., Friedman, C.T. & Calvello, G. (1991). *Learning Together: A Parent Guide to Socially-based Routines for Visually Impaired Infants*. Unpublished guide of the PAVII-project.

Choi, K.H. & Coates, T.J. (1994). Prevention of HIV infection. *AIDS*, 8, 1371–1389.

Chou, C., Montgomery, S., Pentz, M., Rohrbach, L., Johnson, C., Flay, B. & MacKinnon, D. (1998). Effects of a community based prevention program on decreasing drug use in high risk adolescents. *American Journal of Public Health*, 88, 944–948.*

Ciffone, J. (1993). Suicide prevention: A classroom presentation to adolescents. *Social Work*, 38, 196–203.*

Clark, S.L. (2000). *Group Facilitator Manual for Taming Worry Dragons: A Manual for Children, Parents, and other Coaches*. Vancouver, British Columbia: British Columbia Children's Hospital.

Clarke, E.A. & Kiselica, C. (1997). A systematic counselling approach to the problem of bullying. *Elementary School Guidance and Counselling*, 31, 310–325.

Clarke, G., Lewinsohn, P. & Hops, H. (2000). *Leader's Manual for Adolescent Groups. Adolescent Coping with Depression Course*. Portland, OR: Center for Health Research. *http://www.kpchr.org/*

Clarke, G., Lewinsohn, P. & Hops, H. (2000). *Students' Workbook. Adolescent Coping with Depression Course*. Portland, OR: Center for Health Research. *http://www.kpchr.org/*.

Clark-Stewart, K. (1973). Interactions between mothers and their young children: Characteristics and consequences. *Monograph of Social Research on Child Development*, 153, 1–100.

Classen, C., Kooperman, C., Hales, R. & Spiegel, D. (1998). Acute stress disorder as a predictor of posttraumatic stress symptoms. *American Journal of Psychiatry*, 155, 620–624. (Contains the revised version of the Stanford Acute Stress Reaction Questionnaire, SARSQ.)

Coco, N. & Sharpe, L. (1993). An auditory variant of eye-movement desensitization in cases of childhood post-traumatic stress disorder. *Journal of Behaviour Therapy and Experimental Psychiatry*, 24, 373–377.

Coen, E., Huser, J., Beach, D. & Rappaport, J. (1970). Parents' perceptions of their young children and their relationship to indexes of adjustment. *Journal of Consulting and Clinical Psychology*, 34, 97–103.

Cohen, D. & Volkmar, F. (1997). *Handbook of Autism and Pervasive Developmental Disorders* (Second Edition). New York: Wiley.

Cohen, J. & Mannarino, A. (1993). A treatment model for sexually abused preschoolers. *Journal of Interpersonal Violence*, 8, 115–131.

Cohen, J. & Mannarino, A. (1996). A treatment outcome study for sexually abused preschool children: Initial findings. *Journal of the American Academy of Child and Adolescent Psychiatry*, 35, 42–50.*

Cohen, J. & Mannarino, A. (1997). A treatment study for sexually abused preschool children: outcome during a one year follow-up. *Journal of the American Academy of Child and Adolescent Psychiatry*, 36, 1228–1235.*

Cohen, J. & Mannarino, A. (1998). Interventions for sexually abused children: initial treatment findings. *Child Maltreatment*, 3, 17–26.*

Cohen, Y., Spirito, A. & Brown, L. (1996). Suicide and suicidal behaviour. In R. Di Clemente, W. Hansen & L. Ponton (Eds.), *Handbook of Adolescent Health Risk Behaviour* (pp. 193–224). New York: Plenum.

Coleman, G.J., King, J.A. & Reddihough, D.S. (1995). A pilot evaluation of conductive education-based intervention for children with cerebral palsy: The Tongala Project. *Journal of Paediatric Child Health*, 31, 412–417.*

Coleman, J. (1995). *Teenagers and Sexuality*. London: Hodder and Stoughton.

Coleman, J. & Roker, D. (1998). *Teenage Sexuality: Health Risk and Education*. Amsterdam: Harwood.

Coley, R. & Chase-Lansdale, P. (1998). Adolescent pregnancy and parenthood: Recent evidence and future directions. *American Psychologist*, 53, 152–166.

Colland, V. (1993). Learning to cope with asthma: A behavioral self management program for children. *Patient Education and Counselling*, 22, 141–152.*

Colland, V. & Fournier, E. (1990). The Asthma Coping Test. *Gedrag Gezondheid*, 18, 68–77.

Committee for Children (1983). *Talking About Touching: A Personal Safety Curriculum*. (Available from Committee for Children, PO Box 15190, Seattle, WA98115.)

Condon, R. (1979). Pre-language Development: Communication training for the deaf-blind. In O. Peak (Ed.), *Educational Methods for Deaf-blind and Severely Handicapped Students*, Volume 1 (pp. 125–134). Austin, TX: Texas Education Agency, Department of Special Education, Special Education Developmental Services Centre for Deaf-Blind.

Conte, J., (1985). An evaluation of a program to prevent the sexual victimisation of young children. *Child Abuse and Neglect*, 9, 319–328.*

Coolman, R., Bennett, F., Sells, C., Sweanson, M., Andrews, M. & Robinson N. (1985). Neuromotor development of graduates of the neonatal intensive care unit. Patterns encountered in the first two years of life. *Journal of Developmental and Behavioural Pediatrics*, 6, 327–333.

Copeland, M.E. & Copans, S.M. (1998). *The Adolescent Depression Workbook*. New Harbinger Publications.

Corcoran, C. (1987). *Take Care. Preventing Child Sexual Abuse – A Handbook For Parents*. Dublin: Poolbeg Press.

Cormack, C. & Carr, A. (2000). Chapter 7. Drug abuse. In A. Carr (Ed.), *What Works with Children and Adolescents? A Critical Review of Psychological Interventions with Children, Adolescents and Their Families* (pp. 155–177). London: Routledge.

Cox, D.J. & Gonder-Frederick, L. (1992). Major developments in behavioural diabetes research. *Journal of Consulting and Clinical Psychology*, 60(4), 628–638.

Crabtree, C.R. (1990). *When Friends are Hurting.* (Available from C.R. Crabtree, Texas Tech University, Department of Sociology, Anthropology, and Social Work, P.O. Box 41012, Lubbock, TX, 79409–1012, USA.)

Creer, T.L. & Levstek, D. (1997). Adherence to asthma regimens. In D.S. Gochman (Ed.), *Handbook of Health Behavior Research II: Provider Determinants* (pp. 131–148). New York: Plenum Press.

Creer, T.L., Marion, R.J. & Creer, P.P. (1983). Asthma problem behavior checklist: Parental perceptions of the behavior of asthmatic children. *Journal of Asthma,* 20(2), 97–104.

D'Angelo, L. & Di Clemente, R. (1996). Sexually transmitted diseases including Human Immunodeficiency Virus Infection. In R. Di Clemente, W. Hansen & L. Ponton (Eds.), *Handbook of Adolescent Health Risk Behaviour* (pp. 333–367). New York: Plenum.

Dadds, M.R., Spence, S.H., Holland, D.E., Barrett, P.M. & Laurens, K.R. (1997). Prevention and early intervention for anxiety disorders: A controlled trial. *Journal of Consulting and Clinical Psychology,* 65, 627–635.

Dahl, J., Gustaffson, D. & Melin, L. (1990). Effects of a behavioral treatment program on children with asthma. *Journal of Asthma,* 27 (1), 41–46.*

Davidson, P. & Harrison, G. (1997). The effectiveness of early intervention for children with visual impairments. In M. Guralnick (Ed.), *The Effectiveness of Early Intervention* (pp. 483–495). Baltimore: Brookes.

Davis, C. (1980). *Perkins–Binet Tests of Intelligence for the Blind.* Watertown, MA: Perkins School for the Blind.

Dawson, G. & Osterling, J. (1997). Early intervention in autism. In M.J. Guralnick (Ed.), *The Effectiveness of Early Intervention.* (pp. 307–326). Baltimore: Brookes.

DCCT (Diabetes Control and Complications Trial Research Group) (1994). Effect of intensive diabetes treatment on the development and progression of long-term complications in adolescents with insulin-dependent diabetes mellitus: Diabetes Control and Complications Trial. *Journal of Paediatrics,* 125(2), 177–188.

Deblinger, E. & Hefin, A.H. (1996). *Treating Sexually Abused Children And Their Non-Offending Parents: A Cognitive Behavioural Approach.* Thousand Oaks, CA: Sage.

Deblinger, E., Lippmann, J. & Steer, R. (1996). Sexually abused children suffering posttraumatic stress symptoms: initial treatment outcome findings. *Child Maltreatment,* 1, 310–321.*

Delamater, A.M., Bubb, J., Davis, S., Smith, J.A., Schmidt, L., White, N.H. & Santiago, J.V. (1990). Randomized prospective study of self-management training with newly diagnosed diabetic children. *Diabetes Care,* 13(5), 492–498.*

Delamater, A.M., Smith, J.A., Bubb, J., Davis, S.G., Gamble, T., White, N.H. & Santiago, J.V. (1991). Family based behavior therapy for diabetic adolescents. In J. Johnson & S. Johnson (Eds.), *Advances in Child Health Psychology* (pp. 100–120). Florida: University of Florida Press/Gainesville.

Department of Education (1994). *Don't Suffer in Silence. An Anti-bullying Pack for Schools.* London: HMSO. Resource pack and video based on the Sheffield Project Available from the Department of Education, London, UK.

Deutsch, M., Deutsch, C.P., Jordan, T.J. & Grallo, R. (1983). The IDS programme: An experiment in early and sustained enrichment. In The Consortium for Longitudinal Studies (Eds.), *As The Twig Is Bent . . . Lasting Effects Of Pre-School Programmes.* (pp. 377–410)., Hillsdale, NJ: Lawrence Erlbaum Associates Inc.*

Di Clemente, R. & Peterson, J. (1994). *Preventing Aids: Theories, Methods and Behavioural Interventions*. New York: Plenum.

Di Clemente, R.J., Pies, C.A., Stoller, E.J., Straits, C., Olivia, G.E., Haskin, J. & Rutherford, G.W. (1989). Evaluation of school-based AIDS education curricula in San Francisco. *Journal of Sex Research*, 26(2), 188–198.*

Di Clemente, R., Hansen, W. & Ponton, L. (1996), *Handbook of Adolescent Health Risk Behaviour*. New York: Plenum.

Didden, R., Duker, P.C. & Korzilius, H. (1997). Meta-analytic study on treatment effectiveness for problem behaviors with individuals who have mental retardation. *American Journal of Mental Retardation*, 101(4), 387–399.

Dolan Savage, E. (1996). *Winning over Asthma*. Amherst, MA: Pedipress.

Doll, E. (1965). *Vineland Social Maturity Scale*. Circle Pines, MN: American Guidance Service.

Duesenbury, L. & Falco, M. (1997). School based drug abuse prevention strategies. From research to policy to practice. In P. Weissberg, T. Gullotta, R. Hamptom, B. Ryan & G. Adams (Eds.), *Enhancing Children's Wellness* (pp. 47–75). Thousand Oaks, CA: Sage.

Duker, P.C., Didden, R., Korzilius, H. et al. (1996). Database problem behavior: a literature retrieval system for professionals dealing with problem behaviours of individuals with intellectual disabilities. *International Journal of Disability, Development and Education*, 43(3), 197–202.

Dunn, L.M. (1965) *Peabody Picture Vocabulary Test Manual*. Minneapolis, MN: American Guidance Service.

Dunn, L.M., Chun, L.T., Crowell, D.C., Dunn, L.M., Alexy, L.G. & Yachel, E.R. (1976). *Peabody Early Experience Kit*. Circle Pines, MN: American Guidance Services.

Durand, V.M. (1990). *Severe Behaviour Problems: A Functional Communication Training Approach*. New York: Guilford.

Durand, V.M. (1993). Functional communication training using assistive devices: effects on challenging behavior and affect. *Augmentative and Alternative Communication*. 9, 168–178.*

Durand, V.M. & Crimmins, D. (1992). *Motivation Assessment Scale*. Topeka, KS: Monaco & Associates.

Eggleston, P. (1999). Asthma. In J. McMillan, C. DeAngelis, R. Feigin & J. Warshaw (Eds.), *Oski's Pediatrics: Principles and Practice* (Third Edition, pp. 2041–2048). Philadelphia, PA: Lippincott, Williams & Wilkins.

Eilers, R.E., Fishmna, L.M., Oller, D.K. & Steffens, M.L. (1993). Tactile vocoders as aids to speech production in young hearing-impaired children. *Volta Review*, 95, 265–293.

Elias, M., Larcen, S.W., Zlotwow, S.P. & Chinsky, J.H. (1978). An innovative measure of children's cognition in problematic interpersonal situations. Paper presented at the American Psychological Association; Totonto, Canada.

Elliott, M. (1994). *Bullying: A Practical Guide to Coping for Schools*. Harlow: Longman.

Ellis, C.R., Singh, Y.N. & Singh, N. (1997). Use of behavior modifying drugs. In N. Singh (Ed.), *Prevention and Treatment of Severe Behavior Problems: Models and Methods in Developmental Disabilities*. Pacific Grove: Brooks/Cole.

Emerson, E. (1995). *Challenging Behaviour: Analysis and Intervention in People with Learning Disabilities*. Cambridge: University Press.

ETR Associates (1998). *Safer Choices: Preventing HIV, Other STD and Pregnancy.* Santa Cruz, CA: ETR Associates.

Evans, P.M. & Alberman, E. (1985). Recording motor defects of children with cerebral palsy. *Developmental Medicine and Child Neurology,* 27, 401–406.

Farrell, M. & Taylor. E. (1994). Drug and alcohol use and misuse. In M. Rutter, E. Taylor & L. Hersov (Eds.), *Child and Adolescent Psychiatry: Modern Approaches* (Third Edition, pp. 529–545). Oxford: Blackwell.

Farrington, D.P. (1993) Understanding and preventing bullying. In M. Tonry & N. Morris (Eds.), *Crime and Justice: An annual review of research,* Vol. 17. Chicago: University of Chicago Press.

Fawole, I.O., Asuzu, M.C., Oduntan, O. & Brieger, W.R. (1999). A school-based AIDS education programme for secondary school students in Nigeria: a review of effectiveness. *Health Education Research Theory and Practice,* 14(5), 675–683.*

Fenske, E., Stanley, Z., Krantz, P. & McClannahan, L. (1985). Age at intervention and treatment outcome for autistic children in a comprehensive intervention program. *Analysis and Intervention in Developmental Disabilities,* 5, 49–58.*

Ferrell, K. (1985). *Reach out and Teach. Materials for Parents of Visually Handicapped and Multihandicapped Young Children.* New York, NY: American Foundation for the Blind.

Field, T., Widmayer, S., Greenberg, R. & Stoller, S. (1982). Effects of parent training on teenage mothers and their infants. *Paediatrics,* 69, 703–707.*

Field, T., Schanberg, S., Scafidi, E., Bauer, C., Vega-Lahr, N., Garcia, R., Nystrom, J. & Kuhn, C. (1986). Tactile/kinesthetic stimulation effects of preterm neonates. *Pediatrics,* 77, 654–658.*

Film Fair Communications (1979). *Better Safe than Sorry II.* Ventura, CA. Author. (Available from Film Fair Communications, 900 Ventura Blvd, Box 1278, Studio, CA, 91604.)

Finkelhor, D. (1984). *Child Sexual Abuse: New Research and Theory.* New York: Free Press.

Finkelhor, D. & Dziuba-Leatherman, J. (1995). Victimization prevention programmes: A national survey of children's exposure and reactions. *Child Abuse and Neglect,* 19, 129–139.

Finkelhor, D. & Strapko, N. (1992). Sexual abuse prevention education: A review of evaluation studies. In D. Willis, E. Holden & M. Rosenberg (Eds.), *Child Abuse Prevention.* New York: John Wiley.

Fireman, P., Friday, G.A., Gira, C., Viertaler, W.A. & Michaels, L. (1981). Teaching self management skills to asthmatic children and their parents in an ambulatory care setting. *Pediatrics, 68* (3), 341–345.*

Fisher, W.W., Adelinis, J.D., Thompson, R.H. et al. (1998). Functional analysis and treatment of destructive behavior maintained by termination of 'don't' (and symmetrical 'do') requests. *Journal of Applied Behaviour Analysis,* 31, 339–356.*

Fletcher, K. (1997). The Childhood PTSD Interview-Child Form. In E. Carlson (Ed.), *Trauma Assessments: A Clinician's Guide* (pp. 248–250). New York: Guilford Press.

Foa, E.B. & Meadows, E.A. (1997). Psychological treatments for post-traumatic stress disorder: a critical review. *Annual Review of Psychology,* 48, 449–480.

Folio, R., Fewell, R. & Dubose, R.F. (1983). *Peabody Developmental Motor Scales.* Toronto: Teaching Resources Co.

Fonagy, P. & Moran, G.S. (1990). Studies of the efficacy of child psychoanalysis. *Journal of Consulting and Clinical Psychology,* 58 (6), 684–695.*

Ford, J.D. & Rogers, K. (1997). Empirically based assessment of trauma and PTSD with children and adolescents. In: *Proceedings From the International Society of Traumatic Stress Studies Annual Meeting*, Montreal, November, 1997. (Contains the Traumatic Events Screening Inventory for Children (TESI-C).)

Forehand, B. & McMahon, R. (1981). *Helping the Non-compliant Child: A Clinician's Guide to Parent Training*. New York: Guilford.

Fraiberg, S. (1977). *Insights from the Blind: Comparative Studies of Blind and Sighted Children*. New York: Basic Books.

Frankenburg, W.K., Dodds, J.B. & Fandal, A.W. (1970). *The Denver Developmental Screening Test Manual (Revised)*. Denver, CO: University of Colorado Medical Centre.

Franklin, C., Grant, D., Corcoran, J., Miller, P.O. & Bultman, L. (1997). Effectiveness of prevention programs for adolescent pregnancy: A meta-analysis. *Journal of Marriage and the Family*, 59, 551–567.

Freeman, N. (1985). *The Deaf-blind Baby: A Programme of Care*: London: William Heinemann Medical Books.

Freeman, R., Carbin, C. & Boese, R. (1981). *Can't your Child Hear?: A Guide for those who Care about Deaf Children*. Baltimore, MD: University Park Press.

French, J.L. (1964). *The Pictorial Test of Intelligence*. Boston: Houghton Mifflin.

Friedrich, W.N., Grambsch, P., Damon, L., Hewitt, S.K., Koverola, C., Lang, R.A., Wolfe, V. & Broughton, D. (1992). The Child Sexual Behaviour Inventory: Normative and clinical comparisons. *Psychological Assessment*, 4, 303–311.

Friedrich, W.N., Greenberg, M.T. & Crnic, K. (1983). A short form of the Questionnaire on Resources and Stress. *American Journal of Mental Deficiency*, 88, 41–48.

Frith, U. & Happé, F. (1994). Autism: Beyond 'Theory of mind'. *Cognition*, 50, 115–132.

Frostig, M. & Horne, D. (1964), *The Frostig Program for the Development of Visual Perception*. Chicago: Follett.

Fryer, Jr, G.E., Kraizer, S.K. & Miyoshi, T. (1987a). Measuring actual reduction of risk to child abuse: a new approach. *Child Abuse and Neglect*, 11, 173–179.*

Fryer, Jr, G.E., Kraizer, S.K. & Miyoshi, T. (1987b). Measuring children's retention of skills to resist stranger abduction: use of the simulation technique. *Child Abuse and Neglect*, 11, 181–185.*

Galante, R. & Foa, D. (1986). An epidemiological study of psychic trauma and treatment effectiveness for children after a natural disaster. *Journal of the American Academy of Child Psychiatry*, 25, No. 3, 357–363.*

Galatzer, A., Amir, S., Gil, R., Karp, M. & Laron, Z. (1982). Crisis intervention program in newly diagnosed diabetic children. *Diabetes Care*, 5(4), 414–419.*

Garber, H.L. (1988). *The Milwaukee Project: Preventing Mental Retardation in Children At Risk*. Washington, DC: American Association on Mental Retardation.*

Garland, A., Shaffer, D. & Whittle, B. (1989). A national survey of school-based suicide prevention programs. *Journal of the American Academy of Child and Adolescent Psychiatry*, 28(6), 931–934.

Garland, A. & Zigler, E. (1993). Adolescent suicide prevention: Current research and social policy implications. *American Psychologist*, 48(2), 169–182.

Garland, E.J. & Clark, S.L. (1996). *Taming Worry Dragons: A Manual for Children, Parents and other Coaches*. Vancouver, British Columbia: British Columbia Children's Hospital.

Garretson, M. (1994). *Deafness: Life and Culture*. Silver Spring, MD: National Association of the Deaf.

Gebert, N., Hümmelink, R., Könnig, J., Staab, D., Schmidt, S., Szczepanski, R., Runde, B. & Wahn, U. (1998). Efficacy of a self management program for childhood asthma: A prospective study. *Patient, Education and Counseling*, 35, 213–220.*

Geers, A.E., Kuehn, G. & Moog, J.S. (1981). 'Evaluation and Results' in EPIC-Experimental Project in Instructional Concentration. *American Annals of the Deaf*, 126, 8.

Gelles, F. (1987). *The Violent Home* (Updated edition). Beverly Hills, CA: Sage.

Gersten, E.L. (1976). A Health Resources Inventory: The development of a measure of personal and social competence of primary grade children. *Journal of Consulting and Clinical Psychology*, 44, 775–786.

Gesell Institute of Human Development (1985). *Gesell Development Schedules*. New Haven, CT: Author.

Gillberg, C. & Coleman, M. (2000). *The Biology of Autistic Syndromes* (Third Edition). London: MacKeith Press.

Gilliam, J. (1991). *Gilliam Autism Rating Scale*. Odessa, FL: Psychological Assessment Resources. (PAR, PO Box 998, Odessa, Florida, 33556.)

Giovacchini, P. (1983). *The Urge to Die: Why Young People Commit Suicide*. New York: Penguin.

Goenjian, A.K., Karayan, I., Pynoos, R.S., Minassian, B.S., Najarian, L.M., Steinberg, A.M. & Faribanks, L.A. (1997). Outcome of psychotherapy among early adolescents after trauma. *American Journal of Psychiatry*, 154, 536–542.*

Gonen, B., Rubenstein, A., Rochman, H. et al. (1977). Haemoglobin A1: An indicator of the metabolic control of diabetic patients. *Lancet*, ii. 734–737.

Goodman, M., Rothberg, A., Houston-Mcmillan, J., Cooper, P.A., Cartwright, J.D. & Van Der Velde, M.A. (1985). Effect of early neurodevelopmental therapy in normal and at risk survivors of neonatal intensive care. *Lancet*, ii, 1327–1330.*

Goodman, R. (1994). Brain disorders. In M. Rutter, E. Taylor & L. Hersov (Eds.), *Child and Adolescent Psychiatry: Modern Approaches*. (Third Edition, pp. 172–190). London: Blackwell.

Gordon, I.J. (1970). *Baby Learning Through Baby Play*. New York: St Martin's Press.

Gordon, I. & Lally, R. (1967). *Intellectual Stimulation for Infants and Toddlers*. Gainsville, FA: Institute of Development of Human Resources.

Gordon, I.J., Guinagh, B.J. & Jester, R.E. (1972). *Child Learning Through Play*. New York: St Martin's Press.

Grandin, T. & Scariano, M. (1986). *Emergence, Labelled Autistic*. London: Costello. (Biographical account of autism.)

Gray, J., Cutler, C., Dean, J. & Kempe, C. H. (1979). Prediction and prevention of child abuse and neglect. *Journal of Social Issues*, 35, 127–139.*

Gray, S. & Klaus, R. (1965). An experimental preschool program for culturally deprived children. *Child Development*, 36, 887–898.*

Gray, S. & Klaus, R. (1970). The early training project: A seventh-year report. *Child Development*, 41, 909–924.*

Greco, P., La Greca, A.M., Auslander, W.F., Speter, D., Skyler, J.S., Fisher, E. & Santiago, J.V. (1990). Assessing adherence in IDDM: A comparison of two methods. *Diabetes*, 40 (Suppl. 3), 108A (abstract).

Green, G. (1996). Early behavioral intervention for autism. What does the research tell us? In C. Maurice (Ed.), *Behavioral Intervention for Young Children with Autism* (pp. 29–44). Austin, TX: Pro-Ed.

Greenberg, M. (1983). Family stress and child competence: The effects of early intervention for families with deaf infants. *American Annals of the Deaf*, 128, 407–417.*

Greenberg, M. & Kusche, C. (1993). *Promoting Social and Emotional Development of Deaf Children: The PATHS Project*. Seattle: Washington Press.*

Greenberg, M. & Kusche, C. (1998). Preventative intervention for school age deaf children. The PATHS curriculum. *Journal of Deaf Studies and Deaf Education*, 13(1), 49–63.

Greenberg, M., Calderon, R. & Kusche, C. (1984). Early intervention using simultaneous communication with deaf infants. The effects on communicative development. *Child Development*, 55, 607–616.*

Greenberg, P. & Epstein, B. (1973). *Bridges to Reading*. Morristown, NJ: General Learning Corp.

Greenwald, R. (1994). Applying eye-movement desensitization and reprocessing (EMDR) to the treatment of traumatized children: five case studies. *Anxiety Disorders Practice Journal*, 1, 83–97.

Gresham, F. & MacMillan, D. (1998). Early Intervention Project: Can its claims be substantiated and its effects replicated? *Journal of Autism and Developmental Disorders*, 28(1), 5–13.

Grey, M., Boland, E., Davidson, M., Yu, C., Sullivan-Bolyai, S. & Tamborlane, W.V. (1998). Short-term effects of coping skills training as adjunct to intensive therapy in adolescents. *Diabetes Care*, 21(6), 902–908.*

Grey, M., Kanner, S. & Lacey, K.O. (1999). Characteristics of the Learner: Children and adolescents. *The Diabetes Educator*, 25 (6), (suppl), 25–33.

Grey, M., Boland, E.A., Davidson, M. & Tamborlane, W.V. (2000). Coping skills training for youth with diabetes mellitus has long-lasting effects on metabolic control and quality of life. *Journal of Paediatrics*, 137(1), 107–113.*

Griffiths, R. (1954). *The Abilities of Babies: A Study in Mental Measurement*. Thetford, Norfolk: Lowe and Brydone for The Association For Research in Infant and Child Development.

Grossman, H.Y., Brink, S. & Hauser, S.T. (1987). Self-efficacy in adolescent girls and boys with insulin-dependent diabetes mellitus. *Diabetes Care*, 10, 324–329.

Group for the Advancement of Psychiatry (1996). *Adolescent Suicide*. Report No. 140. Washington, DC: APA.

Guralnick, M. (1997). *The Effectiveness of Early Intervention*. Baltimore: Brookes.

Guralnick, M.J. (1998). Effectiveness of early intervention for vulnerable children: A developmental perspective. *American Journal on Mental Retardation*, 102, 4, 319–345.

Guralnick, M. & Bennet, F. (1987). *The Effectiveness of Early Intervention for at Risk and Handicapped Children*. New York: Academic Press.

Gustaffson, P.A., Kjellman, N-I.M. & Cederblad, M. (1986). Family therapy in the treatment of severe childhood asthma. *Journal of Psychosomatic Research*, 30 (3), 369–374.*

Gutelius, M.F., Kirsch, A.D., MacDonald, S., Brooks, M.R., McErlean, T. & Newcomb, C. (1972). Promising results from a cognitive stimulation program in infancy. *Clinical Pediatrics*, 11, 585–593.*

Guterman, N. (1997). Early prevention of physical child abuse and neglect: Existing evidence of future directions. *Child Maltreatment*, 2, 12–34.

Hageman, W. & Arrindell, W. (1993). A further refinement of the reliable change (RC) index by improving the pre-post difference score: Introducing RC-ID. *Behaviour Research and Therapy*, 31, 693–700.

Hagopian, L.P., Fisher, W.W., Sullivan, M.T. et al. (1998). Effectiveness of functional communication training with and without extinction and punishment: a summary of 21 inpatient cases. *Journal of Applied Behavior Analysis*, 31(2), 211–235.

Hansen, W. & Graham, J. (1991). Preventing alcohol, marijuana and cigarette use among adolescents: Peer pressure resistance training versus establishing conservative norms. *Preventive Medicine*, 20, 414–430.*

Hansen, W. & O'Malley, P. (1996). Drug abuse. In R. Di Clemente, W. Hansen & L. Ponton (Eds.), *Handbook of Adolescent Health Risk Behaviour* (pp. 161–192). New York: Plenum.

Hansen, W. and colleagues (1989). *ALL STARS Drug Abuse Prevention Programme*. Contact Dr William Hansen, Department of Public Health Sciences, Bowman Gray School of Medicine, Winston Salem, North Carolina, 27157.

Hansen, W. and colleagues (1991). *Project SMART Drug Abuse Prevention Programme*. Contact Dr William Hansen, Department of Public Health Sciences, Bowman Gray School of Medicine, Winston Salem, North Carolina, 27157.

Hansen, W., Johnson, C., Flay, B., Graham, J. & Sobel, J. (1988). Affective and social influence approaches to the prevention of multiple substance abuse among seventh grade students: Results from Project SMART, *Preventive Medicine*, 17, 135–154.*

Hansen, W., Graham, J., Wolkenstein, B. & Rohrbach, L. (1991). Program integrity as a moderator of prevention program effectiveness: Results for fifth-grade students in the adolescent alcohol prevention trial. *Journal of Studies on Alcohol*, 52, 568–579.*

Hardy, J.B. & Street, R. (1989). Family support and parenting education in the home: An effective extension of clinic-based preventive health care service for poor children. *Journal of Paediatrics*, 115, 927–931.*

Hari, M. & Akos, K. (1988). *Conductive Education*. London: Routledge.

Hari, M. & Tillemans, T. (1984). Conductive Education. In D. Scrutton (Ed.), *Management of the Motor Disorders of Children with Cerebral Palsy* (pp. 19–35). Oxford: Blackwell.

Harris, J. (1992). Neurobiological factors in self-injurious behaviour. In J.K. Luiselli, J.L. Matson & N.N. Singh (Eds.), *Self-injurious Behaviour: Analysis, Assessment and Treatment* (pp. 59–92). New York: Springer-Verlag.

Harris, J. (1996). Physical restraint procedures for managing challenging behaviours presented by mentally retarded adults and children. *Research in Developmental Disabilities*, 17(2), 99–134.

Harris, S. (1976). *Teaching Speech to a Non-verbal Child*. Lawrence, KS: H & H Enterprises.

Harris, S. (1987). Early intervention for children with motor handicaps. In M.J. Guralnick & F.C. Bennett (Eds.), *The Effectiveness of Early Intervention for At-Risk and Handicapped Children* (pp. 175–212). Orlando, FL: Academic Press.

Harris, S. (1994). *Siblings of Children with Autism. A Guide for Families*. Bethesda, MD: Woodbine House.

Harris, S. (1997). The effectiveness of early intervention for children with cerebral palsy and related motor difficulties. In M.J. Guralnick (Ed.), *The Effectiveness of Early Intervention* (pp. 327–347). Baltimore: Brookes.

Harris, S. & Handleman, J. (1997). Helping children with autism enter the mainstream. In D. Cohen & F. Volkmar (Eds.), *Handbook of Autism and Pervasive Developmental Disorders* (Second Edition, pp. 665–676). New York: Wiley.

Harris, S., Wolchik, S.A. & Milch, R.E. (1983). Changing the speech of autistic children and their parents. *Child and Family Behavior Therapy*, 4, 151–173.*

Harris, S., Handleman, J., Kristoff, B., Bass, L. & Gordon, R. (1990). Changes in language development among autistic and peer children in segregated and integrated preschool settings. *Journal of Autism and Developmental Disorders*, 20, 23–31.*

Harvey, P. (1988). The prevention of sexual abuse: Examination of the effectiveness of a program with kindergarten-age children. *Behaviour Therapy*, 19, 429–435.*

Hawkins, J., Catalano, R. & Miller, J. (1992). Risk and protective factors for alcohol and their drug problems in adolescence and early adulthood: Implications for substance abuse prevention. *Psychological Bulletin*, 112, 64–105.

Hazlewood, M.E., Brown, J.K., Rowe, P.J. & Salter, P.M. (1994). The use of therapeutic electrical stimulation in the treatment of hemiplegic cerebral palsy. *Developmental Medicine and Child Neurology*, 36, 661–673.*

Hazzard, A. (1999). *What I Know about Touching Scale*. Atlanta, GA: Grady Memorial Hospital. (Available from Dr Ann Hazzard, Box 26065, Grady Memorial Hospital, 80 Butler Street, S.E., Atlanta, GA 30335.)

Hazzard, A., Webb, C., Kleemeier, C., Angert, L. & Pohl, J. (1991). Child sexual abuse prevention: Evaluation and one-year follow-up. *Child Abuse and Neglect*, 15, 123–138.*

Helfer, R., Hoffmeister, J. & Schneider, C. (1978). *The Michigan Screening Profile of Parenting*. Boulder, CO: Manual Test Analysis and Development Corporation.

Hennig, C.W., Crabtree, R.C. & Baum, D.B. (1998). Mental Health CPR: Peer contracting as a response to potential suicide in adolescents. *Archives of Suicide Research*, 4, 169–187.*

Herbert, J.D., Lilienfeld, S.O., Lohr, J.M., Montgomery, R.W., O'Donohue, W.T., Rosen, G.M. & Tolin, D.F. (2000). Science and pseudoscience in the development of eye movement desensitization and reprocessing: implications for clinical psychology. *Clinical Psychology Review*, 20, 945–971.

Hermelin, B. & O'Connor, N. (1970). *Psychological Experiments with Autistic Children*. London: Pergamon Press.

Hindley. P. & Brown. H. (1994). Psychiatric aspects of specific sensory impairments. In M. Rutter, E. Taylor & L. Hersov (Eds.), *Child and Adolescent Psychiatry: Modern Approaches* (Third Edition, pp. 720–736). London: Blackwell.

Hindley, P. & Reed, H. (1999). Promoting Alternative Thinking Strategies (PATHS): Mental health promotion with deaf children in school. In S. Decker, S. Kirby, A. Greenwood & D. Moore (Eds.), *Taking Children Seriously. Applications of Counselling and Therapy in Education*. London: Cassell.

Hobson, R. (1993). *Autism and the Development of Mind*. Hillsdale, NJ: Lawrence Erlbaum Associates Inc.

Hoffman, J. (Producer) & Life, R. (Director) (1989). *Seriously Fresh (film)*. (Available from SELECT Media, 225, Lafayette St., Suite 1102, New York, NY 10012.)

Holroyd, J. (1973). *Manual for the Questionnaire on Resources and Stress*. Los Angeles: UCLA Neuropsychiatric Institute.

Holroyd, J. (1974). The Questionnaire on Resources and Stress: An instrument to measure family response to a handicapped family member. *American Journal of Community Psychology*, 2, 92–94.

Holzheimer, L. (1993). *What's That Noise?* Brisbane: Queensland University of Technology.

Holzheimer, L., Mokay, H. & Masters, I.B. (1998). Educating young children about asthma: Comparing the effectiveness of a developmentally appropriate asthma education video tape and picture book. *Child Care Health and Development*, 24(1), 85–99.*

Horn, E., Warren, S. & Jones, H. (1995). An experimental analysis of neurobehavioural intervention. *Developmental Medicine and Child Neurology*, 37, 679–714.

Horner, R.H., Sprague, J.R., O'Brien, M. & Heathfield, L.T. (1990). The role of response efficiency in the reduction of problem behaviors through functional equivalence training: a case study. *Journal of the Association for Persons with Severe Handicaps*, 15(2), 91–97.*

Horner, R.H., Day, H.M. & Day, J.R. (1997). Using neutralizing routines to reduce problem behaviors. *Journal of Applied Behavior Analysis*, 30, 601–614.*

Horowitz, M.J., Wilner, N. & Alvarez, W. (1979). Impact of Events Scale: a measure of subjective stress. *Psychosomatic Medicine*, 41, 209–218.

Hovell, M., Hillman, E., Blumberg, E., Sipan, C., Atkins, C., Hofstetter, C. & Myers, C. (1994). A behavioural-ecological model of adolescent sexual development: A template for AIDS prevention. *Journal of Sex Research*, 31, 267–281.

Howard, M. & McCabe, J.B. (1990). Helping teenagers postpone sexual involvement. *Family Planning Perspectives*, 22(1), 21–26.*

Howlin, P. (1997). Prognosis in autism: Do specialist treatments affect long-term outcome? *European Child and Adolescent Psychiatry*, 6, 65–72.

Howlin, P. (1998). Practitioner review: psychological and educational treatments for autism. *Journal of Child Psychology and Psychiatry*, 39, 307–322.

Howlin, P. & Rutter, M. (1987). *Treatment of Autistic Children*. New York: Wiley.

Hubbard, B.M., Giese, M.L. & Rainey, J. (1998). A replication study of reducing the risk, a theory-based sexuality curriculum for adolescents. *Journal of School Health*, 68(6), 243–247.*

Hughes, D.M., McLeod, M., Garner, B. & Goldbloom, R.B. (1991). Controlled trial of a home and ambulatory program for asthmatic children. *Pediatrics*, 87(1), 54–61.*

Hur, J.J. (1997). Skills for independence for children with cerebral palsy: A comparative longitudinal study. *International Journal of Disability and Education*, 44(3), 263–274.*

Huszti, H.C., Clopton, J.R. & Mason, P.J. (1989). Acquired Immunodeficiency Syndrome educational program: Effects on adolescents' knowledge and attitudes. *Pediatrics*, 84(6), 986–994.*

Infant Health and Development Program (1990). Enhancing the outcomes of low birth weight, premature infants. *Journal of the American Medical Association*, 263, 3035–3042.

Infante-Rivard, C., Filion, G., Baumgarten, M., Bourassa, M., Labelle, J. & Messier, M. (1989). A public health home intervention among families of low socio-economic status. *Children's Health Care*, 18, 102–107.*

Institute of Medicine (1985). *Preventing Low Birth Weight. Summary*. Washington, DC: National Academy Press.

Isenberg, S., Lehrer, P. & Hochron, S. (1992). The effects of suggestion and emotional arousal on pulmonary functions in asthma: A review and a hypothesis regarding vagal mediation. *Psychosomatic Medicine*, 54, 192–216.

Iwata, B.A., Wong, S.E., Riordan, M.M., Dorsey, M.F. & Lou, M.M. (1982).

Assessment and training of clinical interviewer skills: analogue analysis and field replication. *Journal of Applied Behavior Analysis*, 15, 191–203.

Iwata, B.A., Dorsey, J.R., Slifer, K.J. et al. (1994a). Towards a functional analysis of self-injury. *Journal of Applied Behavior Analysis*, 27(2), 197–209.

Iwata, B.A., Pace, G.M., Dorsey, J.R. et al. (1994b). The functions of self-injurious behaviour: an experimental-epidemiological analysis. *Journal of Applied Behavior Analysis*, 27(2), 215–240.

Jacobs, D. (Ed.) (1999). *The Harvard Medical School Guide to Suicide Assessment and Intervention*. San Francisco, CA: Jossey Bass.

Jacobson, N., Follette, W. & Revenstorf, D. (1984). Psychotherapy outcome research: Methods for reporting variability and evaluating clinical significance. *Behaviour Therapy*, 15, 336–352.

Jemmott, J., Jemmott, L. & Fong, G. (1992). Reductions in HIV risk-associated sexual behaviours among black male adolescents: Effects of an AIDS prevention intervention. *American Journal of Public Health*, 82(3), 372–377.*

Jester, R.E. & Guinagh, B.J. (1983). The Gordon parent education infant and toddler program. In The Consortium for Longitudinal Studies (Eds.), *As The Twig Is Bent . . . Lasting Effects Of Pre-School Programmes* (pp. 103–132). Hillsdale, NJ: Lawrence Erlbaum Associates Inc.*

Joan, P. (1986). *Preventing Teenage Suicide: The Living Alternative Handbook*. New York: Human Sciences Press.

Johnson, C., Pentz, M., Weber, M., Dwyer, J., Bear, N., MacKinnon, D., Hansen, W. & Flay, B. (1990). Relative effectiveness of comprehensive community programming for drug abuse prevention with high risk and low risk adolescents. *Journal of Consulting and Clinical Psychology*, 58, 447–456.*

Johnson, D. & Walker, T. (1991). A follow-up evaluation of the Houston Parent-Child Development Centre: School Performance. *Journal of Early Intervention*, 15(3), 226–236.

Johnson, S., Rosenbloom, J., Rosenbloom, A., Carter, R. & Cunningham, W. (1986). Assessing daily management in childhood diabetes. *Health Psychology*, 5, 545–564.

Johnstone, M., Munn, P. & Edwards, L. (1991). *Action Against Bullying: A Support Pack for Schools*. Edinburgh: SCRE.

Jordon, R. & Jones, G. (1996). *Educational provision for Children with Autism in Scotland*. Birmingham, UK: School of Education, University of Birmingham.

Jordon, R. & Powell, S. (1995). *Understanding and Teaching Children with Autism*. New York: Wiley.

Kaiminer, Y., Wagner, E., Plummer, E. & Seifer, R. (1993). Validation of the Teen Addiction Severity Index (T-ASI). Preliminary Findings. *American Journal of Addictions*, 3, 250–254.

Kalafat, J. (1997). Prevention of youth suicide. In R.P. Weissberg, T.P. Gullotta, R.L. Hampton, A.R. Bruce & G.R. Adams, *Enhancing Children's Wellness* (pp. 175–213). Thousand Oaks, CA: Sage Publications.

Kalafat, J. & Elias, M. (1994). An evaluation of a school based suicide awareness intervention. *Suicide and Life-Threatening Behavior*, 24, 224–233.*

Kalafat, J. & Gagliano, C. (1996). The use of simulations to assess the impact of an adolescent suicide response curriculum. *Suicide and Life-Threatening Behavior*, 26, 359–364.*

Kalafat, J. & Underwood, M. (1989). *Lifelines: A School-Based Adolescent Suicide Response Program*. Dubuque, IA: Kendall/Hunt.

Kaplan, R.M., Chadwick, M.W., Schimmel, L.E. (1985). Social learning intervention to promote metabolic control in Type 1 diabetes mellitus: Pilot experiment results. *Diabetes Care*, 8(2), 152–155.*

Karnes, M.B., Teska, J.A. & Hodgins, A.S. (1970). The effects of four programs of classroom intervention on the intellectual and language development of 4-year-old disadvantaged children. *American Journal of Orthopsychiatry*, 40(1), 58–78.*

Kates, L. & Schein, J.D. (1980). *A Complete Guide to Communication with Deaf-blind Persons*. Silver Spring, MD: National Association of the Deaf.

Kaufman, A. & Kaufman, N. (1983). *Kaufman Assessment Battery for Children*. Circle Pines, MN: American Guidance Service.

Kaufman, J., Birmaher, B., Brent, D., Rao, U., Flynn, C., Moreci, P., Williamson, D. & Ryan, N. (1997). Schedule for Affective Disorders and Schizophrenia for School-Age Children-Present and Lifetime Versions, (K-SADS-PL), PTSD Scale. Initial reliability and validity data. *Journal of the American Academy of Child and Adolescent Psychiatry*, 36, 980–988.

Kazdin, A. (1982). *Single-Case Design Research Designs: Methods for Clinical and Applied Settings*. New York: Oxford University Press.

Kazdin, A., Rodgas, A. & Colbus, D. (1986). The Hopelessness Scale for Children: psychometric characteristics and concurrent validity. *Journal of Consulting and Clinical Psychology*, 54, 241–245.

Keane, T. (1998). Psychological and behavioural treatments for post-traumatic stress disorder. In P. Nathan & J. Gorman (Eds.), *A Guide To Treatments That Work* (pp. 398–407). New York: Oxford University Press.

Kelleher, M. (1998). Youth suicide trends in the Republic of Ireland. *British Journal of Psychiatry*, 173, 196–197.

Kelly, J. (1983). *Treating Abusive Families: Interventions Based on Skills Training Principles*. New York: Plenum.

Kelly, J. (1995). *Changing HIV Risk Behaviour: Practical Strategies*. New York: Guilford.

Kelly, J.A., St Lawrence, J.S., Hood, H.V. & Brasfield, T.L. (1989). An objective test of AIDS risk behaviour knowledge: Scale development, validation, and norms. *Journal of Behaviour Therapy and Experimental Psychiatry*, 20, 227–234.

Kempe, H., Silverman, F.N., Steele, B.F., Droegmueller, W. & Silver, H.K. (1962). The battered child syndrome. *Journal of the American Medical Association*, 181, 17–24.

Kendall-Tackett, K., Williams, L. & Finkelhor, D. (1993). Impact of sexual abuse on children. *Psychological Bulletin*, 113, 164–180.

Kibby, M., Tyc, V. & Mulhern, R. (1998). Effectiveness of psychological intervention for children and adolescents with chronic medical illness: A meta-analysis. *Clinical Psychology Review*, 18, 103–117.

Kidscape: *Stop Bullying*, booklet available through the International Society for the Prevention of Cruelty for Children (ISPCC).

Kienhorst, C.W.M., DeWilde, E.J. & Diekstra, R.F.W. (1995). Suicide behavior in adolescents. *Archives of Suicide Research*, 1, 185–209.

Kim, N., Stanton, B., Dickersin, K. & Galbraith, J. (1997). Effectiveness of the 40 adolescent AIDS-Risk reduction interventions: A Quantitative Review. *Journal of Adolescent Health*, 20, 204–215.

King, K. (1988). Heterosexual transmission of HIV: current evidence and future prospects. Presented at the *Fourth International Conference on AIDS*, Stockholm, Sweden, June.

King, S., Rosenbaum, P. & King, G. (1995). *The Measure of Process of Care: A Means to Assess Family Centred Behaviours of Healthcare Providers*. Hamilton, Ontario: Neurodevelopmental Research Unit, McMaster University.

Kipke, M.D., Boyer, C. & Hein, K. (1993). An evaluation of an AIDS risk reduction education and skills training (ARREST) Program. *Journal of Adolescent Health*, 14, 533–539.*

Kirby, D. (1992). School-based programs to reduce sexual risk-taking behaviours. *Journal of School Health*, 62(7), 280–287.

Kirby, D. (1997). *No Easy Answers. Research Findings on Programmes to Reduce Teen Pregnancy*. Washington, DC: National Campaign to Prevent Teen Pregnancy.

Kirby, D., Barth, R.P., Leland, N. & Fetro, J.V. (1991). Reducing the risk: impact of a new curriculum on sexual risk-taking. *Family Planning Perspectives*, 23(6), 253–263.*

Kirby, D., Short, L., Rugg, D., Kolbe, L., Howard, M., Sonenstein, F. & Zabin, L. (1994). School-based programs to reduce sexual risk behaviours: A review of Effectiveness. *Public Health Reports*, 109(3), 339–360.

Kirk, S.A., McCarthy, J.J. & Kirk, W.D. (1968). *The Illinois Test of Psycholinguistic Abilities*. Urbana, IL: The University of Illinois Press.

Klingelhofer, E.L. & Gershwin, M.E. (1988). Asthma self-management programs: Premises, not promises. *Journal of Asthma*, 25(2), 89–101.

Klingman, A. & Hochdorf, Z. (1993). Coping with distress and self-harm: The impact of a primary prevention program among adolescents. *Adolescence*, 16, 121–140.*

Knobloch, H. & Pasamanick, B. (1974). *Gesell and Amatruda's Developmental Diagnosis*. Hagerstown, MD: Harper & Row.

Knobloch, H., Stevens, F. & Malone, A. (1980). Manual of Developmental Diagnosis: The Administration and Interpretation of the Revised *Gesell and Amatruda's Developmental and Neurologic Examinations*. Hagerstown, MD: Harper & Row.

Kohen, D.P. (1996). Relaxation/mental imagery (self hypnosis) for childhood asthma: Behavioural outcomes in a prospective controlled study. *Australian Journal of Clinical and Experimental Hypnosis*, 24(1), 21–28.*

Kolb, B. & Whishaw, I.Q. (1990). *Fundamentals of Human Neuropsychology* (3rd Edition). New York: W.H. Freeman.

Kolko, D., Moser, J., Litz, J. & Hughes, J. (1987). Promoting awareness and prevention of child sexual victimization using the red flag/green flag program: An evaluation with follow-up. *Journal of Family Violence*, 2(1), 11–35.*

Kotses, H., Glaus, K.D., Bricel, S.K., Edwards, J.E. & Crawford, P.L. (1978). Operant muscle relaxation and peak expiratory flow rate in asthmatic children. *Journal of Psychosomatic Research*, 22, 17–23.*

Kovacs, M. (1992). *Children's Depression Inventory (CDI) Manual*. North Tonawanda, NY: Multi-Health Systems.

Kovacs, M. & Beck, A. (1977). An empirical clinical approach towards definition of childhood depression. In J. Schulterbrandt et al. (Eds.), *Depression in Children* (pp. 1–25). New York: Raven.

Kraizer, S. (1981). *Children Need to Know Personal training Programme*. New York: Health Education Systems.

Krug, D., Arick, J. & Almond, P. (1980). Behaviour checklist for identifying severely handicapped children with high levels of autistic behaviour. *Journal of Child Psychology and Psychiatry*, 21, 221–229.

Krug, D., Arick, J. & Almond, P. (1996). *Autism Screening Instrument For Educational*

Planning (Second Edition). Odessa, FL: Psychological Assessment Resources. (PAR, PO Box 998, Odessa, Florida, 33556.)

Kubly, L.S. & McClellan, M.S. (1984). Effects of self care instruction on asthmatic children. *Issues in Comprehensive Pediatric Nursing*, 7, 121–130.

Kusche, C.A. (1984). *The Understanding of Emotion Concepts by Deaf Children: An Assessment of an Effective Education Curriculum.* Unpublished doctoral dissertation, University of Washington.

Kusche, C.A. & Greenberg, M.T. (1994). *The PATHS Curriculum.* Seattle, WA: Developmental Research and Programs.

Larson, C.P. (1980). Efficacy of prenatal and postpartum visits on child health and development. *Paediatrics*, 66, 191–197.*

Lask, B. & Matthew, D. (1979). Childhood asthma. A controlled trial of family psychotherapy. *Archives of Diseases in Childhood*, 54, 116–119.*

Law, M., Cadman, D., Rosenbaum, P., Walter, S., Russell, D. & Dematteo, C. (1991). Neurodevelopmental therapy and upper-extremity casting for children with cerebral palsy. *Developmental Medicine and Child Neurology*, 33, 379–387.*

Lealman, G.T., Haigh, D., Phillips, J.M., Stone, J. & Ord-Smith, C. (1983). Prediction and prevention of child abuse – An empty hope? *Lancet*, i, 1423–1424.*

Lee, L. (1971). *Northwestern Syntax Screening Test.* Evanston, IL: Northwestern University Press.

Lee, V.E., Schnur, E. & Brooks-Gunn, J. (1988). Does Head Start work? A 1-year follow-up of disadvantaged children attending head start, no preschool, and other preschool programs. *Developmental Psychology*, 24(2) 210–222.*

Lee, V.E., Brooks-Gunn, J., Schnur, E. & Liaw, F. (1990). Are Head Start effects sustained? A longitudinal follow-up comparison of disadvantaged children attending head start, no preschool, and other preschool programs. *Child Development*, 61, 495–507.*

Leib, S.A., Benfield, G. & Guidubaldi, J. (1980). Effects of early intervention and stimulation on the preterm infant. *Pediatrics*, 66, 83–90.*

Lester, D. (1992). *The Cruelest death: The Enigma of Adolescent Suicide.* New York: Charles Press Publishers.

Levenstein, P. (1970). Cognitive growth in preschoolers through verbal interaction with mothers. *American Journal of Orthopsychiatry*, 40, 426–432.

Levenstein, P. & Sunley, R. (1968). Stimulation of verbal interaction between disadvantaged mothers and children. *American Journal of Orthopsychiatry*, 38, 116–121.*

Levine, M. (1986). *Leiter International Performance Scale: A Handbook.* Los Angeles, CA: Western Psychological Services.

Levy, S.R., Perhats, C., Weeks, K., Handler, A.S., Zhu, C. & Flay, B.R. (1995). Impact of a school-based AIDS prevention program on risk and protective behaviour for newly sexually active students. *Journal of School Health*, 65(4), 145–151.*

Lewis, C.E., Rachelefsky, G., Lewis, M.A., De La Sota, A. & Kaplan, M. (1984). A randomized trial of A.C.T. (Asthma Care Training) for Kids. *Pediatrics*, 74(4), 478–486.*

Linscheid, T.R., Pejeau, C., Cohen, S. & Footo-Lenz, M. (1994). Positive side effects in the treatment of SIB using the self-injurious behaviour inhibiting system (SIBIS): implications for operant and biochemical explanations of SIB. *Research in Developmental Disabilities*, 15(1), 81–90.*

London, J. & Westcott, N. (1997). *The Lion who had Asthma*. New York: Albert Whitman.

Lord, C. & Rutter, M. (1994). Autism and pervasive developmental disorders. In M. Rutter, E. Taylor & L. Hersov (Eds.), *Child and Adolescent Psychiatry: Modern Approaches* (Third Edition, pp. 569–593). Oxford: Blackwell.

Lord, C., Rutter, M., Goode, S., Heemsbergen, J., Jordan, H. & Mawhood, L. (1989). Autism diagnostic observation schedule: A standardized observation of communicative and social behaviour. *Journal of Autism and Developmental Disorders*, 19, 185–212. (Training is required for ADOS & ADI-R. Contact Catherine Lord, Child and Adolescent Psychiatry, University of Chicago, 5841 S. Marylan Avenue, Chicago, Illinois 60637.)

Lord, C., Rutter, M. & Le Couteur, A. (1994). Autism Diagnostic Interview-Revised. *Journal of Autism and Developmental Disorders*, 24, 659–685.

Lovaas, O.I. (1987). Behavioral treatment and normal educational and intellectual functioning in young autistic children. *Journal of Consulting and Clinical Psychology*, 55, 3–9.*

Lovaas, O.I. & Leaf, R.I. (1981). Five video tapes for teaching developmentally disabled children. Baltimore: University Park Press.

Lovaas, O.I., Ackerman, A.B., Alexander, D., Firestone, P., Perkins, J. & Young, D. (1980). *Teaching Developmentally Disabled Children: The Me Book*. Austin, TX: Pro-Ed.

Luiselli, J.K. (1986). Modification of self-injurious behavior: an analysis of the use of contingently applied protective equipment. *Behavior Modification*, 10(2), 191–204.*

Luiselli, J.K., Suskin, L. & McPhee, D.F. (1981). Continuous and intermittent application of overcorrection in a self-injurious autistic child: Alternating treatments design and analysis. *Journal of Behaviour Therapy and Experimental Psychiatry*, 12(4), 355–358.*

Luiselli, J.K., Maston, J. & Singh, N. (1992). *Self Injurious Behaviour: Analysis, Assessment and Treatment*. New York: Springer Verlag.

Luterman, D. & Ross, M. (1991). *When your Child is Deaf. A Guide for Parents*. Parkton, MD: New York Press.

Lutzker, J. & Rice, J. (1984). Project 12-Ways: Measuring outcome of a large in-home service for treatment and prevention of child abuse and neglect. *Child Abuse and Neglect*, 8, 519–524.*

McBrien, J. & Felce, D. (1992). *Working with People who have Severe Learning Difficulty and Challenging Behaviour*. England: The Cookley Printers, A BIMH Publication.

McCarthy, D. (1972). *Manual: McCarthy Scales of Children's Abilities*. New York: Psychological Corporation.

McCarton, C., Wallace, I. & Bennett, F. (1995). Preventive interventions with low birth weight premature infants: an evaluation of their success. *Seminars in Perinatology*, 19(4), 330–340.

McCarton, C., Brooks-Gunn, J., Wallace, I.F. et al. (1997). Results at age 8 years of early intervention for low birth weight premature infants. *Journal of the American Medical Association*, 277, 126–132.*

McConaughay S.H. & Achenbach T.M. (1988). *Practical Guide for the Child Behavior Checklist and Related Materials*. Burlington: University of Vermont Department of Psychiatry.

McCormick, M.C., McCarton, C., Tonascia, J. & Brooks-Gunn, J. (1993). Early educational intervention for very low birth weight infants: Results from the Infant Health and Development Programme. *Journal of Pediatrics*, 123, 527–533.*

McDaniel, S.H., Hepworth, J. & Doherty, W. (1992). *Medical Family Therapy*. New York: Basic Books.

McEachin, J.J., Smith,T. & Lovaas, O.I. (1993). Long-term outcome for children with autism who received early intensive behavioural treatment. *American Journal of Mental Retardation*, 97(4), 359–372.*

MacIntyre, D. & Carr, A. (2000). *Prevention of Child Sexual Abuse in Ireland: The Development and Evaluation of the Stay Safe Programme*. Wales: Edwin Mellin.

MacIntyre, D. & Lawlor, M. (1991). *The Stay Safe Programme*. Dublin: Department of Health, Child Abuse Prevention Programme.

McKeown, K. & Gilligan, R. (1991). Child sexual abuse in the Eastern Health Board region of Ireland: An analysis of 512 confirmed cases. *Economic and Social Review*, 22, 101–134.

MacMillan, H.L., MacMillan, J.H., Offord, D.R., Griffith, L. & MacMillan, A. (1994a). Primary prevention of child physical abuse and neglect: A critical review. Part 1. *Journal of Child Psychology and Psychiatry*, 35(5), 835–856.

MacMillan, H., MacMillan, J., Offord, D., Griffith, L. & MacMillan, A. (1994b). The primary prevention of child sexual abuse: A critical review. Part 2. *Journal of Child Psychology and Psychiatry*, 35, 857–876.

McNabb, W. (1990). *In Control*. Chicago, IL: Centre for Research in Medical Education and Health Care.

McNabb, W., Quinn, M.T., Murphy, D.M., Thorp, F.K. & Cook, S. (1994). Increasing children's responsibility for diabetes self-care: The In Control Study. *Diabetes Educator*, 20(2), 121–124.*

McQuaid, E.L. & Nassau, J.H. (1999). Empirically supported treatments of disease related symptoms in pediatric psychology: asthma, diabetes and cancer. *Journal of Pediatric Psychology*, 24(4), 305–328.

Madaras, L. (1989*). What's Happening to My Body? A Growing up Guide for Parents and Sons*. London: Penguin.

Madden, R., Gardner, E., Rudman, H., Karlsen, B. & Merwin, J. (1972). *Stanford Achievement Test for Hearing Impaired Students*. New York: Harcourt Brace Jovanovich.

March, J.S., Parker, J., Sullivan, K., Stallings, P. & Conners, C. (1997a). The Multidimensional Anxiety Scale for Children (MASC): Factor structure, reliability and validity. *Journal of the American Academy of Child and Adolescent Psychiatry*, 36, 554–565.

March, J., Parker, J., Sullivan, K., Stallings, P. & Connors, C. (1997b). The Multidimensional Anxiety Scale for Children (MASC): factor structure, reliability and validity. *Journal of the American Academy of Child and Adolescent Psychiatry*, 36, 554–565.

March, J.S., Amaya-Jackson, L., Murray, M.C. & Schulte, A. (1998). Cognitive behavioural psychotherapy for children and adolescents with post-traumatic stress disorder after a single incident stressor. *Journal of the American Academy of Child and Adolescent Psychiatry*, 37, 585–593.*

Marchenko, M. O. & Spence, M. (1994). Home visitation services for at-risk pregnant and postpartum women: A randomized trial. *American Journal of Orthopsychiatry*, 64, 468–478.*

Marvel Comics (1984) *Spiderman & Power Pack Comic Book on Sexual Abuse.*

Available from: National Committee for the Prevention of Child Abuse, P.O. Box 94283, Chicago, IL 60990.

Maurice, C. (Ed.) (1992). *Behavioral Intervention for Young Children with Autism. A Manual for Parents and Professionals.* Austin, TX: Pro-Ed.

Maurice, C. (1993). *Let Me Hear Your Voice.* New York: Knopf. (A mother's story of children's recovery following behavioural treatment.)

Mayer, J. & Filstead, W. (1979). The adolescent alcohol involvement scale: An instrument for measuring adolescent use and misuse of alcohol. *Journal of Studies in Alcohol*, 40, 291–300.

Mayo, N.E. (1991). The effect of physical therapy for children with motor delay and cerebral palsy. A randomised clinical trial. *American Journal of Physical and Medical Rehabilitation*, 70, 258–267.*

Meadow, K.P. (1983). *Revised Manual. Meadow/Kendall Social-Emotional Assessment Inventory for Deaf and Hearing-Impaired Children.* Washington, DC: Pre-College Programs, Gallaudet Research Institute.

Meadow-Orlans, K. (1987). An analysis of the effectiveness of early intervention programmes for hearing-impaired children. In M.J. Guralnick & F.C. Bennet (Eds.), *The Effectiveness of Early Intervention for at Risk and Handicapped Children* (pp. 325–357). New York: Academic Press.

Meichenbaum, D. (1985). *Stress Inoculation Training.* New York: Pergamon Press.

Mellor, A. (1993). *Bullying and How to Fight it: A Guide for Families.* Edinburgh: SCRE.

Mendez, F. & Belendez, M. (1997). Effects of a behavioural intervention on treatment adherence and stress management in adolescents with IDDM. *Diabetes Care*, 20(9), 1370–1375.

Mesibov, G., Schopler, E. & Caison, W. (1989). *Adolescent and Adult Psycho-Educational Profile (AAPEP).* Austin, TX: Pro-ed.

Meyer, E., Coll, C., Lester, B., Boukydis, C., McDonough, S. & Oh, W. (1994). Family-based intervention improves maternal psychological well-being and feeding interaction of preterm infants. *Pediatrics*, 93(2), 241–246.*

Miller, B. & Wood, B. (1991). Childhood asthma in interaction with family, school and peer systems: A developmental model of primary care. *Journal of Asthma*, 28, 405–414.

Miller, B., Card, J., Paikoff, R. & Peterson, J. (1992). *Preventing Adolescent Pregnancy.* Newbury Park, CA: Sage.

Miller, D.N. & DuPaul, G.J. (1996). School-Based Prevention of Adolescent Suicide: Issues, Obstacles, and Recommendations for Practice. *Journal of Emotional and Behavioral Disorders*, Oct, 4, 221–230.

Miller, W.R. & Lief, H.L. (1979). The Sex Knowledge and Attitude Test (SKAT). *Journal of Sex and Marital Therapy*, 5, 282–287.

Milner, J.S. (1980). *The Child Abuse Inventory: Manual.* Webster, NC: Psytec.

Minuchin, S., Baker, L., Rosman, B.L., Liebman, R., Milman, L. & Todd, T.C. (1975). A conceptual model of psychosomatic illness in children. *Archives of General Psychiatry*, 32, 1031–1038.

Mirenda, P. (1997). Supporting individuals with challenging behavior through functional communication training and AAC: research review. *Augmentative and Alternative Communication*, 13 (Dec.), 207–225.

Mohay, H. & Masters, B. (1993). *Young Children Managing Asthma* [Video recording]. Brisbane: TSNII.

Monsen, R.B. (1983). Towards measuring how well hearing-impaired children speak. *Journal of Speech and Hearing Research*, 21(2), 197–219.

Moog, J. & Geers, M.A. (1985). EPIC: A programme to accelerate academic learning in profoundly deaf children. *Volta Review*, 87, 259–277.*

Moog, J.S., Kozak, V.J. & Geers, A.E. (1983). *Grammatical Analysis of Elicited Language: Pre-sentence Level (GAEP-P)*. St Louis, MO: Central Institute for the Deaf.

Mooij, T. (1993). Working towards understanding and prevention in the Netherlands. In D. Tattum (Ed.), *Understanding and Managing Bullying* (pp. 31–44). Oxford: Heinemann.

Moores, D. (1978). *Educating the Deaf. Psychology Principles and Practices*. Boston, MA: Houghton Mifflin.

Moran, G., Fonagy, P., Kurtz, A., Bolton, A. & Brook, C. (1991). A controlled study of the psychoanalytical treatment of brittle diabetes. *Journal of the American Academy of Child and Adolescent Psychiatry*, 30(6), 926–935.*

Morgan, E. & Watkins, S. (1989). *Assessment of Developmental Skills for Young Multi-handicapped Sensory-impaired Children*. Logan, UT: HOPE.

Mufson, L., Moreau, D., Weissman, M. & Kerman, G. (1993). *Interpersonal Psychotherapy for Depressed Adolescents*. New York: Guilford.

Munn, P. (1993). *Schools Action Against Bullying: Involving Parents and Non Teaching Staff*. Edinburgh: SCRE.

Munthe, E. (1989). Bullying in Scandinavia. In E. Roland & E. Munthe (Eds.), *Bullying, an International Perspective* (pp. 66–78). London: David Fulton.

Muris, P. & deJongh, A. (1996). Eye movement desensitization and reprocessing: a new treatment method for trauma related anxiety complaints (in Dutch) *Kind en Adolescent*, 17, 190–199.

Murphy, S. (1994). Asthma etiology and management: Primary to tertiary prevention. *Preventive Medicine*, 23, 688–692.

Murphy, S., Orkow, B. & Nicola, R. (1985). Prenatal prediction of child abuse and neglect: A prospective study. *Child Abuse and Neglect*, 9, 225–235.

Murray, M. & Keane, C. (1998). *The ABC of Bullying*. Dublin: Mercier.

Nader, K.O., Blake, D., Kriegler, J. & Pynoos, R. (1994). *Clinician Administered PTSD Scale for Children (CAPS-C), Current and Lifetime Diagnosis Version*. Los Angeles: UCLA Neuropsychiatric Institute and National Centre for PTSD.

Nader, K.O., Kriegler, J.A., Blake, D.D., Pynoos, R.S., Newman, E. & Weather, F.W. (1996). *Clinically Administered PTSD Scale, Child and Adolescent Version*. White River Junction, VT: National Centre for PTSD.

National Autistic Society (1993). *Approaches to Autism* (Second Edition). London: National Autistic Society.

National Film Board of Canada (1985). *Feeling Yes–Feeling No Programme*. Canada: National Film Board of Canada.

Neimeyer, R.A. & MacInnes, W.D. (1981). Assessing paraprofessional competence with the Suicide Intervention Response Inventory. *Journal of Counseling Psychology*, 28, 176–179.

Neisser, U., Boodoo, G., Bouchard, T. et al. (1996). Intelligence Knowns and Unknowns (Report of a Task Force Established by the American Psychological Association). *American Psychologist*, 51, 77–101.

Nelson, F.C. (1987a). Evaluation of a youth suicide prevention program. *Adolescence*, 88, 813–825.*

Nelson, F. (1987b). *Curriculum Assessment Instrument*. (Available from Dr Franklyn

Nelson, Director of clinical training, The Institute for Studies of Destructive Behaviors and the Suicide Prevention Center, 1041 South Menlo Avenue, Los Angeles, California 90006.)

Nemerofsky, A.G., Sanford, H.J., Baer, B., Cage, M. & Wood, D. (1986). *The Children's Primary Prevention Training Programme*. Baltimore, MD: Authors.

Nemerofsky, A., Carran, D. & Rosenberg, L. (1994). Age variation in performance among preschool children in a sexual abuse prevention program. *Journal of Child Sexual Abuse*, 3(1), 85–102.*

Neufeld, A. & Fantuzzo, J.W. (1984). Contingent application of a protective device to treat the severe self-biting behavior of a disturbed autistic child. *Journal of Behaviour Therapy and Experimental Psychiatry*, 15(1), 79–83.*

Newcomb, M. & Bentler, P. (1988). *Consequence of Adolescent Drug Abuse; Impact on the Lives of Young Adults*. Newbury Park, CA: Sage.

Newland, T. (1971). *Blind Learning Aptitude Test*. Champaign, IL: University of Illinois Press.

Nitz, K. (1999). Adolescent pregnancy prevention: a review of interventions and programs. *Clinical Psychology Review*, 19, 457–471.

Norris, M., Spaulding, P. & Brodie, F. (1957). *Blindness in Children*. Chicago: University of Chicago Press.

Novaco, R.W. (1975). *Anger Control: the Development and Evaluation of an Experimental Treatment*. Lexington, MA: Heath.

O'Connor, R. & Sheehy, N. (2000). *Understanding Suicidal Behaviour*. Leicester, UK: British Psychological Society Books.

O'Connor, S., Vietze, P.M., Sherrod, K.B., Sandler, H.M. & Altemeier, W.A. (1980). Reduced incidence of parenting inadequacy following rooming-in. *Paediatrics*, 66, 176–182.*

Oetting, E.R., Beauvais, F., Edwards, R. & Waters, M. (1984). *The Drug and Alcohol Assessment System*. Western Behavioural Studies, Colorado State University, Fort Collins, Colorado.

Oldfield, D., Hays, B.J. & Megel, M.E. (1996). Evaluation of the effectiveness of project Trust: An elementary school-based victimization prevention strategy. *Child Abuse & Neglect*, 20, 821–832*.

Olds, D.L., Henderson, C.R., Chamberlin, R. & Tatelbaum, R. (1986). Preventing child abuse and neglect: A randomized trial of nurse home visitation. *Paediatrics*, 78, 65–78.*

Ollendick, T.H. (1983). Reliability and validity of the revised Fear Survey Schedule for Children (FSSC-R). *Behaviour Research and Therapy*, 21, 77–84.

Olsen, J.L. & Widom, C.S. (1993). Prevention of child abuse and neglect. *Applied and Preventive Psychology*, 2, 217–229.

Olson, M. (1987). Early intervention for children with visual impairments. In M.J. Guralnick & F.C. Bennet (Eds.), *The Effectiveness of Early Intervention for at Risk and Handicapped Children* (pp. 325–357). New York: Academic Press.

Olweus, D. (1989). *Questionnaire for Students* (Junior and senior versions). Unpublished manuscript.

Olweus D. (1991). Bully/Victim school problems among school children: Basic effects of a school based intervention program. In D. Pepler & K. Rubin (Eds.), *The Development and Treatment of Childhood Aggression*. Hillsdale, NJ: Lawrence Erlbaum Associates Inc.*

Olweus, D. (1992). Bullying among school children: Intervention and prevention. In

R.D. Peters, R.J. McMahon & V.L. Quincy (Eds.), *Aggression Throughout the Life Span*. Newbury Park, CA: Sage.*

Olweus, D. (1993). *Bullying in Schools: What We Know and What We Can Do*. Oxford: Blackwell.*

Olweus, D. (1997). Bully/victim problems in school: Knowledge base and an effective intervention program. *Irish Journal of Psychology*, 18(2), 170–190.*

Olweus D. & Alsakar, F.D. (1991). Assessing change in a cohort longitudinal study with hierarchical data. In D. Magnusson, L. Bergman, G. Rudiger & B. Torestad (Eds.), *Problems and Methods in Longitudinal Research*. New York: Cambridge University Press.*

Olweus D. & Roland, E. (1983). *Mobbing – Bakgrunn og Tiltik*. Oslo, Norway: Kirke-og undevisnigdepartmentet.

Olweus, D. & Smith, P.K. (in press). *Manual for the Olweus Bully/Victim Questionnaire*. Oxford: Blackwell.

O'Moore, A.M., Kirkham, C. & Smith, M. (1997). Bullying behaviour in Irish schools: A Nation-wide study. *Irish Journal of Psychology*, 18(2), 141–169.

O'Neill, R.E., Horner, R.H., Albin, R.W., Storey, K. & Sprague, J. (1990). *Functional Analysis: A Practical Assessment Guide*. Pacific Grove, CA: Brookes Cole.

O'Neill, R.E., Horner, R.H., Albin, R.W., Sprague, J., Storey, K. & Newton, J. (1997). *Functional Assessment and Programme Development for Problem Behaviour: A Practical Handbook* (Second Edition). Pacific Grove, CA: Brookes Cole.

Orbach, I. (1988). *Children Who Don't Want to Live*. San Francisco: Jossey Bass.

Orbach, I. & Bar-Joseph, H. (1993). The impact of a suicide prevention program for adolescents on suicidal tendencies, hopelessness, ego-identity and coping. *Suicide and Life-Threatening Behavior*, 23, 120–129.*

Overholser, J.C., Hemstreet, A.H., Spirito, A. & Vyse, S. (1989). Suicide awareness programs in the schools: Effects of gender and personal experience. *Journal of the American Academy of Child and Adolescent Psychiatry*, 28(6), 925–930.*

Ozonoff, S. (1994). Executive functions in autism. In E. Schopler & G. Mesibov (Eds.), *Learning and Cognition in Autism* (pp. 220–230). New York: Plenum Press.

Ozonoff, S. & Cathcart, K. (1998). Effectiveness of a home programme intervention for young children with autism. *Journal of Autism and Developmental Disorders*, 28, 25–32.*

Padgett, D., Mumford, E. & Hynes, M. (1988). Meta-analysis of the effects of educational and psychosocial interventions on management of diabetes mellitus. *Journal of Clinical Epidemiology*, 41, 1007–1030.

Pagliaro, A. & Pagliaro, L. (1996). *Substance Use among Children and Adolescents*. New York: Wiley.

Palmer, F. (1971). *Concept Training Curriculum For Children Ages Two to Five*. Stony Brook, NY: State University of New York, Stony Brook.

Palmer, F.B., Shapiro, B.K., Wachtel, R.C., Allen, M.C., Hiller, J.E., Harryman, S.E., Mosher, B.S., Meinert, C.L. & Capute, A.J. (1988). The effects of physical therapy on cerebral palsy, a controlled trial in infants with spastic diplegia. *New England Journal of Medicine*, 318(13), 803–808.*

Palmer, F.B., Shapiro, B.K., Allen, M.C., Mosher, B.S., Bilker, S.A., Harryman, S.E., Meinert, C.L. & Capute, A.J. (1990). Infant stimulation curriculum for infants with cerebral palsy: effects on infant temperament, parent-infant interaction, and home environment. *Paediatrics*, 85, 411–415.*

Palumba, D., Davidson, P., Peloquin, L.J. & Gigliotti, F. (1995). Psychological effects of paediatric infectious diseases. In M. Roberts (Eds.), *Handbook of Paediatric Psychology* (Second Edition, pp. 437–447). New York: Guilford Press.

Parcel, G.S. & Meyer, M.P. (1978). Development of an instrument to measure children's health locus of control. *Health Education Monograph*, 6, 149.

Parcel, G.S. & Nadar, P.R (1997). Evaluation of a pilot school health education program for asthmatic children. *Journal of School Health*, 47, 453.*

Parcel, G.G., Tiernan, K. & Nadar, P.R. (1979). *Teaching Myself about Asthma.* St Louis, MO: CV Mosby.

Parcel, G.S., Nadar, P.R. & Tiernan, K. (1980). A health education program for children with asthma. *Developmental and Behavioral Pediatrics*, 1(3), 128–133.*

Parker, S., Zahr, L., Cole, J. & Brecht, M. (1992). Outcome after developmental intervention in the neonatal intensive care unit for mothers of preterm infants with low socioeconomic status. *Journal of Pediatrics*, 120, 780–785.

Pearlin, I. & Schooler, C. (1978). The structure of coping. *Journal of Health and Social Behaviour*, 19, 2–21.

Pechacek T., Fox B., Murray D. & Leupker, A. (1984). Review of techniques for measurement of smoking behaviour in behavioural health. In J. Matazarro, J. Herd, N. Miller & S. Weiss (Eds.), *A Handbook of Health Enhancement and Disease Prevention* (pp. 729–754). New York: Wiley.

Pellegrino, L. (1997). Cerebral palsy. In M. Batshaw (Ed.), *Children with Disabilities* (Fourth Edition. pp. 499–528). Baltimore, MD: Brookes.

Pentz, M., Trebow, E., Hansen, W., MacKinnon, D., Dwyer, J., Johnson, C., Flay, B., Daniels, S. & Cormack, C. (1990). Effects of program implementation on adolescent drug use behaviour: The Midwestern Prevention. *Project Evaluation Review*, 14, 264–289.*

Pepler, D.J., Craig, W.M., Ziegler, S. & Charach, A. (1993). A school-based anti-bullying intervention program. In D. Tattum (Ed.), *Understanding and Managing Bullying* (pp. 76–91). Oxford: Heinemann.*

Pepler, D.J., Craig, W.M., Ziegler, S. & Charach, A. (1994). An evaluation of an anti-bullying intervention in Toronto schools. *Canadian Journal of Community, Mental Health*, 13(2), 95–110.*

Perez, M.G., Feldman, L. & Caballero, F. (1999). Effects of a self management educational program for the control of childhood asthma. *Patient Education and Counseling*, 36, 47–55.*

Perrin, J.M., Maclean, W.E., Gortmaker, S.L. & Asher, K.N. (1992). Improving the psychological status of children with asthma: A randomized controlled trial. *Developmental and Behavioural Pediatrics*, 13(4), 241–247.*

Perrin, S., Smith, P. & Yule, W. (2000). Practitioner review: The assessment and treatment of post-traumatic stress disorder in children and adolescents. *Journal of Child Psychology and Psychiatry*, 41, 277–289.

Perry, B.P. & Azad, I. (1999). Posttraumatic stress disorders in children and adolescents. *Current Opinion in Paediatrics*, 11, 310–316.

Perry, C., Willliams, C., Veblen-Mortenson, S., Toomey, T., Komro, K., Anstine, P., McGovern, P., Finnegan, J., Forster, J., Wagenaar, A. & Wolfson, M. (1996). Project Northland: Outcomes of a community wide alcohol use prevention programme during early adolescence. *American Journal of Public Health*, 86, 956–965.*

Perry, C., Willliams, C., Komro, K., Veblen-Mortenson, S. et al. (2000). Project Northland: Outcomes of a community wide alcohol use prevention programme during early adolescence. *American Journal of Public Health*, 86, 956–965.*

Perry, D.G., Kusel, S.J. & Perry, L.C. (1988). Victims of peer aggression. *Developmental Psychology*, 24, 801–814.

Pfefferbaum, B. (1997). Post-traumatic stress disorder in children: a review of the past 10 years. *Journal of the American Academy of Child and Adolescent Psychiatry*, 36, 1503–1511.

Pikas, A. (1989). The common concern method for the treatment of mobbing. In E. Roland & E. Munthe (Eds.), *Bullying an International Perspective*. London: David Fulton.

Piper, M.C. (1990). Efficacy of physical therapy: rate of motor development in children with cerebral palsy. *Pediatric Physical Therapy*, 2, 126–130.

Pirner, C. & Westcott, N. (1994). *Even Little Kids get Diabetes*. New York: Albert Whitman.

Plant, T.F. (1988). *Children with Asthma: A Manual for Parents*. Amherst, MA: Pedipress.

Platt, S. (1992). Parasuicide in Europe: the WHO/EURO multicentre study on parasuicide. *Acta Psychiatrica Scandinavica*, 85, 97–104.

Plotnick, I. (1999). Type 1 (Insulin dependent) diabetes. In J. McMillan, C. DeAngelis, R. Feigin & J. Warshaw (Eds.), *Oski's Pediatrics: Principles and Practice* (pp. 1793–1802) Philadelphia, PA: Lippincott, Williams & Wilkins.

Powell, C. & Grantham-McGregor, S. (1989) Home visiting of varying frequency and child development. *Pediatrics*, 84, 1.*

Powell, L.F. (1974). The effect of extra stimulation and maternal involvement on the development of low birth weight infants and on maternal behavior. *Child Development*, 45, 106–113.*

Pratt, W.E., Stouffer, G.A. & Yanuzzi, J.R. (1975). *American School Achievement Tests*. Indianapolis, IN: Bobbs-Merrill.

Psychological Society of Ireland: Learning Disability Group (April 1998). *Responding to Behaviour that Challenges*. Dublin: PSI.

Pynoos, R. & Eth, S. (1986). Witness to violence: The child interview. *Journal of the American Academy of Child and Adolescent Psychiatry*, 25, 306–319.

Pynoos, R.S., Frederick, C., Nader, K., Arroyo, W., Steinberg, A., Eth, S., Nunez, F. & Fairbanks, L. (1992). Life threat and posttraumatic stress in school-age children. *Archives of General Psychiatry*, 44, 1057–1063. (Contains the Child Posttraumatic Stress Reaction Index.)

Quigley, S. & Kretschmer, R. (1982). *The Education of Deaf Children*. Baltimore, MD: University Park Press.

Quigley, S.P., Steinkamp, M.W., Power, D.J. & Jones, B.W. (1978). *Test of Syntactic Abilities*. Beaverton, OR: Dormac.

Radler, G.A., Plesa, C., Senini, K. & Reicha, J. (1985). Treatment of self-injurious behaviour in a severely handicapped adolescent: A case study. *Australia and New Zealand Journal of Developmental Disabilities*, 11(2), 107–112.*

Radloff, L. (1977). The CES-D Scale: A self report depression scale for use in the general population. *Journal of Applied Psychological Measurement*, 1, 385–401.

Rakos, R.F., Grodek, M.V. & Mack, K.K. (1985). The impact of self-administered behavioral intervention program on pediatric asthma. *Journal of Psychometric Research*, 29(1), 101–108.*

Ramey, C.T. & Campbell, F.A. (1991). Poverty, early childhood education, and academic competence: The Abecedarian experiment. In A.C. Huston (Ed.), *Children in Poverty*. Cambridge University Press.*

Ramey, C.T. & Smith, B.J. (1977) Assessing the intellectual consequences of early intervention with high-risk infants. *American Journal of Mental Deficiency*, 81, 318–324.

Ramey, C.T., Bryant, D.M., Wasik, B.H., Sparling, J.J., Fendt, K.H. & LaVange, L.M. (1992). Infant health and development program for low birth weight, premature infants: Program elements, family participation, and child intelligence. *Pediatrics*, 3, 454–465.*

Rauh, V., Achenbach, T., Nurcombe, B., Howell, C. & Teti, D. (1988). Minimizing adverse effects of low birth weight: Four year results of an early intervention program. *Child Development*, 59, 544–553.*

Reddihough, D.S., King, J., Coleman, G. & Catanese, T. (1998). Efficacy of programmes based on conductive education for young children with cerebral palsy. *Developmental Medicine and Child Neurology*, 40, 763–770.*

Reichle, J., York, J. & Sigafoos, J. (1991). *Implementing Augmentative and Alternative Communication.* Baltimore: Paul H Brookes.

Resnick, G. (1985). Enhancing parental competencies for high risk mothers: An evaluation of prevention effects. *Child Abuse and Neglect*, 9, 479–489.*

Resnick, M. & Packer, A. (1990). *Infant Development Activities for Parents.* New York: St Martins Press.

Resnick, M., Eyler, F.D., Nelson, R.M., Eitzman, D.V. & Bucciarelli, R.L. (1987). Developmental intervention for low birth weight infants: Improved early developmental outcome. *Pediatrics*, 80, 68–74.*

Resnick, M., Armstrong, S. & Carter, R. (1988). Developmental intervention for high risk premature infants. Effects of development and parent-infant interactions. *Journal of Developmental and Behavioural Pediatrics*, 9, 73–78.*

Reynell, J. (1979). *Manual for the Reynell-Zinkin Scales, Developmental Scales for Visually Handicapped Children. Part 1: Mental Development.* Windsor, Berks: NFER.

Reynolds, C.R. & Richmond, B.O. (1985). *Revised Children's Manifest Anxiety Scale Manual, (RCMAS).* Los Angeles: Western Psychological Services.

Riestenberg, N. (1993). *Trust: Teaching Reaching Using Students & Theatre: A Manual To Train Child Sexual Abuse Prevention Peer Educators.* Minneapolis, MN: Illusion Theatre.

Rigby, K. (1996). *Bullying In Australia Schools – And What to Do About it.* Melbourne: ACER.

Rigby, K. (1997). Attitudes and beliefs about bullying among Australian school children. *Irish Journal of Psychology*, 18 (2), 202–220.

Rispens, J., Aleman, A. & Goudena, P. (1997). Prevention of child abuse victimization: A meta-analysis of school programs. *Child Abuse and Neglect*, 21(10), 975–987.

Robinson, E.A., Eyeberg, S. & Ross, A.W. (1980). The standardisation of an inventory of child conduct problem behaviours. *Journal of Clinical Child Psychology*, 9, 22–28.

Robinson, G. & Jan, J. (1993). Acquired ocular visual impairment in children: 1960–1989. *American Journal of Diseases of Children*, 147, 325–328.

Roderick, T. (1988). Jonny can learn to negotiate. *Educational Leadership*, 45(4), 86–90.

Rogers, S.J. (1998). Empirically supported comprehensive treatments for young children with autism. *Journal of Clinical Child Psychology*, 27, 168–179.

Roland, E. (1989a). Bullying: The Scandinavian research tradition. In D.P. Tattum & D.A. Lane (Eds.), *Bullying in Schools*. Stoke-on Trent: Trentham Books.*

Roland, E. (1989b). A system oriented strategy against bullying. In E. Roland & E. Munthe (Eds.), *Bullying: An International Perspective* (pp. 143–151). London: David Fulton.*

Roland, E. & Munthe E. (1989). *Bullying: An International Perspective*. London: David Fulton.

Roland, E. & Munthe, E. (1997). The 1996 Norwegian program for preventing and managing bullying schools. *Irish Journal of Psychology*, 18(2), 233–247.*

Rosenbaum, A. (1986). A schedule for assessing self-control behavior. *Behavior Therapy*, 17, 132–142.

Rosenthal, S., Cohen, S. & Biro, F. (1994). Sexually transmitted diseases. In R. Simeonson (Ed.), *Risk, Resilience and Prevention* (pp. 239–264). New York: Brooks.

Rowland, C. (1990, 1996). *Communication Matrix*. Portland, OR: Oregon Health Sciences University.

Rowland, C. & Schweigert, P. (1997). *Hands-on Problem-Solving for Children with Deafblindess (SIPPS, HIPSS, TAPPS and Guide to Assessment and Teaching Strategies)*. Portland, OR: Oregon Health Sciences University.

Rowland, C. & Schweigert, P. (2000). *Time to Learn*. Portland, OR: Oregon Health Sciences University.

Rubin, R. & Peyrot, M. (1992). Psychosocial problems and interventions in diabetes. *Diabetes Care*, 15 (11), 1649–1657.

Rubin, R., Young-Hyman, D. & Peyrot, M. (1989). Parent-child responsibility and conflict in diabetes care. *Diabetes*, 38 (suppl. 2), 28 A (abstract).

Rudd, M. & Joiner, T. (1998). The assessment management and treatment of suicidality; towards clinically informed and balanced standards of care. *Clinical Psychology: Science and Practice*, 5, 135–150.

Rumsey, J. & Vitiello, B. (2000). Treatments for people with autism and other pervasive developmental disorders. Special issue of *Journal of Autism and Developmental Disorders*, Volume 30, Whole of Number 5, 369–508.

Russell, D.J., Rosenbaum, P.L., Cadman, D.T., Gowland, C., Hardy, S. & Jarvis, S. (1989). The Gross Motor Function Measure: A means to evaluate the effects of physical therapy. *Developmental Medicine and Child Neurology*, 31, 341–352.

Ryden, O., Nevander, L., Johnson, P., Hansson K., Kronvali, P., Sjöblad, S. & Westborn, L. (1994). Family therapy in poorly controlled juvenile IDDM: effects on diabetic control, self-evaluation and behavioural symptoms. *Acta Paediatrica*, 83, 285–291.

Sacco, W.P., Levine, B., Reed, D.L. & Thompson, K. (1991). Attitudes about condom use as an AIDS-relevant behaviour: Their factor structure and relation to condom use. *Psychological Assessment: A Journal of Consulting and Clinical Psychology*, 3, 276–292.

Saigh, P.A. (1989). The validity of DSM-III post traumatic stress disorder classification as applied to children. *Journal of Abnormal Psychology*, 198, 189–192.

Sarno, J. & Wurtele, S. (1997). Effects of a personal safety program on preschoolers' knowledge, skills, and perceptions of child sexual abuse. *Child Maltreatment*, 2(1), 35–45.*

Saslawsky, D.A. & Wurtele, S.K. (1986). Educating children about sexual abuse: Implications for pediatric intervention and possible prevention. *Journal of Pediatric Psychology*, 11, 235–245.*

Satin, W., La Greca, A.M., Zigo, M.A. & Skyler, N. (1989). Diabetes in adolescence: Effects of multifamily group intervention and parent stimulation of diabetes. *Journal of Pediatric Psychology*, 14(2), 259–275.*

Scarr-Salapatek, S. & Williams, M.L. (1973). The effects of early stimulation on low-birth-weight infants. *Child Development*, 44, 94–101.*

Schaalma, H.P., Kok, G., Bosker, R.J., Parcel, G.S., Poelman, J. & Reinder, J. (1996). Planned development and evaluation of AIDS/STD education for secondary school students in the Netherlands: Short-term effects. *Health Education Quarterly*, 23(4), 469–487.*

Schaefer, C. & Friemeister, J. (1989). *Handbook of Parent Training*. New York: Wiley.

Schaefer, E. & Bell, R. (1958). Development of a Parental Attitudes Research Instrument (PARI). *Child Development*, 29, 337–361.

Schafer, L. (1986). Supportive and non-supportive family behaviours: Relationships to adherence and metabolic control in persons with Type 1 diabetes. *Diabetes*, 9, 179–185. (Contains the Diabetes Family Behaviour Checklist.)

Schinke, S., Blythe, B.J. & Gilchrist, L.D. (1981). Cognitive–behavioural prevention of adolescent pregnancy. *Journal of Counseling Psychology*, 28(5), 451–454.*

Schinke, S., Schilling, R.F., Barth, R.P., Gilchrist, L.D. & Maxwell, J.S. (1986). Stress management intervention to prevent family violence. *Journal of Family Violence*, 1, 13–26.*

Schinke, S.P., Gordon, A.N. & Weston, R.E. (1990). Self-instruction to prevent HIV infection among African-American and Hispanic-American Adolescents. *Journal of Consulting and Clinical Psychology*, 58(4), 432–436.*

Schinke, S., Botvin, G. & Orlandi, M. (1991). *Substance Abuse in Children and Adolescents: Evaluation and Intervention*. Thousand Oaks, CA: Sage.

Schlesinger, H. & Meadow, K.P. (1976). *Studies of Family Interaction, Language Acquisition and Deafness*. Washington, DC: Office of Maternal and Child Health.

Schneider, C., Helfer, R. & Pollock, E. (1972). The predictive questionnaire: A preliminary report. In C. Hempe & R. Helfer (Eds.), *Helping the Battered Child and His Family*. Philadelphia: JB Lippincott.

Schneider, M. & Robin, S. (1978). *Manual for the Turtle Technique*. Unpublished manual, Department of Psychology, State University of New York at Stony Brook.

Schneider, M., Bijam-Schulte, A.M., Jannssen, C.G. & Stolk, J. (1996). The origin of self-injurious behaviour of children with mental retardation. *British Journal of Developmental Disabilities*, 42(2), 136–148.

Schope, J., Copeland, L., Marcoux, B. & Kamp, M. (1996). Effectiveness of a school-based substance abuse prevention program. *Journal of Drug Education*, 26, 323–337.*

Schope, J., Copeland, L., Kamp, M. & Lang, S. (1998). Twelfth grade follow-up of the effectiveness of a middle school-based substance abuse prevention program. *Journal of Drug Education*, 28, 185–197.*

Schope, J., Weimer, M., Dielman, L., Smith, A. et al. (1987). *Substance Use Prevention Education and Alcohol Misuse Prevention: Curricula for 5th, 6th and 7th grades and Booster Sessions*. Ann Arbor: University of Michigan. (Contact Dr Jean Schope, Transportation Institute, University of Michigan, 2901, Baxter Road, Ann Arbor, MI 48109–2150.)

Schopler, E. (1980). *Video of TEACCH Programme for Parents*. Chapel Hill, NC: Health Sciences Consortium Distribution Department.

Schopler, E. (1980). *Demonstration tape on using the Childhood Autism Rating Scale*

(CARS). TEACCH (Treatment and Education of Autistic and related Communication handicapped CHildren) Videotapes. Health Sciences Consortium Distribution Department, 201 Silver Cedar Court, Chapel Hill, NC.

Schopler, E. (1980*). Demonstration videotape on scoring the Psychoeducational Profile (PEP).* Chapel Hill, NC: Health Sciences Consortium Distribution Department.

Schopler, E. (1980). *Video of TEACCH Programme for Teachers.* Chapel Hill, NC: Health Sciences Consortium Distribution Department.

Schopler, E. (1980). *Videotape of an individualised education programme. Conversion of a psychoeducational profile (PEP) into an individualised teaching programmes.* Chapel Hill, NC: Health Sciences Consortium Distribution Department.

Schopler, E. (1997). Implementation of TEACHH philosophy. In D. Cohen & F. Volkmar (Eds.), *Handbook of Autism and Pervasive Developmental Disorders* (Second Edition, pp. 767–795). New York: Wiley.

Schopler, E., Lansing, M. & Reichler, R. (1979). *Individualised Assessment and Treatment for Autistic and Developmentally Disabled Children. Teaching Strategies for Parents and Professionals Volume 11.* Austin, TX: Pro-ed.

Schopler, E., Lansing, M. & Waters, L. (1980). *Individualised Assessment and Treatment for Autistic and Developmentally Disabled Children. Teaching Strategies for Parents and Professionals Volume 111.* Austin, TX: Pro-ed.

Schopler, E., Richler, R. & Renner, B. (1986). *The Childhood Autism Rating Scale (CARS) for Diagnostic Screening and Classification of Autism.* New York: Irvington. (Order CARS from Western Psychological Services 12031 Wilshire Boulevard, Los Angeles, California 90025–1251. Phone 1–800–648–8857. Order a CARS training video from Health Sciences Consortium 201 Silver Cedar Court, Chapel Hill, NC, 27514–1517.)

Schopler, E., Reichler, R.J., Bashford, A., Lansing, M.D. & Marcus, L.M. (1990). *The Psychoeducational Profile-Revised (PEP-R).* Austin, TX: Pro-Ed.

Schweinhart, L.J., Berrueta-Clement, J.R., Barnett, W.S., Epstein, A.S. & Weikert, D.P. (1985). Effects of the Perry Preschool Program on youths through age 19: A summary. *Topics in Early Childhood Education,* 5, 26–35.*

Scott, S. (1994). Mental retardation. In M. Rutter, E. Taylor & L. Hersov (Eds.), *Child and Adolescent Psychiatry: Modern Approaches* (Third Edition, pp. 616–646). London: Blackwell.

Scotti, J.R., Evans, I.M., Meyer, L.H. & Walker, P. (1991). A meta-analysis of intervention research with problem behavior: Treatment validity and standards of practice. *American Journal on Mental Retardation,* 96(3), 233–256.

Scruggs, T.E., Mastropieri, M.A. & Casto, G. (1987). The quantitative synthesis of single-subject research: methodology and validation. *Remedial and Special Education,* 8(2), 24–33.

Scrutton, D. (1984). *Management of the Motor Disorders of Children with Cerebral Palsy.* London: Spastics International Medical Publications.

Shadish, W. (1993). *Effect Size Coding Manual.* Memphis State University.

Shaffer, D. & Piacentini, J. (1994). Suicide and attempted suicide. In M. Rutter, E. Taylor & L. Hersov (Eds.), *Child and Adolescent Psychiatry: Modern Approaches* (Third Edition, pp. 407–424). Oxford: Blackwell.

Shaffer, D., Garland, A., Gould, M., Fisher, P. & Trautman, P. (1988). Preventing teenage suicide: A critical review. *Journal of the American Academy of Child and Adolescent Psychiatry,* 27, 675–687.

Shamoo, T.K., Patros, P.G. & Rinzler, A. (1997). *Helping your Child Cope with Depression and Suicidal Thoughts*. San Francisco, CA: Jossey Bass.

Shapiro, B. & Capute, A. (1999). Cerebral palsy. In J. McMillan, C. DeAngelis, R. Feigin & J. Warshaw (Eds.), *Oski's Pediatrics: Principles and Practice* (Third Edition, pp. 1910–1917). Philadelphia, PA: Lippincott, Williams & Wilkins.

Shapiro, F. (1989). Eye movement desensitization: a new treatment for post-traumatic stress disorder. *Journal of Behavior Therapy and Experimental Psychiatry*, 20, 211–217.

Sharp, S. & Smith, P. (1994). *Tackling Bullying in Your School: A Practical Handbook for Teachers*. London: Routledge.

Sheehan, R. (1979). Mild to moderately handicapped preschoolers: How do you select child assessment instruments. In T. Black (Ed.), *Perspective on Measurement. A Collection of Readings for Educators of Young Handicapped Children* (pp. 29–30). Chapel Hill, NC: Technical Assistance Development system.

Sheeran, P., Abraham, C. & Orbell, S. (1999). Psychosocial correlates of condom use: A meta-analysis. *Psychological Bulletin*, 125, 90–132.

Sheinkopf, S.J. & Siegel, B. (1998). Home-based behavioral treatment of young children. *Journal of Autism and Developmental Disorders*, 28, 15–23.*

Showland, J., Bauchner, H. & Adair, R. (1988). The impact of pediatric asthma education on morbidity: Assessing the evidence. *Chest*, 94, 964–969.*

Siegel, E., Bauman, K.E., Schaefer, E.S., Saunders, M.M. & Ingram, D.D. (1980). Hospital and home support during infancy: Impact on maternal attachment, child abuse and neglect, and health care utilization. *Paediatrics*, 66, 183–190.*

Sigafoos, J. & Meikle, B. (1996). Functional communication training for the treatment of multiply determined challenging behavior in two boys with autism. *Behavior Modification*, 20(1), 60–84.*

Sigman, M. (1995). Behavioural research in childhood autism. In M. Lenzenweger & J. Haugaard (Eds.), *Frontiers of developmental psychopathology* (pp. 190–206). New York: Springer Verlag.

Simonoff, E., Bolton, P. & Rutter, M. (1996). Mental retardation: Genetic findings, clinical implications and research agenda. *Journal of Child Psychology and Psychiatry*, 37, 259–280.

Singh, N. (1997). *Prevention and Treatment of Severe Behavior Problems: Models and Methods in Developmental Disabilities*. Pacific Grove: Brooks/Cole.

Singh, N., Dawson, M.J. & Manning, P.J. (1981). The effects of physical restraint on self-injurious behaviour. *Journal of Mental Deficiency Research*, 25, 207–216.*

Skinner, H. (1982). The drug abuse screening test. *Addictive Behaviour*, 7, 363–371.

Slaughter, D.T. (1983). Early Interventions and its effects on maternal and child development. *Monographs of the Society for Research in Child Development*, 48, 4.*

Smith, P. (1997). Bullying in schools: The UK experience and the Sheffield anti-bullying project. *Irish Journal of Psychology*, 18(2), 191–201.*

Smith, P. & Sharp, S. (Eds.) (1994). *School Bullying: Insights and Perspectives*. London: Routledge.*

Smith, P. & Thompson, D. (1991). *Practical Approaches to Bullying*. London: David Fulton.

Smith, P., Dyregrov, A., Yule, W., Gupta, L., Perrin, S. & Gjestad, R. (1999). *Children and Disaster: Teaching Recovery Techniques*. Bergen, Norway: Children and War Foundation.

Sonksen, P.M., Petrie, A. & Drew, K. (1991). Promotion of visual development of severely visually impaired babies: Evaluation of a developmentally based programme. *Developmental Medicine and Child Neurology*, 33, 320–335*.

Sparling, J. & Lewis, I. (1979) *Learning Games for the First Three Years: A Program for Parent/Center Partnership*. New York: Walker Educational.

Sparling, J. & Lewis, I. (1984a). *Partners for Learning*. Lewisville, NC: Kaplan Press.

Sparling, J. & Lewis, I. (1984b). *Learningames for Threes and Fours: A Guide To Parent–Child Play*. New York: Walker.

Sparling, J., Lewis, I. & Neuwirth, S. (1988). *Early partners Curriculum Kit*. Lewisville, NC: Kaplan Press.

Sparling, J., Lewis, I., Ramey, C., Wasik, B., Bryant, D. & LaVange, L. (1991). Partners: A curriculum to help premature, low birth weight infants get off to a good start. *Top Early Child Special Education*, 11, 36–55.

Sparrow, S.D., Bella, D.A. & Cicchetti, D.V. (1985). *The Vineland Adaptive Behaviour Scales*. Circle Pines, MN: American Guidance Services.

Spielberger, C.D. (1973). *Manual for the State-Trait Anxiety Inventory for Children*. Palo Alto, CA: Consulting Psychologists Press.

Spirito, A., Overholser, J., Ashworth, S., Morgan, J. & Benedict-Drew, C. (1988a). Evaluation of a suicide awareness curriculum for high school students. *Journal of the American Academy of Child and Adolescent Psychiatry*, 27(6), 705–711.*

Spirito, A., Overholser, J., Ashworth, S., Morgan, J. & Benedict-Drew, C. (1988b). *Attitudes Toward Suicide Test* and *Suicide Knowledge Test (SKT)*. (Available from Dr Spirito, Child & Family Psychiatry, Rhode Island Hospital, 593 Eddy St Providence, RI 02903.)

St Lawrence, J.S., Jefferson, K.W., Alleyne, E. & Brasfield, T.L. (1995a). Comparison of education versus behavioral skills training interventions in lowering sexual HIV-Risk behaviour of substance-dependent adolescents. *Journal of Consulting and Clinical Psychology*, 63(1), 154–157.*

St Lawrence, J.S., Brasfield, T.L., Jefferson, K.W., Alleyne, E., O'Bannon, R.E. III & Shirley, A. (1995b). Cognitive-Behavioural intervention to reduce African American adolescents' risk for HIV infection. *Journal of Consulting and Clinical Psychology*, 63, 221–237.*

Standardisation of lung function testing in children (1980). Proceedings and recommendations of the GAP conference committee, Cystic Fibrosis Foundation. *Journal of Pediatrics*, 97, 668–678.

Stark, K. & Kendall, P. (1996). *Treating Depressed Children: Therapists Manual for ACTION*. Ardmore, PA: Workbook Publishing.

Stark, K., Kendall, P., McCarthy, M., Stafford, M., Barron, R. & Thomeer, M. (1996). *A Workbook for Overcoming Depression*. Ardmore, PA: Workbook Publishing.

Steege, M.W., Wacker, D.P., Cigrand, K.C., et al. (1990). Use of negative reinforcement in the treatment of self-injurious behavior. *Journal of Applied Behaviour Analysis*, 23, 459–467.*

Steinbok, P., Reiner, A. & Kestle, J.R.W. (1997). Therapeutic electrical stimulation following selective posterior rhizotomy in children with spastic diplegic cerebral palsy: a randomized clinical trial. *Developmental Medicine and Child Neurology*, 39, 515–520.*

Stevens-Simon, C. & Orleans, M. (1999). Low-birth weight prevention programs: the enigma of failure. *Birth*, 26(3), 184–191.

Stillman, R. & Battle, C. (1985). *Callier-Azusa Scale (H): Scales for the Assessment of*

Communicative Abilities. Dallas: University of Texas at Dallas, Callier Centre for Communication Disorders.

Stoppard, M. (1992). *Everygirl's Life-guide*. London: Dorling Kindersley.

Strong, C.J., Clark, T.C., Barringer, D.G., Walden, B., Williams, S.A. (1992). *SKI*HI Home-based Programming for Children with Hearing Impairments: Demographics, Child Identification and Programme Effectiveness*, 1979–1990: Final report to the US Department of Education, Office of Special Education and Rehabilitative Services. Logan: Utah State University of Communication Disorders. SKI*HI Institute.

Strong, C.J., Clark, T.C., Johnson, D., Watkins, S., Barringer, D.G. & Walden, B.E. (1994). SKI*HI Programming for Children who are Deaf or Hard of Hearing: Recent Research Findings. *Infant-Toddler Intervention: The Transdisciplinary Journal*, 4, 25–36*.

Sullivan, K. (2000). *The Anti-Bullying Handbook*. Oxford: Oxford University Press.

Sutton, A. (1988). Conductive education. *Archives of Disease in Childhood*, 63, 214–217.

Tal, D., Gil-Spielberg, R., Antonovsky, H., Tal, A. & Moaz, B. (1990). Teaching families to cope with childhood asthma. *Family Systems Medicine*, 8(2), 135–144.*

Tattum, D.P. (1993). *Understanding and Managing Bullying*. Oxford: Heinemann Educational Books.

Tattum, D.P. (1997). A whole school response: From crisis management to prevention. *Irish Journal of Psychology*, 18(2), 221–232.

Tattum, D. & Herbert, G. (1993). *Countering Bullying*. Stoke on Trent: Trentham Books.

Tattum, D., Tattum, E. & Herbert, G. (1993). *Cycle of Violence*. Cardiff: Drake Educational Associates.

Taylor, D.K. & Beauchamp, C. (1988). Hospital-based primary prevention strategy in child abuse: A multi-level needs assessment. *Child Abuse and Neglect*, 12, 343–354.*

Taylor, I., O'Reilly, M. & Lancioni, G. (1996). An evaluation of an ongoing consultation model to train teachers to treat challenging behaviour. *International Journal of Disability, Development and Education*, 43(3), 203–218.*

Teens who choose life: The suicidal crisis, part II. Gail chooses life [Video filmstrip]. (1986). Pleasantville, NY: Sunburst Communications. (Available from Sunburst Communications, 39 Washington Avenue, Pleasantville, NY 10570–0040.)

Terman L. & Merrill, M.A. (1972). *Stanford Binet Intelligence Scale: Manual for the Third Revision, Form L-M*. Boston: Houghton-Mifflin.

Terr, L.C. (1991). Childhood traumas: an outline and overview. *American Journal of Psychiatry*, 148, 10–20.

Thorndike, R., Hagen, E. & Sattler, J. (1986). *Stanford-Binet Intelligence Scale: Fourth Edition*. San Antonio: Psychological Corporation.

Tiegs, E.W. & Clark, W.W. (1971). *California Achievement Tests*. Monterey Park, CA: California Test Bureau (McGraw-Hill).

Tinker, R. & Wilson, S. (1999). *Through the Eyes of a Child: EMDR with Children*. London: Norton.

Tirosh, E. & Rabino, S. (1989). Physiotherapy for children with cerebral palsy. *American Journal of Diseases of Children*, 143, 552–555.

Tonelson, S. & Watkins, S. (1979). *Instruction Manual for the SKI*HI Language Development Scale: Assessment of Language Skills for Hearing Impaired Children from Infancy to Five Years of Age*. Logan, UT: SKI*HI institute, Utah State University.

Torabi, M.R. & Yarber, W. (1992). Alternate forms of HIV prevention attitude scale for teenagers. *AIDS Education and Prevention*, 4, 172–182.

Traskman-Bendz, L., Alling, C., Alsen, M., Regnell, G., Simonsson, P. & Ohman, R. (1993). The role of monamines in suicidal behavior. *Acta Psychiatrica Scandinavica Suppl*, 371, 45–47.

Tsai, L. (1987). Pre-, peri, and neonatal complications in autism. In E. Schopler & G. Mesibov (Eds.), *Neurobiological Issues in Autism* (pp. 179–189). New York: Plenum.

Turnbull, J.D. (1993). Early intervention for children with or at risk of cerebral palsy. *American Journal of Diseases of Children*, 147, 54–59.

Tutty, L. (1991). Child sexual abuse: A range of prevention options. *Journal of Child and Youth Care* (Special Issue), 23–41.

Tutty, L. (1992). The ability of elementary school children to learn child sexual abuse prevention concepts. *Child Abuse and Neglect*, 16, 369–384.*

Tutty, L. (1995). The Revised Children's Knowledge of Abuse Questionnaire: Development of a measure of children's understanding of sexual abuse prevention concepts. *Social Work Research*, 19(2), 112–120.

Tutty, L. (1997). Child sexual abuse prevention programs: Evaluating who do you tell. *Child Abuse and Neglect*, 21(9), 869–881.*

Tzuriel, D. (1984). Sex-role typing and ego identity in Israeli, Oriental, and Western adolescents. *Journal of Personality and Social Psychology*, 46, 440–457.

Tzuriel, D. & Bar-Joseph, H. (1989). *The Israeli Index of Potential Suicide (IIPS)*. Ramat-Gan: Bar-Ilan University, Department of Psychology. (Available from Dr Bar-Joseph, Department of Psychology, Bar-Ilan University, Ramat-Gan 52900, Israel.)

University of Edinburgh (1981). *Edinburgh Reading Test: Manual of Instruction*. London: Hodder and Stoughton.

Uzgiris, I.G. & Hunt, J.McV. (1978) *Assessment in infancy: Ordinal scales of Psychological Development*. Chicago, IL: University of Illinois Press.

Van Der Kolk, B., McFarlane, A. & Weiseath, L. (1999). *Traumatic Stress: The Effects of Overwhelming Experience on Mind, Body and Society*. New York: Guilford.

Vazquez, M.I. & Buceta, V.M. (1993). Psychological treatment of asthma: Effectiveness of a self management program with and without relaxation training. *Journal of Asthma*, 30(3), 171–183.*

Vergara, K.C., Miskiel, L.W., Oller, D.K., Eilers, R.E. & Balkany, T. (1993). Hierarchy of goals and objectives for tactual vocoder training with hearing-impaired children. In A. Risberg, S. Felicetti, G. Plant & K.E. Spens (Eds.), *Proceedings of the Second International Conference on Tactile Aids, Hearing Aids and cochlear Implants* (pp. 125–133). Stockholm, Sweden: Akademitryck AB: Edsbruck.

Vulpe, S.G. (1982). *Vulpe Assessment Battery*. Toronto: National Institute of Mental Retardation.

Walker, H.M. (1976). *Walker Problem Behaviour Identification Checklist (manual)*. Los Angeles: Western Psychological Services.

Walt Disney Educational Media (producer) (1986). *AIDS; acquired immunodeficiency syndrome (film)*. Burbank, CA: Walt Disney Educational Media.

Walter, H.J. & Vaughan, R.D. (1993). AIDS risk reduction among a multiethnic sample of urban high school students. *JAMA*, 270(6), 725–730.

Wasik, B. (1984a). *Problem Solving for Parents*. Chapel Hill, NC: Frank Porter Graham Child Development Centre.

Wasik, B. (1984b). *Coping with Parenting Through Effective Problem Solving : A Hand-*

book for Professionals. Chapel Hill, NC: Frank Porter Graham Child Development Centre.

Wasik, B.H. & Karweit, N.L. (1994). Off to a good start. Effects of birth to three interventions on early school succes. In N.L. Slaving & B.A. Wasik (Eds.), *Preventing Early School Failure, Research, Policy & Practice* (pp. 13–57). New York: Allyn & Bacon.*

Wasik, B., Bryant, D. & Lyons, D. (1990a). *Home Visiting*. Newbury Park: Sage.

Wasik, B.H., Ramey, G.T., Bryant, D.M. & Sparling, J.J. (1990b). A longitudinal study of two early intervention strategies: Project CARE. *Child Development*, 61, 1682–1696.*

Watkins, S. (1987). Long-term effects of home intervention with hearing-impaired children. *American Annals of the Deaf*, 132, 267–271*

Watkins, S. & Clark, T.C. (1992). *The SKI*HI model: A Resource Manual for Family-Centred, Home-based Programming for Infants, Toddlers, and Pre-school-aged Children with Hearing Impairment*. Logan, UT: HOPE.

Watkins, S., Clark, T., Strong, C. & Barringer, D. (1993). The effectiveness of an intervener model of services for young deaf-blind Children. *American Annals of the Deaf*, 139, 404–409.*

Watkins, S., Pittman, P. & Walden, B. (1998). The deaf mentor project for young children who are deaf and their families. *American Annals of the Deaf*, 143, 29–34.*

Wechsler, D. (1955). *Wechsler Adult Intelligence Scale*. New York: Psychological Corporation.

Wechsler, D. (1967). *Wechsler Pre-school and Primary Scale of Intelligence*. New York: Psychological Corporation.

Wechsler, D. (1974). *Manual for the Wechsler Intelligence Scale for Children (Rev. ed.)*. New York: Psychological Corporation.

Wechsler, D. (1989). *Wechsler Preschool and Primary Scale of Intelligence-Revised (WPPSI-R)*. San Antonio: Psychological Corporation.

Wechsler, D. (1991). *Wechsler Intelligence Scale for Children. Third Edition (WISC-111)*. San Antonio: Psychological Corporation.

Weindling, A.M., Hallam, P., Gregg, J., Klenka, H., Rosenbloom, L. & Hutton, J.L. (1996). A randomized controlled trial of early physiotherapy for high-risk infants. *Acta Paediatrica*, 85, 1107–1111.*

Weiss, J.B. (1981). *Superstuff. In Self Management Educational Programs for Childhood Asthma* (Vol. 2., pp. 273–294). Bethesda, MD: National Institute of Allergic and Infectious Diseases.

Weissberg, R.P., Gesten, E.L., Liebenstein, N.L., Doherty-Schmid, K.D. & Sutton, H. (1980). *The Rochester Social Problem-Solving (SPS) Program*. Rochester, NY: University of Rochester.

Wellings, K., Field, J., Johnson, A. & Wadsworth, J. (1994). *Sexual Behaviour in Britain*. London: Penguin.

Wessely, S., Rose, S. & Bisson, J. (1998). A systematic review of brief psychological interventions ('debriefing') for the treatment of immediate trauma related symptoms and the prevention of post traumatic stress disorder. *The Cochrane Library*, 1998, (4) 1–13.

White, K.R., Bush, D.W. & Casto, G.C. (1985). Learning from reviews of early intervention. *Journal of Special Education*, 19, 417–428.

Whitman, N., West, D., Brough, F.K. & Welch, M. (1985). A study of a self care rehabilitation program in pediatric asthma. *Health Education Quarterly*, 12(4), 333–342.*

Wilder, D. & Carr, J. (1998). Recent advances in the modification of establishing operations to reduce aberrant behaviour. *Behavioural Interventions*, 13, 43–59.

Williams, C. (2000). Project Northland Alcohol Prevention Curriculum for grades 6–8. Minneapolis, MN: Hazelden. (Available from *www.hazelden.org*. Information on programme materials is available from Professor Cheryl Perry, Division of Epidemiology, School of Public Health, University of Minnesota, 1300 S Second Street, Suite 300, Minneapolis, MN 55454. Email *perry@epivax.epi.umn.edu.*)

Williams, C. & Perry, C. (1998). Lessons from Project Northland. *Alcohol Health and Research World*, 22, 107–116.*

Williams, D. (1992). *Nobody Nowhere*. London: Doubleday. (Biographical account of autism).

Williams, J. (1980). *Red Flag – Green Flag People*. Fargo, ND: Rape and Abuse Crisis Center.

Williams, K. (1995). *A Parents Guide For Suicidal And Depressed Teens: Help for Recognizing if a Child is in Crisis and What to Do*. Hazeldon Information Education.

Williams, M.L. & Scarr, S. (1971). Effects of short term intervention on performance in low-birth-weight, disadvantaged children. *Pediatrics*, 47, 289–298.*

Willis, D., Holden, E. & Rosenberg, M. (1992). *Prevention of Child Maltreatment: Developmental and Ecological Perspectives*. New York: Wiley.

Wing, L. (1996). *The Autistic Spectrum: A Guide for Parents and Professionals*. Constable: London.

Wing, L. (2000). *DISCO: The Diagnostic Interview Schedule for Social and Communication Disorders*. UK: National Autistic Society. (Available from The Centre for Social and Communication Disorders, Elliott House. 113 Masons Hill, Bromley, Kent BR2 9HT. Email: elliot.house@nas.org.uk.)

Winters, K. (1989). *Personal Experience Screening Questionnaire*. Los Angeles, CA: Western Psychological Services.

Winters, K. & Henly, G. (1989). *Personal Experience Inventory*. Los Angeles, CA: Western Psychological Services.

Winton, P. (1998). The family focused interview: An assessment measure and goal setting mechanism. In D. Bailey & R. Simeounson (Eds.), *Family Assessment in Early Intervention* (pp. 195–205). Columbus, OH: Merrill.

Wolery, M. (1983). Proportional change index. An alternative for comparing child change data. *Exceptional Children*, 50(2), 167–170.

Wolfe, D. (1991). *Preventing Physical and Emotional Abuse of Children*. New York: Guilford.

Wolfe, D. A., Edwards, B., Manion, I. & Koverola, C. (1988). Early intervention for parents at risk of child abuse and neglect: A preliminary investigation. *Journal of Consulting and Clinical Psychology*, 56, 40–47.*

Wolfe, D. & McMahon, R. (1997). *Child Abuse: New Directions in Prevention and Treatment Across the Lifespan*. Thousand Oaks, CA: Sage.

Wolfe, V. (1998). Child Sexual Abuse. In E. Mash & R. Barkley (Eds.), *Treatment of Childhood Disorders* (Second Edition, pp. 545–597). New York: Guilford.

Wolfe, V. & Birt, J. (1995). The psychological sequalae of child sexual abuse. In T. Ollendick & R. Prinz (Eds.), *Advances in Clinical Child Psychology* (Volume 17, pp. 233–263). New York: Plenum.

Woodcock, R.W. & Johnson, M.B. (1977). *Woodcock-Johnson Psycho-Educational Battery*. Hingham, MA: Teaching Resources Corporation.

World Health Organization (1984). *Strategies for The Prevention of Blindness in National Programmes*. Geneva: WHO.

World Health Organization (1992). *The ICD-10 Classification of Mental and Behavioural Disorders*. Geneva: WHO.

Wurtele, S. (1986). *Teaching Young Children Personal Body Safety: The Behavioural Skills Training Program*. Colorado Springs, CO: Author.

Wurtele, S. (1988a). *'What If' Situations Test* (WIST). Austin, CO: Department of Psychology, University of Colorado. (Dr Sandy Wurtele, Department of Psychology, University of Colorado at Colorado Springs, 1420 Austin Bluffs Parkway, Colorado Springs, CO 80933–7150.)

Wurtele, S. (1988b). *Personal Safety Questionnaire* (PSQ). Austin, CO: Department of Psychology, University of Colorado. (Dr Sandy Wurtele, Department of Psychology, University of Colorado at Colorado Springs, 1420 Austin Bluffs Parkway, Colorado Springs, CO 80933–7150.)

Wurtele, S. (1989a). *Teachers' Perceptions Questionnaire*. Austin, CO: Department of Psychology, University of Colorado. (Dr Sandy Wurtele, Department of Psychology, University of Colorado at Colorado Springs, 1420 Austin Bluffs Parkway, Colorado Springs, CO 80933–7150.)

Wurtele, S. (1989b). *Parents' Perceptions Questionnaire*. Austin, CO: Department of Psychology, University of Colorado. (Dr Sandy Wurtele, Department of Psychology, University of Colorado at Colorado Springs, 1420 Austin Bluffs Parkway, Colorado Springs, CO 80933–7150.)

Wurtele, S. (1990). Teaching personal safety skills to four-year-old children: A behavioural approach. *Behaviour Therapy*, 21, 25–32.*

Wurtele, S. (1997). Sexual Abuse. In R.T. Ammerman & M. Hersen (Eds.), *Handbook of Prevention and Treatment with Children and Adolescents: Intervention in the Real World Context*. Chichester: Wiley.

Wurtele, S. & Sarno-Owens, J. (1997). Teaching personal safety skills to young children: An investigation of age and gender across five studies. *Child Abuse and Neglect*, 21(8), 805–814.*

Wurtele, S., Kast, L., Miller-Perrin, C. & Kondrick, P. (1989). Comparisons of programs for teaching personal safety skills to preschoolers. *Journal of Consulting and Clinical Psychology*, 57(4), 505–511.*

Wurtele, S., Gillispie, E., Currier, L. & Franklin, C. (1992a). A comparison of teachers vs. parents as instructors of a personal safety program for preschoolers. *Child Abuse and Neglect*, 16, 127–137.*

Wurtele, S., Kast, L. & Melzer, A. (1992b). Sexual abuse prevention education for young children: A comparison of teachers and parents as instructors. *Child Abuse and Neglect*, 16, 865–876.*

Wysocki, T., Harris, M.A., Greco, P., Bubb, J., Danda, C.E., Harvey, L.M., McDonell, K., Taylor, A. & White, N.H. (2000). Randomized, controlled trial of behavior therapy for families of adolescents with insulin-dependent diabetes mellitus. *Journal of Pediatric Psychology*, 25(1), 23–33.*

Yehuda, R., Marshall, R. & Giller, E. (1998). Psychopharmacological treatment of post-traumatic stress disorder. In P. Nathan & J. Gorman (Eds.), *A Guide To Treatments That Work* (pp. 377–397). New York: Oxford University Press.

Yule, W. (1992). Posttraumatic stress disorder in childhood survivors of shipping disasters: the sinking of the 'Jupiter'. *Psychotherapy Psychosomatics*, 57, 200–205.*

Yule, W. (1994). Posttraumatic stress disorder, In M. Rutter, E. Taylor & L. Hersov (Eds.), *Child and Adolescent Psychiatry: Modern Approaches*. (Third Edition, pp. 392–406). London: Blackwell.

Zahr, L., Parker, S. & Cole, J. (1992). Comparing the effects of neonatal intensive care unit interventions of premature infants of different weights. *Journal of Developmental and Behavioural Pediatrics*, 13, 165–172.

Ziegler, S., Charach, A. & Pepler, D.J. (1992). *Bullying at School*. Unpublished manuscript.

Zimmerman, I.L., Steiner, V. & Pond, R. (1979). *Preschool Language Scale*. Columbus, OH: Charles Merrill.

Zimmerman, J. & Asnis, G. (Eds.) (1995). *Treatment Approaches with Suicidal Adolescents*. New York: Wiley.

Zung, W.W.K. (1974). Index of potential suicide (IPS): A rating scale for suicide prevention. In T. Beck, H. Resnick & D. Lettieri (Eds.), *The Prediction of Suicide* (pp. 221–249). Bowie, MD: Charles Press.

Index